Infection Prevention and Control

at a Glance

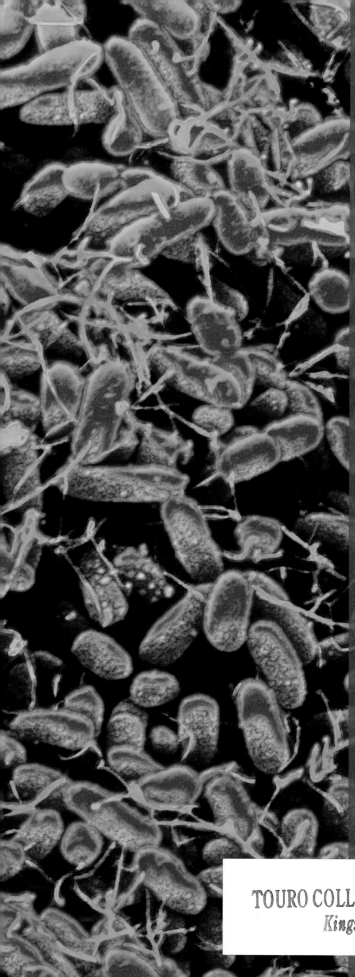

Infection
Prevention
and Control
at a Glance

Debbie Weston
Assistant Director
Infection Prevention and Control
Dartford and Gravesham NHS Trust

Alison Burgess
Health Protection Practitioner
Public Health England

Sue Roberts
Deputy Director
Lead Nurse, Infection Prevention and Control
East Kent Hospitals University NHS
Foundation Trust

Series Editor: Ian Peate

WILEY Blackwell

Library of Congress Cataloging-in-Publication Data

Names: Weston, Debbie, author. | Burgess, Alison, 1963- , author. | Roberts, Sue, 1955- , author.
Title: Infection prevention and control at a glance / Debbie Weston, Alison Burgess, Sue Roberts.
Other titles: At a glance series (Oxford, England)
Description: Chichester, West Sussex: John Wiley and Sons, Ltd, 2017. | Series: At a glance series | Includes bibliographical references and index.
Identifiers: LCCN 2016012192 (print) | LCCN 2016013004 (ebook)
ISBN 9781118973554 (pbk.) | ISBN 9781118973547 (pdf) | ISBN 9781118973523 (epub)
Subjects: | MESH: Cross Infection—nursing | Cross Infection—prevention & control | Infection Control | Handbooks
Classification: LCC RC112 (print) | LCC RC112 (ebook) | NLM WY 49
DDC 616.9/04231—dc23
LC record available at http://lccn.loc.gov/2016012192

A catalogue record for this book is available from the British Library.

Set in 9.5/11.5 Minion Pro by Aptara, India
Printed and bound in Singapore by Markono Print Media Pte Ltd

1 2017

9/15/17

Contents

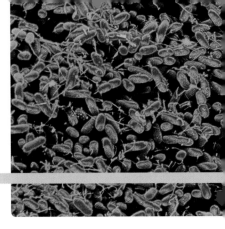

Part 4 Infections and infectious diseases 67

Preface

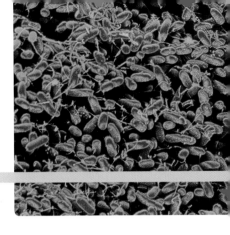

The idea for this book emerged from the recognition that whilst there are a number of excellent infection prevention and control textbooks available, the concise 'at a glance' format is unique and there was therefore a gap in the market for presenting infection prevention and control (IP&C) in this way.

The book has been written by three Senior Infection Prevention and Control Clinical Nurse Specialists with a wealth of experience, still working in a clinical setting, who are alert to and understand the difficulties of clinical staff adhering to infection prevention principles, with many other competing priorities. With this in mind, the concise nature of this book is aimed at a wide range of healthcare professionals, from student nurses embarking on their first exploration of microbiology and the principles of infection prevention and control, to more experienced healthcare professionals working in a high-pressure environment who may have limited time on their hands, find it hard to read the guidance and policies in depth, and simply require a quick revision of the pertinent points.

The book, consisting of 45 short chapters (all of which are based on the most up-to-date guidance), takes the reader on a journey, initially introducing basic microbiology and the body's immune response before moving on to the practical management of patients with infections caused by specific microorganisms (including current highly resistant microorganisms). Each chapter outlines the characteristics of *specific* microorganisms, method of diagnosis and the key points of patient management, as well as the pathogenesis of infection where appropriate. Student nurses may find it useful to refer to an anatomy and physiology textbook where appropriate, particularly where aspects of the pathogenesis of infection are described.

The book is *not* intended to be read from cover to cover in one sitting, although the understanding of the reader may be enhanced if the basic microbiology chapters are read first. Rather, each chapter is written as a separate entity, which can be read on its own or in combination with chapters that are linked. On completion of the book, the reader should have an excellent knowledge of basic microbiology and immunology, which underpins the principles of infection prevention and control, and feel more confident regarding their own management of patients with infections. Hopefully, the book will encourage the reader to want to expand their knowledge still further.

We very much hope that you enjoy reading this book in whichever way is suitable for you.

Bold type is used in the text for emphasis of important terms and points. Terms that appear and are defined in the Glossary are in colour.

Debbie, Ali and Sue

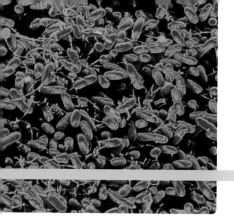

Acknowledgements

Ali and Sue would like to thank Debbie for all her support and encouragement in the development of this book.

The authors would like to thank their families for their support in the creation of this book, along with grateful thanks to Karen Moore and the team at Wiley for their invaluable support and guidance. Ali would like to acknowledge Clive Burgess, who drew several of the original drawings, Eric Grafman from the CDC, who assisted her with obtaining images for some of the chapters, and her colleagues at Public Health England. Sue would like to thank Tina Dunstall for her assistance, and also East Kent Hospitals University NHS Foundation Trust for permission to reproduce some of the figures. Debbie would like to thank Sue and Ali for their hard work, support and commitment.

Introduction to infection prevention and control

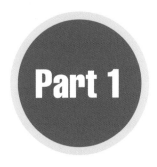

Part 1

Chapters

1 Infection prevention and control (IP&C)

Figure 1.1 Healthcare associated infections (HCAIs)

Box 1 HCAIs – patient risk factors

- Extremes of age
- Emergency admission to an intensive care unit
- Hospital inpatient stay > 7 days
- Insertion of an invasive device (see Chapters 20 and 30)
- Surgery/trauma-induced immunosuppression
- Neutropenia
- Impaired functional status
- Colonisation with an antibiotic-resistant organism (e.g. carbapenemase-producing organisms (see Chapter 29); MRSA (see Chapter 43)
- Any co-morbidities
- Antibiotics
- Obesity
- Malnutrition
- Loss of mobility

References: Golden et al (1999); Hirsch et al (2008); World Health Organization (2011)

Box 2 Other HCAI risk factors

- Increase in patients undergoing invasive procedures
- Increasing age of the population
- Confused, wandering and/or 'non-compliant patients', and patients with reduced mental capacity
- Increased bed occupancy rates, patient turnaround and delayed discharges
- Increased staff : patient ratios
- Lack of isolation facilities/poor isolation practices (see Chapter 21)
- Poor cleaning/decontamination practices (equipment)
- Poor standards of environmental cleanliness (see Chapter 17)
- Antibiotic resistance and poor antimicrobial stewardship (see Chapters 10 and 11)
- Poor infection and prevention control (IP&C) practice – non-compliance with the application of standard precautions (see Chapters 14, 16 and 18) and local IP&C policies

References: Department of Health (2002; 2004; 2007a); Cunningham et al (2005); Wigglesworth and Wilcox (2006); Griffiths et al (2008)

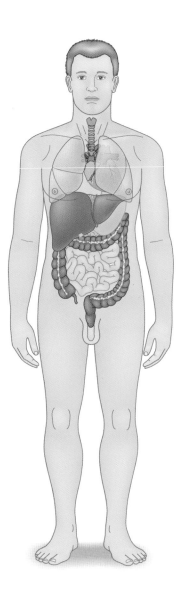

Box 3 The six commonest HCAIs (Health Protection Agency, 2012a)

1 Pneumonia/lower respiratory tract infections (see Chapter 32)
2 Urinary tract infections (see Chapter 30)
3 Surgical site infections (see Chapter 24)
4 Clinical sepsis (see Chapter 25)
5 Gastrointestinal infections (see Chapters 22 and 31)
6 Bloodstream infections (see Chapter 26)

Box 4 'Alert organisms'

- MRSA (see Chapter 43)
- Panton–Valentine leukocidin (PVL) producing strains of MRSA/ *Staphylococcus aureus* (see Chapter 43)
- *Clostridium difficile* (see Chapter 31)
- *Streptococcus pyogenes* (see Chapter 36)
- Group B haemolytic streptococci
- *Legionella* (see Chapter 37)
- Extended-spectrum beta lactamases (ESBLs) and carbapenemase-producing organisms (see Chapter 29)
- Glycopeptide-resistant enterococci (GRE)
- Resistant Gram-negative bacilli
- *Campylobacter* species (see Chapter 28)
- *Salmonella* species (see Chapter 42)
- *Escherichia coli* 0157

Box 5 'Alert conditions'

- Infectious diarrhoea (see Chapter 22)
- Food poisoning (see Chapters 28 and 42)
- Scabies and infestations (see Chapter 34)
- Tuberculosis (see Chapter 44)
- Chickenpox and shingles (see Chapter 45)
- Meningococcal disease (see Chapter 39)
- Typhoid and paratyphoid fever
- Viral hepatitis
- Post-operative surgical site infections (see Chapter 24)
- Creutzfeldt–Jakob disease (CJD)

Box 6 IP&C standard precautions

- Hand hygiene (see Chapter 14)
- Personal protective equipment (PPE) (see Chapter 16)
- Cleaning/decontamination of the environment and equipment (see Chapter 17)
- The safe use and disposal of sharps (see Chapter 18)
- The management of waste
- The management of linen

Figure 1.2 The role of the Infection Prevention and Control Team (IP&CT)

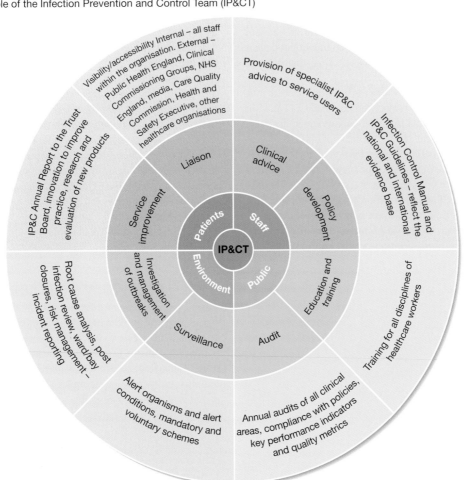

Table 1.1 The Code of Practice (The Health and Social Care Act, 2008 – Department of Health, 2015)

Compliance criterion	What the registered provider will need to demonstrate
1	Systems to manage and monitor the prevention and control of infection. These systems use risk assessments and consider the susceptibility of service users and any risks that their environment and other users may pose to them.
2	Provide and maintain a clean and appropriate environment in managed premises that facilitates the prevention and control of infections
3	Ensure appropriate antimicrobial use to optimise patient outcomes and to reduce the risk of adverse events and antimicrobial resistance
4	Provide suitable accurate information on infections to service users, their visitors and any person concerned with providing further support or nursing/medical care in a timely fashion
5	Ensure prompt identification of people who have or are at risk of developing an infection so that they receive timely and appropriate treatment to reduce the risk of transmitting infection to other people
6	Systems to ensure that all care workers (including contractors and volunteers) are aware of and discharge their responsibilities in the process of preventing and controlling infection
7	Provide or secure adequate isolation facilities
8	Secure adequate access to laboratory support as appropriate
9	Have and adhere to policies designed for the individual's care and provider organisations that will help to prevent and control infections
10	Providers have a system in place to manage the occupational health needs and obligations of staff in relation to infection

Source: Department of Health. Used under OGL

A healthcare associated infection (HCAI) can be defined as 'an infection occurring in a patient during the process of care in a hospital or other healthcare facility, which was not present or incubating at the time of admission. This includes infections acquired in the hospital but appearing after discharge and also occupational infections among staff of the facility' (WHO, 2011). Figure 1.1, Boxes 1 and 2, describes individual patient and other risk factors for the development of HCAIs; Box 3 lists the top six HCAIs.

HCAIs are **significant harm events** and healthcare staff have to be aware of their implications, not just from an individual patient perspective (patients can, and do, die from infections that they did not come into hospital with, or contracted as a result of hospital or other healthcare intervention), but also in the wider context. It is important to have a high awareness of the possibility of HCAI in both patients and healthcare staff to ensure early and rapid diagnosis resulting in effective treatment and containment of infection.

The introduction of national reduction, and local 'stretch', targets for MRSA bloodstream infections (see Chapter 43) and *Clostridium difficile* (see Chapter 31) , has kept these organisms at the top of the Department of Health agenda and in the media spotlight since 2004. These targets have largely been successful.

The focus has been on the implementation of evidence-based best practice and adherence to sound infection prevention and control practice, supported by a large number of Department of Health / NHS England / Public Health England drives, initiatives and legislation. MRSA and *C. difficile*, however, are just the tip of the iceberg, as the nature of infections and infectious diseases is constantly evolving. At the time of writing, the greatest 'infection control' threat that the NHS is facing is not from pandemic influenza (see Chapter 41) or another outbreak of Ebola virus disease (see Chapter 33) but from **multi-drug resistant Gram-negative bacteria** (see Chapter 29), which presents a global public health threat and, perhaps, the beginning of a world without antibiotics. The application of, and compliance with, infection prevention and control as part of everyday practice is going to become more crucial to patient care than ever, given the risk of patients dying from infections that previously could have been treated.

Organisms causing HCAIs

Figure 1.1, Box 4, lists the 'alert organisms' that are commonly implicated in HCAIs, as they can cause cross-infection and outbreaks in healthcare settings. There are also a number of 'alert conditions' that have wider public healthcare implications (see Figure 1.1, Box 5).

While HCAIs are, on the majority of occasions, acquired as a result of cross-infection arising from exposure to other colonised or infected patients or staff, they can arise endogenously from the patient's own resident microbial population, particularly where invasive devices (see Chapters 20 and 30) are inappropriately managed. Communicable diseases (see Chapter 2) acquired in healthcare settings through exposure to other patients, relatives or healthcare staff, can also be considered to be healthcare associated.

The Health and Social Care Act (Code of Practice)

The Code of Practice on the prevention and control of infections and related guidance (DH, 2015) came into being in 2008 as part of the Health and Social Care Act, which established the Care Quality Commission (CQC) (http://cqc.org.uk).The Health and Social Care Act 2008 and its regulations **are law, and must be complied with**.

Since April 2009, NHS Trusts have been legally required to register with the Care Quality Commission (CQC) under the Health and Social Care Act, 2008, and as a legal requirement of their registration must protect patients, workers and others who may be at risk of a healthcare associated infection. This has since extended to encompass other NHS bodies, independent healthcare and social care providers, primary dental care and independent sector ambulance providers and primary medical care providers.

In relation to HCAI, the CQC will monitor compliance with the statutory requirements of registration and will judge whether the requirement is met with reference to the *Code of Practice*. In cases of failure to comply with the registration requirements, the CQC has a range of enforcement powers that it can use to respond to breaches and which are proportionate to the risk of infection. It may draw the breach to the registered provider's attention and give the provider an opportunity to put it right within a reasonable period of time. In extreme cases the CQC has the power to cancel registration.

Table 1.1 lists the 10 Compliance Criteria of the *Code of Practice*.

IP&C – everybody's business

Infection prevention and control is an integral part of an effective risk management and patient safety programme and as such must be embedded in every aspect of patient care in every conceivable patient / healthcare setting by all healthcare staff. It is important to note that Registered Nurses and Midwives are bound by the Nursing and Midwifery Council (NMC) *Professional Standards of practice and behaviour for Nurses and Midwives (The Code)* (NMC, 2015), and medical staff registered with the General Medical Council (GMC) and licensed to practise medicine have to abide by the GMC's *Good Practice Guidance* (2013) (http://www.gmc-uk.org/guidance/good_medical_practice.asp).

Good management and organisation are crucial to establishing high standards of infection control. All healthcare providers must ensure that they have systems in place that address:
- leadership
- management arrangements
- design and maintenance of the environment and devices
- application of evidence-based protocols and practices for both users and staff
- education, training, information and communication.

All staff are responsible for the care that they give, and are **accountable** or answerable to someone for their actions. They also have a **duty of care**, which is a legal obligation to ensure that patients in their care come to no harm as a consequence of any act or omission by the healthcare worker. The Infection Prevention and Control Team (IP&CT) are required to hold staff to account and to challenge poor practice and non-compliance (compliance essentially means acting in accordance with agreed standards or guidelines). Therefore it is essential that staff understand that they are responsible for their practice in relation to IP&C, and for protecting the patients in their care as far it is practically and reasonably possible from HCAIs, and that they are answerable to someone if they are non-compliant. For example, failure to record the visual infusion phlebitis (VIP) scores for two days on a patient with a peripheral cannula in situ (see Chapter 20) leading to a bloodstream infection (BSI – bacteraemia or septicaemia; see Chapter 25) could be viewed as negligent, meaning that harm has been caused to the patient through careless omission (as opposed to a deliberate act), and that the duty of care has been breached.

Holding staff to account however is not about apportioning blame. It is about encouraging responsibility, ownership and engagement, and the IP&CT and healthcare staff working together to reduce, prevent, control and manage HCAIs and the risk to patients. IP&C is an integral component of patient centred care, and all aspects of IP&C clinical practice must be viewed as being *as* important as *all other aspects* of patient care, *not* as add-ons.

Staff must have the **competency** or ability to undertake tasks or clinical interventions; part of this ability means possessing the necessary knowledge and skills. To undertake clinical activities / interventions without the appropriate knowledge or skills or training places patients and healthcare workers at risk. Staff must also be aware that if there are omissions or gaps in a patient's paperwork in relation to the **documentation** of IP&C interventions, the legal interpretation is that care was not given.

Avoidable versus unavoidable infections

Avoidable HCAIs are essentially those where poor clinical practice and non-compliance with IP&C can be evidenced / demonstrated. Any successful reduction in HCAIs requires a zero tolerance approach by all healthcare staff with regard to poor infection control practice, non-compliance with policies, protocols and evidence-based best practice recommendations, and avoidable infections.

HCAIs and the Duty of Candour

All NHS provider bodies registered with the Care Quality Commission (CQC) have to comply with the new Statutory Duty of Candour as a requirement of their registration.

The Duty of Candour is **legal duty** on hospital, community and mental health Trusts to inform and apologise to patients if there have been mistakes in their care that have led to significant harm. It is therefore applicable to all healthcare professionals in all settings who have a professional responsibility to be honest with patients when things go wrong. This includes reporting incidents and near misses, being open and honest with patients / clients and their carers, and apologising. With regard to applying the Duty of Candour in relation to HCAIs, the onus is on the medical team responsible for the patient's care, not the IP&CT.

The role of the Infection Prevention and Control Team

The Code of Practice on the prevention and control of infections and related guidance (DH, 2015), part of the Health and Social Care 2008, requires healthcare organisations to have, or have access to, 'an appropriate mix of both nursing and consultant medical expertise (with specialist training in infection prevention and cleanliness)'. The IP&CT are the nursing and medical experts responsible for providing the organisation within which they work with evidence-based best practice advice on all aspects of infection prevention and control, and are the only specialist nursing and medical team with responsibility for patients, staff, the public and the environment. The IP&CT are the authors of the Infection Prevention and Control Annual Report, which is presented to the Trust Board of Directors and describes the activities undertaken by the IP&CT during that year in relation to the prevention and control of healthcare associated infections (HCAIs). Activities undertaken by the IP&CT are described in Figure 1.2, and are all focused on ensuring that the organisation is compliant with the Code of Practice.

The application of IP&C outside an acute NHS Trust setting

The risk of HCAIs is generally considered to be greater to patients within an acute healthcare setting (i.e. NHS Trusts) given the types of interventions / invasive procedures that patients typically undergo, and other HCAI risk factors (see Figure 1.1, Boxes 1 and 2), although, in theory, infections / outbreaks should be easier to prevent and manage given that the hospital environment is more 'controlled'.

There are some patient/client groups in whom the prevention and control of infection poses particular challenges, such as those who are confused and wandering, and/or have reduced mental capacity, or disabilities.

Staff education and training in the application of standard precautions (see Figure 1.1, Box 6) is paramount, and staff may need to be creative in how they actually apply or practice IP&C. When caring for elderly, confused and wandering patients who are colonised or who have an infection for example (and this is just as applicable to an acute care setting), there will need to be an increased focus on patient / client hand hygiene (i.e. by using patient hand hygiene 'wet wipes'), and additional / enhanced cleaning of the environment, particularly frequent 'touch points' (areas that the patients' / clients' hands are most likely to come into contact with) and communal areas such as toilets and bathrooms.

NICE (2012) and the DH/HPA (2013) have published specific guidance for the prevention and control of infection in community care, and the HPA/DH have also published specific guidance for staff working in prisons and places of detention (HPA/DH, 2011).

2 Communicable diseases

Figure 2.1 List of notifiable diseases

Diseases notifiable to local authority proper officers under the Health Protection (Notification) Regulations 2010	
• Acute encephalitis	• Malaria
• Acute infectious hepatitis	• Measles (see Chapter 38)
• Acute meningitis (see Chapter 39)	• Meningococcal septicaemia (see Chapter 39)
• Acute poliomyelitis	• Mumps (see Chapter 38)
• Anthrax	• Plague
• Botulism	• Rabies
• Brucellosis	• Rubella (see Chapter 38)
• Cholera	• Severe acute respiratory syndrome (SARS)
• Diphtheria	
• Enteric fever (typhoid or paratyphoid fever)	• Scarlet fever
• Food poisoning (See Chapters 28 and 42)	• Smallpox
• Haemolytic uraemic syndrome (HUS)	• Tetanus
• Infectious bloody diarrhoea	• Tuberculosis (see Chapter 44)
• Invasive group A streptococcal disease (see Chapter 36)	• Typhus
	• Viral haemorrhagic fever (VHF) (see Chapter 33)
• Legionnaires' disease (see Chapter 37)	• Whooping cough (see Chapter 27)
• Leprosy	• Yellow fever

Source: www.gov.uk/guidance/notifiable-diseases-and-causative-organisms-how-to-report

Figure 2.2 Vaccine preventable diseases (PHE, 2013c)

- Anthrax
- Cholera
- Diphtheria
- *Haemophilus influenzae* type b (Hib)
- Hepatitis A
- Hepatitis B
- Influenza
- Japanese encephalitis
- Measles
- Meningococcal
- Mumps
- Pertussis
- Pneumococcal
- Polio
- Rabies
- Rubella
- Smallpox and vaccinia
- Tetanus
- Tick-borne encephalitis
- Tuberculosis
- Typhoid
- Varicella
- Yellow fever

Figure 2.3 The prevention of communicable diseases

Vaccination for all vaccine preventable diseases
(see www.gov.uk/government/collections/immunisation-against-infectious-disease-the-green-book)

Screening, i.e.:
- staff on pre-employment (childhood vaccinations, TB, Hepatitis B vaccination)
- at ports/airports during outbreaks. During the West Africa Ebola outbreak, passenger data was used to identify travellers from West Africa These passengers had a temperature check on disembarking and had to complete a health questionnaire (current health, travel history, and potential contact). Individuals were either given advice and allowed to travel onwards, or were referred to hospital for assessment. Passenger screening was also undertaken during the SARS outbreak
- all visa applicants from countries where the incidence of TB is $\geq 40/100\,000$ population and who are intending to stay in the UK for > 6 months, must be certified free from TB before they can apply for a visa
- identification of susceptible 'patient' and staff contacts following a single case of a communicable disease occuring within a healthcare setting; i.e. chickenpox, pertussis, meningococcal diseases, respiratory tuberculosis
- identification of contacts following a decontamination failure (surgical instruments or endoscopy equipment) that has potentially exposed patients to blood-borne viruses (BBVs)
- identification of patient contacts following confirmation of a BBV in a healthcare worker undertaking exposure-prone procedures

Post-exposure prophylaxis/chemo-prophylaxis (through vaccination and/or antibiotics), i.e.:
- close contacts of cases of meningococcal disease
- potential exposure to HIV/hepatitis
- close contacts (i.e. patients/staff) of a case of pertussis
- 'high-risk' individuals following significant exposure to varicella zoster infection
- vaccination against seasonal influenza; administration of anti-viral agents during pandemics (i.e. administration of Tamiflu to close contacts of individuals with 'swine flu' during the 2009–10 H1N1 pandemic)

Education and training on the prevention and control of infections for staff working in hospital/community care settings, including care homes; nurseries, schools and colleges; staff working with prisoners/in detention centres

Information/public health campaigns on the benefits of vaccination; hand hygiene; respiratory hygiene

Infection Prevention and Control at a Glance, First Edition. By Debbie Weston, Alison Burgess and Sue Roberts.
© 2017 John Wiley & Sons, Ltd. Published 2017 by John Wiley & Sons, Ltd.

Communicable diseases are **contagious or infectious diseases** spread by **pathogenic** microorganisms that can be transmitted from one person to another and that generally have significant public health implications for the **wider community and global public health**. In 2002, the Chief Medical Officer published *Getting Ahead of the Curve* (DH, 2002) which emphasised the inevitability of the global emergence of, and subsequent threat from, new infectious diseases, given that 30 such diseases had emerged since the 1970s. Among these diseases were Ebola (see Chapter 33), HIV and HCV (see Chapter 26) and Legionnaires' disease (see Chapter 37). Ebola and HIV, along with severe acute respiratory syndrome (SARS) which first emerged in China in 2003 (caused by a novel coronavirus), and Middle East respiratory syndrome coronavirus (MERS-CoV) which was first identified in Saudi Arabia in 2012, are known or strongly suspected to have originated in animals (zoonotic infections). Some communicable diseases are particularly associated with children, such as measles, mumps and rubella (Chapter 38), whooping cough (pertussis) (Chapter 27), varicella (Chapter 45) and meningococcal disease (Chapter 39).

Responsibility for public health

In England, Public Health England (PHE) is an external agency sponsored by the Department of Health (DH) whose overarching aim is to protect and improve the nation's health and wellbeing and reduce health inequalities. One of its key roles is the provision of specialist advice in relation to outbreaks and incidences of infectious diseases, including preparedness planning and local and national responses to infectious disease threats (www.gov.uk/government/organisations/public-health-england). (See www.healthscotland.com, www.publichealthwales.wales.nhs.uk and www.publichealth.ie for public health arrangements in Wales, Scotland and Ireland.) The Centers for Disease Control and Prevention (CDC) is the public health agency in America (www.cdc.gov). The World Health Organization (WHO) is the directing and coordinating authority on international health within the United Nations system.

Notification and surveillance

Under the Health Protection (Notification) Regulations (2010), there are 32 notifiable infectious diseases (www.gov.uk/guidance/notifiable-diseases-and-causative-organisms-how-to-report) and 60 notifiable bacteria and viruses (see Figures 2.1 and 2.2).

The doctor looking after the patient (hospital or GP) has a statutory duty (legal requirement) to notify the 'Proper Officer' (the Consultant in Communicable Disease Control (CCDC) at the local Public Health England (PHE) Health Protection Team) if s/he **suspects a single case of a notifiable infection**; therefore notification must *not* be delayed until positive laboratory confirmation has been received. The main purpose of the notification system is that of **surveillance** in order to detect, as early as possible, potential outbreaks. Communicable disease surveillance has four key functions (Hawker et al, 2012). It:

- identifies individual cases of infection and allows action to be taken to prevent spread

- monitors the **incidence** of infections / infectious diseases and can detect outbreaks
- tracks changes in the occurrence and risk factors
- evaluates existing control measures.

Global risk factors for the spread of communicable diseases

- Mass gatherings, particularly those that bring people together from different countries and cultures and that facilitate the importation of a communicable disease from its host country and subsequent amplification and spread (Heymann, 2015).
- Movement across borders (a factor in the spread of Ebola in West Africa) / displaced persons.
- Poverty.
- Environmental factors in developing countries (water, sanitation, food, climate).
- International travel and trade. SARS affected 4300 people in 32 countries, with over 8000 probable cases and more than 800 deaths (WHO, 2003). Pandemic influenza (see Chapter 41) has the potential to circle the globe within three months.
- High-risk life styles (i.e. blood-borne virus transmission (see Chapter 26) and sexually transmitted diseases).
- Unavailability of vaccination (Figure 2.2) in some developing countries.
- The emergence of more **virulent** forms of microorganisms.

Under the International Health Regulations (IHR) (part of a global agreement under the WHO constitution and adopted by all member states), communicable diseases are monitored by global surveillance, alert and response activities, and public health infrastructures are strengthened, or in some cases re-established, in order to ensure that emerging disease threats, whether 'old' or new, are identified early in order that a rapid public health response can be initiated (Heymann, 2015). There are four communicable diseases that are considered to have such significant public health implications that the **emergence of just a single case poses a public health emergency of international concern** and must be notified to the WHO (Heymann, 2015). These diseases are:

- **Smallpox** – eradicated in 1979. Outbreaks can only occur through accidental or deliberate release. There are 'legitimate' stocks of the smallpox virus held in two WHO-approved high-security locations.
- **Poliomyelitis due to wild-type poliovirus**. Only two countries are polio endemic (Afghanistan and Pakistan). However, according to WHO 'As long as a single child remains infected, children in all countries are at risk of contracting polio. Failure to eradicate polio from these last remaining strongholds could result in as many as 200 000 new cases every year, within 10 years, all over the world' (www.who.int/mediacentre/factsheets/fs114/en/).
- **Human influenza caused by a new virus subtype** (see Chapter 41).
- **SARS** – declared eradicated in 2005 but has the potential to re-emerge.

Figure 2.3 describes some essential key measures in the prevention of communicable diseases applicable to healthcare and other settings.

3 Bacterial classification and structure

Figure 3.1 Bacterial cell structure

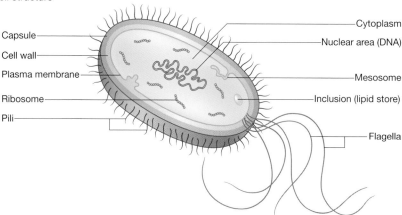
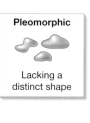

Capsule

Cell wall

Plasma membrane

Ribosome

Pili

Cytoplasm

Nuclear area (DNA)

Mesosome

Inclusion (lipid store)

Flagella

Figure 3.2 Common bacterial shapes

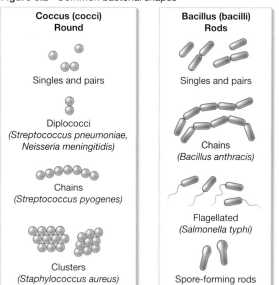
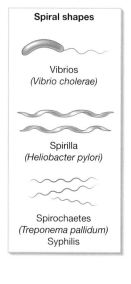

Coccus (cocci) Round

Singles and pairs

Diplococci
(*Streptococcus pneumoniae, Neisseria meningitidis*)

Chains
(*Streptococcus pyogenes*)

Clusters
(*Staphylococcus aureus*)

Bacillus (bacilli) Rods

Singles and pairs

Chains
(*Bacillus anthracis*)

Flagellated
(*Salmonella typhi*)

Spore-forming rods

Spiral shapes

Vibrios
(*Vibrio cholerae*)

Spirilla
(*Heliobacter pylori*)

Spirochaetes
(*Treponema pallidum*)
Syphilis

Pleomorphic

Lacking a
distinct shape

Figure 3.3 Examples of Gram-positive bacteria

- *Staphylococcus aureus*, including meticillin-resistant *Staphylococcus aureus* (MRSA) (see Chapter 43)
- *Staphylococcus epidermidis*
- *Streptococcus pyogenes* (Group A Strep) (see Chapter 36)
- *Bacillus cereus*
- *Clostridium difficile* (see Chapter 31)
- *Corynebacterium diphtheriae*
- *Listeria monocytogenes*

Figure 3.4 Examples of Gram-negative bacteria

- *Escherichia coli*
- *Klebsiella*
- *Salmonella* (see Chapter 42)
- *Shigella*
- *Pseudomonas aeruginosa*
- *Campylobacter jejuni* (see Chapter 28)
- *Helicobacter pylori*
- *Neisseria meningitidis* (see Chapter 39)
- *Haemophilus influenzae*
- *Bordetella pertussis* (see Chapter 27)
- *Legionella pneumophilia* (see Chapter 37)
- *Treponema pallidum* (syphilis)

Infection Prevention and Control at a Glance, First Edition. By Debbie Weston, Alison Burgess and Sue Roberts.
© 2017 John Wiley & Sons, Ltd. Published 2017 by John Wiley & Sons, Ltd.

In order to understand the role of different microbes in causing infection, it is important to understand the way in which their genetic material and cellular components are organised. All organisms other than viruses (see Chapter 5) and **prions** are made up of cells (Mims et al, 2004a). There are two major divisions of cellular organisms, **prokaryotes** and **eukaryotes**, and many differences between the two. Bacteria are classed as prokaryotes whilst all other organisms (animals, plants, algae, fungi and protozoa) are classed as eukaryotes. Bacteria are all around us in huge numbers but only a few of them actually cause disease.

Bacterial (prokaryote) cell structure

Figure 3.1 shows the structure of a bacterial cell. Bacteria are single-celled microorganisms, smaller and much less complex than eukaryote cells, with a much simpler internal structure. The main components of bacterial cells are as follows:

Capsules: Some bacteria have capsules, which lie outside the cell wall, made out of **glycocalyx** to protect them from white blood cells (see Chapter 4).

Flagella, fimbriae and pili: These are often present on the exterior of the cell (see Chapter 4).

Cell wall: The cell wall is located outside the plasma membrane and is made up of a rigid matrix of **peptidoglycan**, which gives the cell shape and provides a rigid structural support. The thickness of the cell wall varies and determines whether bacteria are classed as **Gram-positive** or **Gram-negative**. Gram-positive bacteria have a thick peptidoglycan wall (20–80 nm), with extensive cross-linking of amino acid chains, whereas Gram-negative bacteria have thinner cell walls (5–10 nm) with a much simpler cross-linking pattern (Mims et al, 2004b). As bacteria are colourless, the process of Gram staining in the laboratory is used to identify both the type of cell wall and whether a bacterium is round or rod-shaped (Gladwin and Trattler, 2006a). Gram-positive bacteria stain blue and Gram-negative bacteria stain red (see Chapter 9). **NB:** Some bacteria do not clearly fit into either category. Mycobacteria, which cause tuberculosis (see Chapter 44), whilst weakly Gram-positive, can be identified more efficiently in the laboratory using an acid-fast stain. Spirochaetes, whilst Gram-negative, are very tiny so better seen with a special microscope. Mycoplasma do not have a cell wall so are neither Gram-positive nor Gram-negative (Gladwin and Trattler, 2006a).

Cytoplasmic / plasma membrane: This forms the outer structure of the cell and provides a 'selective' barrier that allows certain substances and chemicals to move into and out of the cell (Betsy and Keogh, 2012a).

Cytoplasm: This contains water, enzymes, waste products, nutrients, proteins, carbohydrates and lipids, all of which are required for the cell's metabolic functions. In addition, the cytoplasm contains the cell chromosomes and the DNA molecule (Weston, 2013).

Ribosomes: These synthesise polypeptides (proteins).

Mesosomes: These are folded areas of membrane thought to be involved in protein secretion, transport and chromosome separation during cell division and, in some bacteria, contain the enzymes for respiration (Wilson, 2006).

Inclusion bodies: These are areas within the cytoplasm used for the storage of lipids, nitrogen, phosphate, starch and sulphur (Betsy and Keogh, 2012a).

The main differences between prokaryote and eukaryote cells are discussed in more detail in Chapter 4.

Understanding bacterial taxonomy / classification of bacteria

Taxonomy or classification of organisms is a scientific way of classifying organisms based on common properties. The top layer of classification is the five **kingdoms**, of which bacteria is one (the four remaining kingdoms are Animalia (including eukaryotes), Fungi, Plantae and **Protozoa**). The kingdom of bacteria is further broken down into the **genus** of the bacteria, followed by the **species**, for example, *Clostridium* (genus) *difficile* (species).

Bacterial shapes

There are four main shapes of bacteria (see Figure 3.2): **cocci**, which are spherical; **bacilli**, which are rod-shaped; **spiral-shaped** (or comma-shaped, 'S'-shaped); and **pleomorphic**, which lack a distinct shape (Gladwin and Trattler, 2006a).

There are six classic Gram-positive bacteria that cause disease in humans, and almost every other organism is Gram-negative (Gladwin and Trattler, 2006a). The six Gram-positive bacteria are Streptococci (forming chains of cocci), and Staphylococci (forming clusters); two rods that produce spores, Bacillus and Clostridium; and finally two non-spore-forming rods – Corynebacterium and Listeria. Listeria is the only genus of Gram-positive bacteria that produces an endotoxin (see Chapter 4).

There is only one group of Gram-negative cocci- *Neisseria*, which is a diplococcus (coffee-bean shaped). There is one group of spiral-shaped organisms known as Spirochaetes, and the remaining Gram-negative bacteria are rod-shaped or pleomorphic (Gladwin and Trattler, 2006a).

Examples of some Gram-positive and Gram-negative bacteria are listed in Figures 3.3 and 3.4.

Other important characteristics of bacteria (see Chapter 9)

Nutrition: All **pathogenic** bacteria are heterotrophic, i.e. they obtain energy by oxidising preformed organic molecules (carbohydrates, lipids and proteins) from their environment (Mims et al, 2004b). Bacteria can also be distinguished by their preference of pH and temperature.

Growth and division: Bacteria rates of growth and division also vary significantly. For example *Escherichia coli* may divide every 20–30 minutes whereas Mycobacterium may only divide every 24 hours. Generally, though, growth and division are faster when the nutritional status of the surrounding environment is good (Mims et al, 2004b).

Bacterial virulence factors

Bacteria have a number of different virulence factors to help them to evade the host's immune system. These are discussed in detail in Chapter 4.

4 Bacterial virulence factors

Figure 4.1 Differences between Gram-positive and Gram-negative bacteria

Gram-positive bacteria	Gram-negative bacteria
Cell wall 2 layers: • Inner cytoplasmic membrane • Outer thick peptidoglycan layer (60–100% peptidoglycan)	Cell wall 3 layers: • Inner cytoplasmic membrane • Thin peptidoglycan layer (5–10% peptidoglycan) • Outer membrane with lipopolysaccharide (LPS)
Low lipid content	High lipid content
No endotoxin (except *Listeria monocytogenes*)	Endotoxin (LPS) – lipid A
No periplasmic space	Periplasmic space
No porin channel	Porin channel
Vulnerable to lysozyme and penicillin attack	Resistant to lysozyme and penicillin attack

Figure 4.4 Examples of bacteria that produce toxins

Neurotoxins	• *Clostridium tetani* • *Clostridium botulinum*
Enterotoxins causing infectious diarrhoea	• *Vibrio cholerae* • *E. coli* • *Campylobacter jejuni* • *Bacillus cereus* • *Shigella dysenteriae*
Enterotoxins causing food poisoning	• *Staphylococcus aureus* • *Bacillus cereus*
Pyrogenic toxins	• *Streptococcus pyogenes* • *Staphylococcus aureus* (toxic shock syndrome)
Tissue invasive toxins	• *Streptococcus pyogenes* • *Staphylococcus aureus* • *Clostridium perfringens*
Miscellaneous toxins	• *Bacillus anthracis* (anthrax) • *Corynebacterium diphtheriae* (diphtheria) • *Bordetella pertussis* – 4 toxins (whooping cough) • *Clostridium difficile* (toxins A and B) • *Pseudomonas aeruginosa* (exotoxin A)

Source: Gladwin and Trattler, 2006b

Figure 4.2 The Gram-negative bacterial cell wall

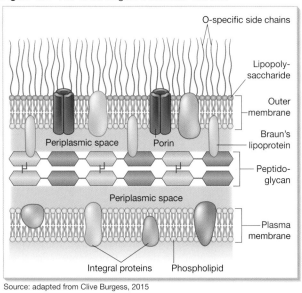

Source: adapted from Clive Burgess, 2015

Figure 4.3 The Gram-positive bacterial cell wall

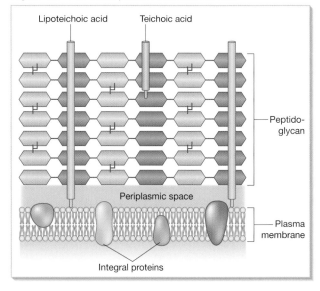

Bacteria have a number of **virulence** factors. These are usually very effective (although their effectiveness varies) in evading the host's immune system. Whilst Gram-positive and Gram-negative bacteria share many of the same virulence factors, Gram-negative bacteria have several unique characteristics present in their cell wall structure that make them generally more pathogenic than Gram-positive bacteria (see Chapter 3), thereby causing a greater number of life-threatening diseases in humans. (see Figures 4.1–4.3)

Flagella

Flagella, present in both Gram-positive and Gram-negative bacteria, assist bacteria in moving freely within their

Infection Prevention and Control at a Glance, First Edition. By Debbie Weston, Alison Burgess and Sue Roberts.
© 2017 John Wiley & Sons, Ltd. Published 2017 by John Wiley & Sons, Ltd.

environment. Flagella are long protein filaments fixed to the basal body of the bacteria, extending from the cell membrane and several times the length of the bacterial cell. The basal body spins around, which has the effect of causing the bacterium to move in a coordinated manner either towards a chemical concentration or away from it by a process called chemotaxis (Gladwin and Trattler, 2006b). There are very different patterns of flagella distribution in bacteria, ranging from a single flagellum (monotrichous) to clusters/tufts of flagella (lophotrichous), and they move in different ways (Prescott et al, 2005a).

Pili (fimbriae)

Pili (fimbriae) are straight filaments, shorter and more rigid than flagella. There are two types of pili: 'sex' pili, which attach to other bacteria (see Chapter 11), and 'common' pili which attach to host cells with adhesins (Mims et al, 2004b). Adhesins are specialised molecules or structures on the bacteria's cell surface that bind to complementary receptor sites on the host cell surface (Prescott et al, 2005a). This is an important factor in causing disease. *Escherichia coli* and Campylobacter (see Chapter 28) use adhesins to bind to intestinal cells, and *Bordetella pertussis* (see Chapter 27) uses adhesins to bind to ciliated epithelial cells (Gladwin and Trattler, 2006b). Although pili are not generally thought to be involved in bacterial motility, they are required in the 'twitching motility' that occurs in some bacteria, for example in *Pseudomonas aeruginosa*, and *Neisseria gonorrhoeae* and some strains of *E. coli* (Prescott et al, 2005a). The presence of many pili may also help to prevent phagocytosis (see Chapter 6), reducing host resistance to bacterial infection (Mims et al, 2004b).

Capsules / slime layer

Capsules are protective walls made of **glycocalyx** that surround the outside of the cell membranes of both Gram-positive and Gram-negative bacteria. Bacterial cells may also be surrounded by a layer of slime, which is also made of glycocalyx but easily washed off (Prescott et al, 2005a). Capsules and slime increase the virulence of bacteria because the body's immune system, in particular the macrophages and neutrophils, is unable to phagocytose these particular bacteria (Gladwin and Trattler, 2006b). Capsules are also able to resist **desiccation** and some bacteria glide through the slime to aid their mobility (Prescott et al, 2005a). Fortunately, certain antibodies are able to bind to capsules (opsonisation), and once the macrophages and neutrophils bind to the antibodies they are able to phagocytose the bacteria (Gladwin and Trattler, 2006b) (see Chapters 6 and 7).

Endospores (Gram-positive bacteria only)

The production of endospores is another way in which bacteria try to outwit the host's immune system. Only two bacterial species, both Gram-positive rods, form spores; these are Bacillus and Clostridium. Endospores are metabolically dormant forms of bacteria that are resistant to heat (boiling), cold, drying and chemical agents. Spores (which have a protective coat of five layers) form when there is a shortage of nutrients and can lie dormant for years until the environment and availability of nutrition improve (Gladwin and Trattler, 2006b).

Facultative intracellular organisms

Some bacteria, called facultative intracellular organisms, are phagocytosed by the macrophages and neutrophils but survive within these cells unharmed because they are able to inhibit phagosome–lysosome fusion (see Chapter 6). Examples include *Listeria monocytogenes, Salmonella typhi, Legionella* and *Mycobacterium tuberculosis (Gladwin and Trattler, 2006b) (see Chapters 37 and 44).*

Exotoxins and endotoxins

Exotoxins are proteins that are released by both Gram-positive and Gram-negative bacteria. All Gram-positive bacteria produce exotoxins (extracellularly), with the exception of *Listeria monocytogenes, which produces endotoxin.* Endotoxins, which are only present in Gram-negative bacteria (except for the Gram-positive *Listeria monocytogenes*) differ from exotoxins in that they are cell bound and form an integral part of the cell wall that is only released during cell lysis (Gladwin and Trattler, 2006b).

Exotoxins

Exotoxins that act on the nerves are called **neurotoxins**, and exotoxins that act on the gastrointestinal tract and cause both infectious diarrhoea and food poisoning are called **enterotoxins** (Gladwin and Trattler, 2006b). Examples of bacteria that produce exotoxins can be found in Figure 4.4.

Endotoxins (lipid A) (Gram-negative bacteria only)

Endotoxins are particularly characteristic of Gram-negative bacteria and form part of the bacterial cell wall, which consists of **lipopolysaccharide** (LPS). LPS is composed of: a lipid portion (**lipid A**) inserted into the cell wall which is responsible for much of the toxic activity; a conserved core polysaccharide; and the highly variable **O-polysaccharide** (Mims et al, 2004b). Lipid A is extremely toxic to humans. When the host immune system **lyses** Gram-negative bacterial cells, lipid A is released into the bloodstream, often causing fever and vascular collapse (septic shock) (see Chapter 25), sometimes with fatal consequences (Gladwin and Trattler, 2006b). The most common example of endotoxin (or 'septic') shock is septicaemia caused by Gram-negative bacteria such as *Escherichia coli or Neisseria meningitidis (see Chapter 39) (Mims et al, 2004c).*

The cell membrane of Gram-negative bacteria is also able to block the entry of substances such as antibiotics to the inner parts of the cell, making it harder to treat Gram-negative infections (Gladwin and Trattler, 2006b) (see Chapter 11).

Release of enzymes

Some bacteria release enzymes that break down the tissues or intercellular substances of the host allowing the infection to spread freely. Examples of such enzymes are hyaluronidase, collagenase, DNase and streptokinase (Mims et al, 2004c) (see Chapter 36).

Plasmids

Plasmids are double-stranded DNA(deoxyribonucleic acid) molecules that often carry antimicrobial resistance genes and are easily transferred from one bacterial cell to another by a mechanism known as conjugation, thus facilitating growth of antimicrobial resistance (Prescott et al, 2005a) (see Chapter 11).

5 Viral classification and structure

Figure 5.1 Structure of a single enveloped virus

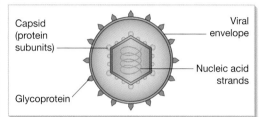

Capsid (protein subunits)

Glycoprotein

Viral envelope

Nucleic acid strands

Figure 5.2 Virus shapes

Cubic symmetry

Enveloped

Herpes virus   Retrovirus

Non-enveloped

Calcivirus   Adenovirus

Helical symmetry

Enveloped

Rabies virus   Paramyxovirus

Complex symmetry

Pox virus

Table 5.1 Common DNA genome viruses that cause disease

Family of DNA virus	Shape of virus	Diseases caused in humans
Adenoviridae Double-stranded (ds) DNA virus	Non-enveloped Icosahedral	Respiratory diseases, e.g. common cold
Herpesviridae Double-stranded (ds) DNA virus	Enveloped Icosahedral	Herpes simplex Varicella zoster (VZV) (chickenpox/shingles) Cytomegalovirus (CMV) Epstein–Barr virus (infectious mononucleosis/ glandular fever)
Papillomaviridae Double-stranded (ds) DNA virus	Non-enveloped Icosahedral	Human papilloma virus (HPV) causing warts and linked to cervical cancer
Poxviridae Double-stranded (ds) DNA virus	Enveloped *Complex* structure	Smallpox

Table 5.2 Common RNA genome viruses that cause disease

Family of RNA virus	Shape of virus	Diseases caused	Family of RNA virus	Shape of virus	Diseases caused
Calciviridae Positive-sense single-stranded (ss) RNA virus	Non-enveloped Icosahedral	Norwalk virus (norovirus) Hepatitis E virus	**Togaviridae** Positive-sense single-stranded (ss) RNA virus	Enveloped Icosahedral	Rubella (German measles)
Coronaviridae Positive-sense single-stranded (ss) RNA virus	Enveloped Helical	Severe acute respiratory syndrome (SARS) Middle East respiratory syndrome coronavirus (MERS-CoV)	**Filoviridae** Negative sense/ ambisense single-stranded (ss) RNA virus	Enveloped Helical	Viral haemorrhagic fever: Ebola/ Marburg
Flaviviridae Positive-sense single-stranded (ss) RNA virus	Enveloped Isometric	Yellow fever Dengue virus Hepatitis C virus (HCV) Japanese encephalitis	**Orthomyxoviridae** Negative-sense/ ambisense single-stranded (ss) RNA virus	Enveloped Helical	Influenza A Influenza B Influenza C
Picornaviridae Positive-sense single-stranded (ss) RNA virus	Non-enveloped Icosahedral	Poliomyelitis Hepatitis A virus Rhinovirus	**Paramyxoviridae** Negative-sense/ ambisense single-stranded (ss) RNA virus	Enveloped Helical	Measles Mumps
Rhabdoviridae Negative-sense/ ambisense single-stranded (ss) RNA virus	Enveloped Helical	Rabies	**Hepadnaviridae** Virus with DNA genome that replicates through an RNA intermediate	Enveloped Isometric	Hepatitis B

Infection Prevention and Control at a Glance, First Edition. By Debbie Weston, Alison Burgess and Sue Roberts.
© 2017 John Wiley & Sons, Ltd. Published 2017 by John Wiley & Sons, Ltd.

Viruses are very different from other microorganisms. Although they are a basic life form – described simply as a piece of genetic material inside a coat of protein – they are highly effective in terms of replicating themselves and infecting other life forms including animals, plants and even bacteria. Unlike bacteria, viruses are not cells, and they do not have cell membranes. On their own viruses are metabolically inert and are therefore reliant on obtaining access to the host cells and using the host machinery for replication of their own kind (Mims et al, 2004d).

Taxonomy / classification of viruses

Viruses are not classified into the same taxonomic groups as bacteria; instead groupings are based on characteristics such as type of nucleic acid present in the genetic material (genome) (**deoxyribonucleic acid (DNA)** or **ribonucleic acid (RNA)**); the number of nucleic acid strands; the mode of replication; the size, structure and symmetry of the virus particle; and the presence or absence of an internal or external envelope (Mims et al, 2004d)

Common structural features of viruses

There are a number of general characteristics that are common to most viruses. These include:

Nucleic acid: The nucleic acid is the genetic material, in the form of single-stranded (ss) *or* double-stranded (ds) RNA or DNA, in a linear (DNA or RNA) or circular (DNA) form, but never both (Mims et al, 2004d).

Capsule / capsid: This is the protein coat that encapsulates the virus, protects the nucleic acid from the environment, determines the shape of the virus and plays a role in attachment of the virus to host cells (Betsy and Keogh, 2012b). The term **nucleocapsid** refers to the complete unit of the nucleic acid and capsid (Mims et al, 2004d).

Envelope: The envelope is the membrane bilayer that some viruses have outside their capsid. A virus that does not have an envelope is called a **naked virus** (Betsy and Keogh 2012b). Naked (non-enveloped) viruses are more resistant than enveloped viruses to heat, acids, drying, and the environment and can survive inside the gastrointestinal (GI) tract. **Enveloped viruses** are more susceptible to environmental factors such as drying, gastric acidity and bile (Mims et al, 2004d). Figure 5.1 shows the structure of an enveloped virus.

Viral shapes and sizes

Viruses range in size from tiny (30 nm) to quite large (at 400 nm the size of small bacteria) and most can only be seen under an electron microscope. Viruses may be **icosahedral** (cubic), **helical** (rod-shaped) or **complex** in shape (Mims et al, 2004d) (see Figure 5.2).

Transmission of viruses

Viruses usually enter the human body via inhaled droplets (e.g. influenza), in food or water (e.g. hepatitis A), by direct transfer from infected hosts (e.g. HIV), and from bites of **vector arthropods** (e.g. yellow fever) (Mims et al, 2004d).

The immune response to viruses

(see Chapter 7)

Virus-infected cells release interferon to signal infection. The innate immune system responds rapidly with the stimulation of natural killer cell lymphocytes. If this does not overwhelm the viral infection the 'adaptive immune response' mobilises specific B lymphocyte antibodies, specific cytotoxic T lymphocytes that kill the infected cells, and memory cells to guard against future infection with the same virus.

Stages of infection and replication of the virus

The first thing the virus does is to attach itself to the host cells. The process of **adsorption (attachment)** is dependent on the virus protein receptors on the cell surface reacting with corresponding receptors on the surface of the host cell. Viruses are only able to invade cells that carry the appropriate receptor on their surface (Wilson, 2008a). Once inside the host cells they are not 'infectious' and are temporarily safe from the host immune system. The viral and host membranes fuse and the virus particle penetrates the plasma membrane and enters the host cell. The capsid is then shed, 'uncoated', and the nucleocapsid released (Mims et al, 2004d).

Replication of the virus then takes place. The process varies depending on whether it is a DNA or RNA virus, and for RNA viruses according to whether they are classed as **positive sense** or **negative sense**. Detailed explanation of the replication process is outside the remit of this book but in summary it involves the processes of **transcription**, **translation** and **replication**. DNA transcription and replication usually occurs in the nucleus, whilst RNA viruses undergo transcription, translation and replication in the cytoplasm (Gladwin and Trattler, 2006c).

Following replication, the viral particles are assembled into capsids and copies of the nucleic acid are inserted into each one (Wilson, 2008a). The enveloped proteins are then released by cell lysis or by 'budding', acquiring their envelope from the host membrane (Mims et al, 2004d). Once outside the cell these **virions** become 'infectious' and are free to infect other cells. Examples of diseases caused by DNA and RNA genome viruses are listed in Tables 5.1 and 5.2.

Cancer-inducing viruses

Some viruses are linked to cancer, for example human papilloma virus (HPV) (cervical cancer), Epstein–Barr virus (Burkett's lymphoma), and herpes simplex virus type 2 (HSV-2) (cervical cancer) (Betsy and Keogh, 2012b).

Treatment

Treatment of viruses is difficult because the virus lives inside the host's own cells. In most cases of acute viral infection, recommended treatment is rest, hydration and symptom control. Antiviral medication is appropriate in some cases, particularly in chronic infections, and aims to inhibit viral replication. Interferons may also be used to stimulate the body's own immune system. Viruses cannot be treated with antibiotics, although these may be used if secondary bacterial infections occur.

6 The innate immune response

Figure 6.1 Physical and biochemical defence mechanisms of the innate immune response

Lysozyme:
• Tears
• Nasal secretions
• Saliva

Mucous membranes:
• Mucus prevents adherence of bacteria to epithelial cells

Lactoperoxide:
• Milk

Flushing action:
• Urine

Spermine and zinc:
• Semen

Flushing action:
• Tears
• Saliva

Ciliary cells:
• Expel microorganisms trapped in mucus by coughing and sneezing

Lactic acid/ fatty acids:
• Sweat
• Skin

Gastric acid:
• Stomach

Source: Mims et al, 2004

Figure 6.2 A macrophage engulfing bacteria

Macrophage

Bacteria

Figure 6.3 The process of phagocytosis

Microbe
Cytoplasm
Pseudopods
Plasma membrane
Phagosome (phagocytic vesicle)
Phagolysosome
Lysosome
Digestive enzymes
Partially digested microbe
Residual body

① ② ③ ④ ⑤ ⑥ ⑦

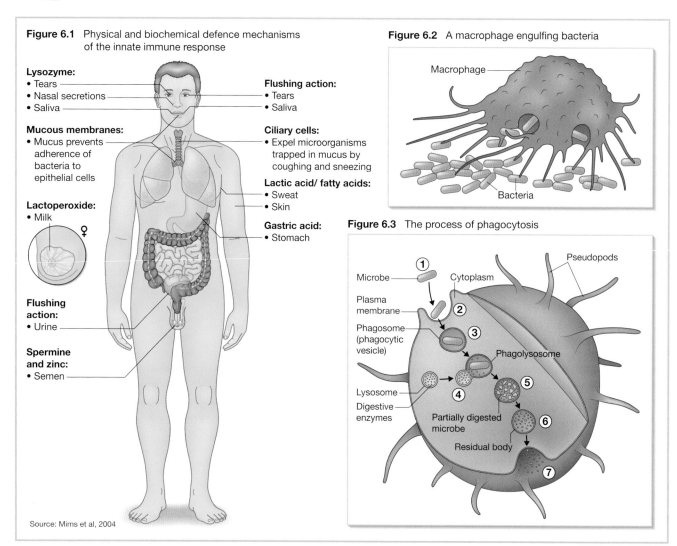

Infection Prevention and Control at a Glance, First Edition. By Debbie Weston, Alison Burgess and Sue Roberts.
© 2017 John Wiley & Sons, Ltd. Published 2017 by John Wiley & Sons, Ltd.

The aim of the immune system is to prevent invasion by microorganisms (bacteria, fungi, protozoa and viruses). It is frequently referred to in relation to how healthy an individual is, with those who have frequent illnesses described as having a 'poor' immune system, whereas those perceived as being healthy are said to have a 'strong' immune system. Whilst this simplistic view is largely true, the human immune system is a much more complex system than most people realise and it is remarkably effective at protecting humans from disease. The success of the immune system is based on its ability to distinguish between 'self' **antigens**, which are molecules on the surface of individual cells that indicate that they belong, and 'non-self' antigens, which the body recognises as being foreign cells/microorganisms that are invading the host. If the immune system recognises antigens as 'self' they will be ignored, but identification of non-self-antigens will initiate the **innate immune response**.

The innate and adaptive (acquired) immune response

There are two main immune responses which are interconnected and overlapping: the **innate response**, which is explained more fully in this chapter, and **the adaptive (acquired) response**, which is explained in Chapter 7. The innate immune response is so called because it is present from birth and unchanging, and is the **first line** of defense against infection. It is also a **non-specific** response that will *not* generate long-lasting immunity (Nairns and Helbert, 2005a).

Mechanical defence mechanisms of the innate immune response

The human body has a number of **non-specific physical and biochemical** defense mechanisms to protect it from infection. The main external barrier is the skin, which is a dry, thick layer of dead, keratinised cells that microorganisms find hard to penetrate. Skin pores, hair follicles and sweat glands are protected by the secretion of toxic chemicals such as fatty acids and lysozyme. Other entry points, such as the gastrointestinal, respiratory and genitourinary tracts, are protected by mucosal membranes that secrete thick layers of mucus, composed of proteins and polysaccharides that prevent penetration of bacteria into epithelial cell surfaces. In addition, there are many **commensal** microorganisms that compete with **pathogenic** bacteria for nutrients and attachment sites. The most common way for microorganisms to enter the body, therefore, is when the natural defences are breached, for example when wounds or burns exist. Figure 6.1 shows some of the biochemical and physical barriers to infection.

Biochemical defence mechanisms of the innate immune response

When microorganisms do successfully penetrate the body, two main defensive strategies are initiated within minutes of the attempted invasion.

First, the non-specific mechanism of **phagocytosis** begins. This involves the engulfment and killing of microorganisms by professional phagocytes which are specialised white blood cells originating in the bone marrow. They are primarily large macrophages, so named from the Greek words '*macros*' and '*phagein*', meaning 'large eaters', and are found in most tissues, particularly the lungs, liver and lymph nodes (Mims et al, 2004d) (see Figure 6.2). The process of phagocytosis is illustrated in Figure 6.3. The macrophage adheres to the microorganism (**1**), ingests it (**2**), forms a phagosome (**3**) that fuses with a lysosome (**4**), digests the microorganism (**5**) and forms a residual body around the indigestible material (**6**), which is then discharged (**7**).

The **neutrophils** (which are the most numerous white blood cells in the blood) then rapidly migrate to the site of infection. When pus is produced at a site of infection it is largely made up of neutrophils. Neutrophils detect structures commonly found on the surface of most bacteria. People who have defective or low counts of neutrophils (neutropenic) are at an increased risk of serious bacterial infection (Nairns and Helbert, 2005a).

Second, there are a number of soluble chemical factors such as bacterial enzymes released which are destructive to microorganisms, including the **complement cascade system**. Complement is a set of proteins circulating in the bloodstream. They are not toxic on their own but are activated by the presence of microorganisms in the host. The innate immune system uses a limited number of these proteins (Nairn and Helbert, 2005a).

The complement system attracts macrophages and neutrophils by chemotaxis and enhances or 'complements' the process of phagocytosis of antigens. It also forms a **membrane-attack complex (MAC)**, which effectively punches holes in the bacterial cell wall – mainly in Gram-negative bacteria. A large group of proteins called **cytokines**, in particular the **interferons (IFNs)**, are utilised. IFNs, which are produced by cells infected with viruses, inhibit the replication of many viruses and are involved in the activation of **natural killer cells (NKCs)**. Some IFNs are thought to have a role in detecting and eliminating cancerous host cells.

The NKCs can also detect certain virally infected cells and lyse them. They do this by using receptors to check the levels of the **major histocompatibility complex (MHC)**, which is a set of molecules found on cell surfaces of vertebrates. If low levels are detected (which is common in abnormal cell function), the NKCs trigger programmed cell death known as apoptosis (Nairn and Helbert, 2005a).

The actions of the innate immune response are often sufficient to destroy invading microbes. However, if it fails to clear the infection rapidly, cytokines are released by the macrophages as a means of signalling that the adaptive (acquired) immune response must be activated (see Chapter 7).

7 The acquired immune response

Table 7.1 Summary of basic differences between the innate and adaptive immune responses

Innate immune response features	Adaptive immune response features
• Present from birth and unchanging • First immune response: Very fast (minutes/hours) • Not specific: recognises general patterns of molecules on bacterial cell surfaces on 'non-self' antigens • Memory cells: No • Complement used: Yes • Able to work independently	• Adapts response permanently according to previous encounters with antigens • Secondary immune response: Slow, 7–10 days • Specific and diverse response: recognises specific 'non-self' antigens • Memory cells: Yes • Complement used: Yes • Will only be activated if innate immune system fails to overwhelm invading microorganisms

Figure 7.2 Examples of diseases with an autoimmune component (there are more than 80 types of autoimmune associated disease)

- Type 1 diabetes
- Hashimoto's thyroiditis
- Guillain–Barré syndrome
- Rheumatoid arthritis
- Reactive arthritis
- Multiple sclerosis
- Systemic lupus erythematosus
- Graves' disease
- Myasthenia gravis
- Pernicious anaemia
- Coeliac disease
- Addison's disease
- Temporal arteritis
- Autoimmune cardiomyopathy
- Narcolepsy
- Sjögren's syndrome

Figure 7.1 Important components involved in the innate and adaptive immune response

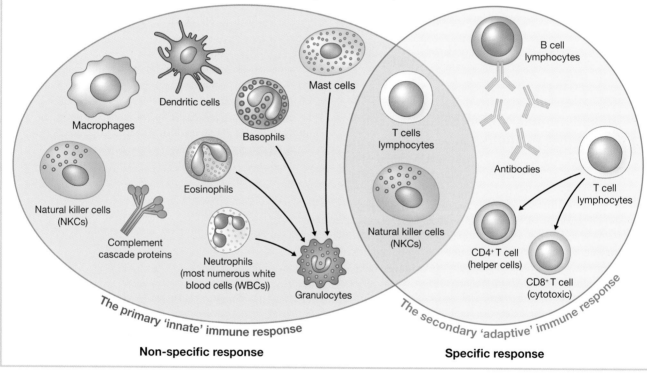

Infection Prevention and Control at a Glance, First Edition. By Debbie Weston, Alison Burgess and Sue Roberts.
© 2017 John Wiley & Sons, Ltd. Published 2017 by John Wiley & Sons, Ltd.

The adaptive system is the secondary immune response, triggered by the innate immune response. It only comes into play if the innate immune response fails to overwhelm the invading microorganism, or if the microorganism has found a way to avoid interaction with the innate system. (See Chapter 4 for information regarding bacterial virulence factors and Chapter 5 for information on the evasion mechanisms employed by viruses.) The adaptive immune system differs from the innate immune system in that it is capable of distinguishing 'self' antigens from 'non-self' antigens (Nairns and Helbert, 2005a). This is accomplished by creating an anticipatory defence system of recognition molecules that interact with foreign, non-self antigens.

Features of the adaptive immune response

The adaptive immune response, whilst highly effective, is much slower than the innate response and may take 7–10 days to mobilise completely (Nairns and Helbert, 2005a). As well as being able to be **specific** in its response, another major feature of the adaptive response is that it is **diverse**, which means it is able to respond to almost any antigen it has previously encountered and has a **memory** of these previous encounters. This helps to prevent the body being re-infected with the same microorganism. Table 7.1 and Figure 7.1 summarise the differences between the innate and immune response systems.

Activation of the adaptive immune response

In addition to macrophages, lymphocytes known as **dendritic cells** (found in the skin) play a critical role in the activation of the adaptive immune response (Nairns and Helbert, 2005a). **Lymphocytes** are white blood cells which also originate in the bone marrow but settle in lymphoid organs such as the thymus (Mims et al, 2004e). The main function of dendritic cells is to present antigens on their cell surface to the T and B cells.

When a foreign antigen enters the body, it eventually encounters a lymphocyte with a matching receptor. The cell that best fits the antigen divides and produces a large number of 'daughter 'cells or clones which are mobilised to attack the invading microorganisms (Nairns and Helbert, 2005b).

Primary antigen-receptor cells active in the adaptive immune response

There are **three** groups of antigen-receptor cells which specifically recognise foreign non-self antigens as part of the adaptive response. They are normally at rest but become activated on encountering non-self antigens or when innate messenger cells signal that assistance in fighting the invading microorganisms is required.

T and B lymphocytes: Unique antigen receptors found on B and T lymphocytes provide *specific* immunity, and B cells also produce soluble antigen receptors known as **antibodies** (Nairns and Helbert, 2005c). Antibodies are proteins or immunoglobulins that react *specifically* with the antigen that originally stimulated their production (Nairns and Helbert, 2005b). The normal circulating antibodies responsible for the immune response to bacteria are IgG and IgM.

The major histocompatibility complex (MHC): The third group of antigen receptors, which is present in all vertebrates, has the function of presenting antigenic peptides to the T cells. B and T cells differ in that B cell antigen receptors can interact directly with antigen, whereas T cell antigen receptors only recognise antigen when it is presented to them on the surface of another cell by MHC molecules. Intracellular pathogens are eliminated by T cells and macrophages, whereas extracellular pathogens are eliminated by B cell antibodies (Nairns and Helbert, 2005c).

NB: The term '**cell-mediated immunity**', which is sometimes used, refers to the function of T cells, phagocytes, and **cytokines**, *without* the involvement of antibodies, whilst **humoral or antibody-mediated immunity** involves the B cells and antibodies.

Complement

In the adaptive immune response, the complement system continues to play a major role by enhancing the effect of antibodies. In summary, complement enhances phagocytosis of antigens (opsonisation), attracts macrophages and neutrophils by chemotaxis, causes cell **lysis** of foreign antigens, and causes agglutination (clumping together) of **pathogens**. There are three ways in which complement can be activated: the lectin pathway, the mannan-binding lectin (MBL) pathway and the classical pathway (Nairns and Helbert, 2005d).

The role of the adaptive immune system in eliminating cancer cells

In addition to recognising non-self antigens, the immune system also recognises alterations of self resulting from certain disease processes, such as modified self-antigens found on tumour cells, and may eliminate the tumour once it is recognised.

The development of autoimmune diseases

Unfortunately, because the adaptive immune system is an anticipatory defence system, it can sometimes generate 'anti-self' receptors which, if not destroyed, can lead to autoimmune (anti-self) diseases (see Figure 7.2 for examples of autoimmune diseases).

Vaccination (see Chapter 13)

The aspect of 'memory' has been used successfully in the formation of **attenuated 'live' vaccines**, which use a less virulent form of a microorganism to stimulate an immune response. This memory ensures that if an identical or similar antigen is encountered, the immune response will be much *faster* and *greater in magnitude*, ensuring that the infection is limited or prevented altogether (Nairns and Helbert, 2005e).

Promoting a healthy immune system

The immune system requires adequate nutrition to function well. Therefore people who are malnourished, as is common with the elderly, may not have a healthy and strong immune system. Eating a balanced diet, particularly one rich in antioxidants, for example vitamins C, E, beta-carotene and selenium, may help to enhance the effectiveness of the immune system.

Principles of specimen collection

Figure 8.1 Best-practice principles of specimen collection

Clinical specimen required to identify infection/disease and ensure appropriate antimicrobial therapy (see Chapter 10), and monitor response to treatment

Correct specimen, from the correct site, taken at the correct time, using the correct technique. The person obtaining the specimen is responsible for its quality and must be competent

Appropriate container for the specimen being collected; shatterproof; not overfilled; lid secure; specimen bag (sealed); secure, rigid, unbreakable container/transport box

Must be accompanied by a Specimen Request Form and labelled as follows:

Patient's full name; date of birth; hospital/NHS number; ward/department or GP

Specimen type and site: Different body sites have different bacterial populations. A poorly labelled clinical specimen will make it harder for laboratory staff to differentiate between organisms which could normally be expected to be resident and those which should not be there

Date and time of specimen collection: The 'age' of the specimen is important. Some organisms are fragile and will die once they have been removed from their normal environment. If the specimen has been contaminated during collection, or if there is mixed growth in the specimen, some organisms may overgrow, making it difficult to single out a particular organism as the cause of the infection

Relevant signs and symptoms

Date of surgery if applicable

Recent history of foreign travel and any vaccinations if appropriate

Current or recently completed courses of antibiotics/other antimicrobial agents: May suppress or inhibit the growth of pathogens

Steroids/immunosuppressive drugs: Can depress the inflammatory response

Investigation required

Danger of Infection labelling: Microorganisms are categorised according to the level of risk they may pose. Specific organisms may be classed as hazardous and will be processed under laboratory conditions accordingly

Figure 8.2 Stool specimens for 'diarrhoea' taking the shape of the pot

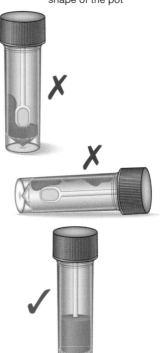

Figure 8.3 Blood culture collection

Indications for collection	Focal signs of infection; core temperature outside normal range; chills or rigors within the previous 24 hours; new or worsening confusion; raised or very low white cell count; signs of sepsis (i.e. acute = circulatory failure, low blood pressure or raised respiratory rate)

Do's and Don'ts

✓ Must only be collected by staff who have been assessed as competent in blood culture collection technique

✓ Use a dedicated blood culture collection pack

✓ If blood is being collected for other tests, collect the blood culture first

✓ If taking blood from an existing central venous catheter (CVC) or a peripherally inserted central catheter (PICC line) if the line is thought to be infected, also obtain a set of cultures from a peripheral stab

✓ Decontaminate hands at the critical points in the procedure (prior to decontaminating the patient's skin; immediately before donning examination gloves; after removing gloves)

✓ Decontaminate the skin around the venepuncture site with 2% chlorhexidine in 70% alcohol

✓ Decontaminate the blood culture bottle tops (which are clean but not sterile) with a 2% chlorhexidine gluconate in 70% alcohol swab and allow to air dry before inoculating the bottles

✓ Inoculate the aerobic bottle first (to prevent any air in the collection set entering the anaerobic bottle)

✓ If collecting more than two sets of blood cultures (i.e. four bottles), take the second set using a fresh stab

✓ Document the procedure in the patient's notes: date; time; site of venepuncture; indication; number of sets/bottles

✗ Do not use existing cannulae, or sites above existing cannulae

✗ Do not take blood from a femoral stab (due to the high risk of contamination)

Source: Department of Health, 2007b

Infection Prevention and Control at a Glance, First Edition. By Debbie Weston, Alison Burgess and Sue Roberts.
© 2017 John Wiley & Sons, Ltd. Published 2017 by John Wiley & Sons, Ltd.

The following clinical specimens are among those that are most commonly requested and collected for microbial culture and sensitivity. Figure 8.1 details the best-practice principles of specimen collection.

Urine

Mid-stream specimen of urine (MSU): The 'first portion' of urine is voided directly into the toilet or a bedpan so that organisms that reside within the distal urethra are flushed out. The 'second portion' is voided into a sterile container, requiring the patient to have sufficient bladder control, and the remainder into the toilet or bedpan. A 'clean-catch' (voided directly into a sterile container) may be the best method for urine collection in some patients. In babies, a self-adhesive urine collection bag can be used. The method used must be recorded on the Specimen Request Form.

Catheter specimen of urine (CSU): Urine specimens from catheterised patients to detect UTI must *only* be sent for laboratory culture if the patient has *clinical signs of sepsis* (see Chapters 25 and 30), *not* because the appearance or smell of the urine suggests that bacteria are present in the urine (Scottish Intercollegiate Guidelines Network, 2012). Urine must be obtained via the sampling port (never directly from the drainage bag) using a strict aseptic technique to avoid contamination of the key parts (see Chapter 19). Urine specimens must be sent to the laboratory within 2 hours of collection, or refrigerated at 4°C for no longer than 24 hours. If left at room temperature, bacteria within the specimen will multiply, making detection of any pathogen(s) difficult.

Sputum

The function of sputum is to trap any foreign material, including bacteria, and it is produced in excess when the lower respiratory tract is inflamed. When infection is present, sputum is generally **purulent**. As the mouth and pharynx host a large resident bacterial population, it can be difficult to detect the pathogen among the residents. A 'good' sputum specimen can yield a high bacterial load, and the 'best' specimen is often produced first thing in the morning following a deep cough. If the patient is physically unable to produce a sputum specimen, or there is no productive cough, sputum induction can be induced by saline nebuliser or bronchoscopy and lavage. As respiratory **pathogens** do not survive for long once they have left the host, sputum specimens must be sent to the laboratory immediately or refrigerated for no longer than 24 hours.

Wounds

Wound specimens should *only* be obtained if there are clinical signs of infection (chronic wounds are often heavily colonised with skin flora). The swab should be moved over the surface of the wound in a zigzag rolling fashion. Any debris on the surface of the wound should be removed before the swab is taken – it may contain high numbers of bacteria but this will not be representative of the organism causing the infection. When taking a specimen from 'deep seated' wounds or abscesses, any pus should be aspirated using a sterile syringe and decanted into a sterile container using an aseptic technique. Wound swabs must not be refrigerated.

Faeces

The colon is home to huge numbers of enteric pathogens, along with resident bowel flora, and with a gram of faeces containing up to 10^{12} organisms, identification of certain organisms may take up to 3–4 days. Stool specimens should be obtained within the first 48 hours of illness, as once the acute stage of the illness passes, the likelihood of identifying the pathogen diminishes. The stool should ideally be passed into a bedpan although it can be 'scraped' off a nappy or incontinence pad given that the stool specimen container has a scoop attached to the inside of the lid. Stool specimens can be tested if mixed with urine (this should be recorded on the Specimen Request Form). If intestinal protozoa are suspected, a 'hot' or fresh stool is required, as the protozoa are more likely to be mobile and therefore more easily identified live in a warm stool. 'Diarrhoeal' specimens, while they should not be described as 'loose stools', will be loose enough to take the shape of the container (see Figure 8.2).

Rectal swabs

Rectal swabs are commonly taken to detect carriage of multi-drug resistant enteric organisms such as **glycopeptide-resistant enterococci (GRE)** and **extended-spectrum beta-lactamases (ESBLs)** and carbapenemase-producing Enterobacteriaceae (CRE) (see Chapter 29). An un-moistened charcoal swab is gently inserted through the rectal sphincter, rotated through one full turn and then withdrawn; faecal matter should be visible on the swab.

Throat swabs

Throat swabs may be taken to identify infection with bacterial or viral pathogens, and asymptomatic carriage of *Streptococcus pyogenes* (see Chapter 36) and *Neisseria meningitidis* (see Chapter 39). The swab should be rolled over any areas of inflammation or exudate, or the tonsillar bed and oral pharynx. The swab should be withdrawn carefully to avoid coming into contact with the teeth, cheeks, tongue or gum, which could result in contamination. For virus detection, the swab should be placed in viral transport medium. Charcoal transport medium is supplied with swabs for bacterial culture.

Pernasal (nose) swabs

Pernasal swabs are taken for the detection of *Bordetella pertussis* (whooping cough), which is covered in Chapter 27. The technique for undertaking pernasal swabs is illustrated in Figure 27.5.

Blood cultures

Figure 8.3 outlines the indications for blood culture collection, along with some essential 'do's and don'ts' in order to avoid contamination of the culture with skin flora.

Cerebrospinal fluid (CSF) (see Chapter 39)

CSF is collected via lumbar puncture (LP) in order to exclude or confirm infection, inflammation and neoplastic disease. 125–150 ml of CSF envelop the brain and spinal cord, and under local anaesthetic and using a strict aseptic technique, approximately 8–15 ml are removed via the insertion of a spinal needle at the level of L3/4, or L4/5, through the ligamentum flavum and the dura mater into the subarachnoid space. Drops of CSF are collected into three sterile specimen pots, which must be labelled in order of collection. Where meningitis is suspected, laboratory staff must be informed in advance of the LP being undertaken so that they are in the laboratory to receive it.

MRSA screens

See Chapter 43.

9 The microbiology laboratory

Figure 9.1 Inoculating solid culture media

(a) The initial inoculum (inoculate) (1) is gradually reduced (2, 3 and 4) as it is 'plated' or 'streaked' onto a solid culture medium

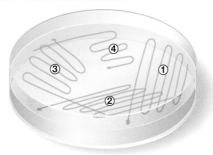

(b) Following incubation, colonies or isolated bacterial cells are visible on inoculated streaks

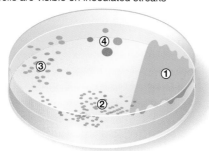

Figure 9.2 Stages in the processing of a clinical specimen

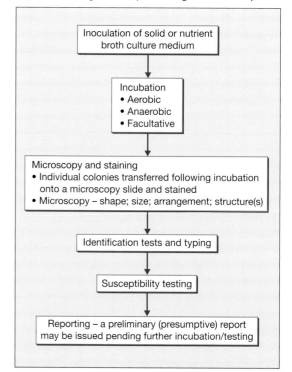

Figure 9.3 Laboratory report

Patient: xxxxxx (hospital or NHS no.)	Surname	Forename	M/F	DOB

Location: (Hospital and Ward or GP)   Dr: (Hospital Consultant or GP)

Tel no:

Specimen No.: xxxxxx (unique specimen identification no.)   Microbiology

Date: Time: Blood culture (specimen type)

Request reason: Temp > 38; cannula site VIP score 3 ?infected

Bacterial culture: (type of test)
Staph.aureus (MRSA) spa type: t002 isolated from 2 bottles (organism isolated and typing)
(Staphylococcus Reference Laboratory Report)

(Antibiotic sensitivities for treatment options)
Resistant: Mupirocin; Co-Amoxiclav; Amoxicillin; Ciprofloxacin; Clindamycin; Erythromycin; Gentamicin; Imipenem; Moxifloxacin; Flucloxacillin; Penicillin; Levofloxacin

Sensitive: Daptomycin; Fusidic acid; Linezolid; Rifampicin; Teicoplanin; Tetracycline; Vancomycin; Fosfomycin; Cotrimoxazole

Infection Prevention and Control at a Glance, First Edition. By Debbie Weston, Alison Burgess and Sue Roberts.
© 2017 John Wiley & Sons, Ltd. Published 2017 by John Wiley & Sons, Ltd.

'Growing' bacteria

In order to isolate organisms within the laboratory, they have to be grown, or cultured, under laboratory conditions that mimic the normal conditions under which they would reach their optimum growth either in the environment or the human host. The aim of growing or culturing bacteria is to grow a population of cells known as a **colony**, which is the product of 20–30 cell divisions of one single cell (Barer, 2007). Bacterial growth, involving an increase in the organism's size and number, is dependent upon a number of factors:

Nutrients: These are broken down by the bacteria and used as an energy source. They include water (a bacterial cell is 70–95% water so moisture is an essential element to ensure that the bacteria remain moist and do not die), oxygen, carbon dioxide, iron, carbohydrates and trace elements. These are provided in various types of solid or liquid culture media, which generally consist of water, sodium chloride and electrolytes, peptone, meat and yeast extracts and blood, to which various nutrients and / or inhibitors (e.g. bile salts and antibiotics) are added. The number of bacterial cells increases exponentially with time. As the nutrient supply becomes depleted, the culture media will become over-populated, and bacterial growth will slow or lag ('lag' phase) and then cease altogether.

Temperature: All bacteria have an optimum growth temperature and will cease to grow if the temperature is below the minimum and above 'their' maximum temperature. Most pathogenic bacteria will grow at normal body temperature 37 °C and multiply rapidly, although it may take 24–48 hours before enough cells have grown to enable further testing. To achieve optimum growth in the laboratory, specimens are placed in incubators.

Oxygen: Some bacteria only grow in an oxygen-rich environment (aerobic bacteria) and others in an oxygen-deprived environment (anaerobic bacteria). Facultative bacteria can grow with or without oxygen, but thrive better in an oxygen-rich environment.

Inoculating culture media (PHE, 2013a)

When inoculating solid culture medium, a swab is rubbed over a quarter, or a third, of the surface of a Petri dish (or plate) containing solid culture medium (i.e. agar). This is the '**inoculum**' or the 'inoculate'. Using either a sterile wire (or plastic loop or a sterile glass spreader), and a completely sterile aseptic technique to avoid contamination, the inoculate is then 'streaked' or 'plated' over the surface of the medium (see Figure 9.1). The lid of the Petri dish is replaced to prevent airborne contamination of the specimen, and the loop / wire is ' flamed' by passing it through the flame of a Bunsen burner until it achieves 'red heat' in order to remove any residual bacteria. This process is repeated and the original inoculate is spread into three sections and reduced with each spread or streak. Bacteria that are well separated from others will grow as isolated colonies and can be assumed to have arisen from a single organism, or an organism cluster which is known as a colony forming unit (cfu).

If a liquid culture medium (nutrient broth) is used, the broth is inoculated from the 'plated' specimen via an inoculating loop or wire.

The specimen is incubated either aerobically or anaerobically for 24–36 hours and then 'read' or visually observed for growth. Millions of bacterial cells will be visible on the agar plate as colonies along the inoculation lines after 24 hours, unless the organism happens to be a slow grower, in which case there will be no visible growth. Nutrient broth will become increasingly cloudy or turbid due to the growth of bacteria. As culture plates normally grow a mix of bacteria, including normal body flora, the colonies can be inoculated onto another culture plate containing a culture medium that is more selective. Bacteria grown in nutrient broth are inoculated onto solid culture medium for bacterial identification.

Gram staining (PHE, 2015a).

Once an organism has been cultured, it needs to be identified (classified). Bacterial classification has a direct impact on the antibiotic therapy required. As bacteria are naturally colourless, the first step in the identification process is Gram staining, which identifies differences in the bacterial cell wall (see Chapter 3). The specimen is 'heat fixed' onto a glass slide. Blue dye (crystal violet) is used to cover the slide and left for 30 seconds. After this the dye is washed off and decolourised with acetone. The acetone is then washed off and a counter stain, a red dye (safranin), is applied. After 60 seconds the slide is washed and blot-dried. If the bacteria are **Gram-positive** they will stain blue / black, having retained the crystal violet; if they are **Gram-negative** then they will stain red / pink, having retained the safranin. Mycobacteria cannot be Gram stained due to the high lipid content of their bacterial cell wall and have to be identified using the Ziehl–Neelsen staining method (see Chapter 44).

Antibiotic susceptibility and sensitivity testing

Isolated bacterial colonies from the culture plate are inoculated onto a new agar plate using an aseptic technique. Antibiotic-impregnated paper discs are placed onto the plate. The antibiotics begin to diffuse into the agar immediately. If the bacteria are sensitive (susceptible) to the antibiotic, a zone of inhibition will form around the disc. If the bacteria are resistant, they will grow right up to the edge of the disc.

Polymerase chain reaction (PCR)

PCR amplifies fragments of DNA millions of times by 'unzipping' DNA fragments through the repeated application of heat, followed by a period of cooling and then re-heating, separating the DNA strands to such a degree that specific detection of a pathogen is possible.

Serology

Antibodies (see Chapter 7) are detected through the examination of blood serum (and bodily fluids such as saliva and semen where appropriate).

Typing

'Typing' , which is undertaken in a specialist Public Health England Reference Laboratory, is used to determine / identify the genus and species of bacteria (see Chapter 3) and differentiate between strains of bacteria within a species based on their phenotype (physical / biochemical characteristics) and genotype (genetic makeup). Typing techniques are also used to identify strain evolution and emerging pathogens / clones.

Figure 9.2 shows the different stages in the processing of a clinical specimen. Figure 9.3 is an illustration of a laboratory report.

10 Antibiotics and prescribing

Figure 10.1 The principles of antimicrobial stewardship

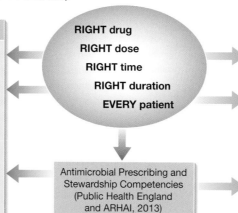

Start Smart

- Do not prescribe antibiotics in the absence of clinical signs of infection

- Obtain appropriate cultures (clinical specimens) before prescribing, but do not delay commencing treatment in the event of potentially life-threatening illness or infection

- The indication for prescribing, duration, route, dose and review date must be recorded on the drug chart

- Make appropriate entries in the medical notes

RIGHT drug
RIGHT dose
RIGHT time
RIGHT duration
EVERY patient

Antimicrobial Prescribing and Stewardship Competencies (Public Health England and ARHAI, 2013)

Then Focus

- Review the patient, check microbiology results and review prescribing decision, at 48 hours

- Document decision
? stop
? *IV/oral switch
? change from broad to narrow spectrum agent
? continue for a further 24 hours and then review
? outpatient parenteral therapy

*IV route only if:
- Severe infection (i.e. septicaemia, meningitis, endocarditis)
- Immunocompromised
- Unable to tolerate orally
- Drug isn't absorbed via the gut
- If adequate blood levels aren't achieved
- If given as surgical prophylaxis

*Switch to oral when:
- Temperature 38°C for 48 hours
- WCC normal/returning to normal
- Able to tolerate oral fluids
- No absorption problems

Source: Department of Health Advisory Committee on Antimicrobial Resistance and Healthcare Associated Infections (ARHAI) (2011)

The definition of 'antibiotic' is 'a substance produced by a microorganism that is effective in killing or inhibiting the growth of another microorganism' (Engelkirk and Duben-Engelkirk, 2011). It was originally applied to naturally occurring compounds such as penicillin that lysed bacteria without harming the host, but with advances in medicine and science, antibiotics have been manufactured synthetically and semi-synthetically through the chemical manipulation of these compounds. Although the term 'antibiotic' is still used to describe the agents used to treat bacterial infections, the broader term 'antimicrobial agents' is now applied to both natural and synthetic compounds used in the treatment of bacterial, viral, fungal, protozoal and helminth infections in humans and animals. They also come under the broader heading of chemotherapeutic agents (any chemical (drug) used to treat any condition or disease).

Characteristics of antibiotics

Selective toxicity: They must be able to kill or inhibit bacteria without adversely harming the host.

Degree of toxicity: Measured by the therapeutic index – the therapeutic dose (the level / amount required for treatment), and the toxic dose (the level at which it is too toxic for the patient). When antibiotics such as intravenous (IV) vancomycin, gentamicin and amikacin are prescribed, doses are based on the patient's renal function and weight.

Therapeutic drug monitoring (TDM): This is required at determined intervals over the course at treatment, pre and post dose, in order to determine 'trough levels' (the level of drug in the bloodstream). The timing of the trough levels and their values / range are specific to each antibiotic. If the trough level pre dose is low, this could be because a dose has been missed and there has been a prolonged time interval between doses, so the level of antibiotic may not be within the therapeutic range. If the trough level is too high, the antibiotic will become toxic to the patient and will be outside the therapeutic range.

Narrow spectrum: Effectiveness is limited to either specific Gram-positive or Gram-negative bacteria (see Chapter 3).

Broad spectrum: Effective against a wide range of Gram-positive and Gram-negative bacteria. The disadvantage of broad-spectrum agents is that they are indiscriminate, and as well as destroying the pathogen(s) they will also destroy or disrupt the resident flora.

Bactericidal: Bacteria are killed

Bacteriostatic: Bacterial growth is slowed or inhibited. The host immune system is able to take over the 'killing' of the pathogen(s). Bacteriostatic agents should never be prescribed for individuals with an impaired immune response, particularly where neutrophil production and response is impaired (see Chapter 6).

Choice / route of administration

The choice of antibiotic is dependent upon: the organism / likely organism and its antibiotic sensitivities; site of infection (not all antibiotics are able to penetrate bone, joints, or cerebrospinal fluid (CSF)); patient history (e.g. allergy or other contraindications).

Certain antibiotics have a synergistic effect when used in combination with another. Combination therapy may be indicated in the initial treatment of systemic infections before the causative organism is known; if the organism cannot be isolated; if the infection is caused by more than one organism (polymicrobial); and in the treatment of infections caused by antibiotic-resistant organisms. The route of administration also depends on the organism and the site of infection. Some antibiotics can only be prescribed orally or IV. The IV route is used where it is particularly important that adequate concentrations of the antibiotic have been achieved for the treatment of serious systemic infections, or where the patient cannot tolerate oral medication.

Classes of antibiotics / actions

Antibiotics that interfere with bacterial cell wall synthesis

The bacterial cell wall is prevented from forming, or is weakened so that the osmotic pressure exerted outside the cell causes it to swell and burst.

Penicillins: Either naturally occurring or semi-synthetic, e.g. benzylpenicillin (penicillin G), amoxicillin, Augmentin (co-amoxyclav), Timentin (ticarcillin / clavulanate) and flucloxacillin. They are bactericidal and belong to a class of antibiotics known as the beta-lactams. They possess in their structure a beta-lactam ring, which is essential for antibacterial activity and specifically targets transpeptidase, a bacterial enzyme responsible for cross-linkage of the peptidoglycan layers in the cell wall (see Chapter 3) (Ryan and Drew, 2010a).

Cephalosporins (beta-lactams): Bactericidal.
- First generation cephalosporins, e.g. cefradine. Narrow spectrum – highly effective against Gram-positive bacteria.
- Second generation, e.g. cefuroxime. Extended spectrum; increased activity against Gram-negative bacteria.
- Third generation, e.g. cefotaxime, ceftazidime, ceftriaxone. Broad spectrum, potent and low toxicity.

Carbapenems (beta-lactams): Bactericidal and broad spectrum, e.g. meropenem, imipenem, doripenem and ertapenem. Their molecular structure makes them highly resistant to enzymes (beta-lactamases) produced by beta-lactam resistant antibiotics, but susceptible to carbapenemases, produced by carbapenem-resistant bacteria (see Chapter 29).

Glycopeptides: Bactericidal, e.g. vancomycin and teicoplanin. Narrow spectrum – Gram-positive bacteria; highly effective against staphylococci and enterococci.

Glycyclines: Tigecycline. Bacteriostatic and broad spectrum. Effective against most medically important bacteria.

Antibiotics that inhibit bacterial protein synthesis

These antibiotics work by 'shutting down' the ribosome, where proteins essential for the cell's function are manufactured.

Macrolides: Bacteriostatic, but bactericidal at high doses, e.g. clarithromycin and erythromycin.

Antibiotics that inhibit nucleic acid synthesis

These antibiotics prevent DNA from being transcribed into RNA, or disrupt the coiling / uncoiling of DNA.

Fluoroquinolones: Bactericidal, e.g. ciprofloxacin, moxifloxacin and levofloxacin.

Oxazolidinone: Bacteriostatic; narrow spectrum – Gram-positive infections only, particularly those caused by MRSA.

Nitroimidazole: Metronidazole. Effective against anaerobic bacteria.

Perforation of bacterial cell membrane

Cyclic lipopeptide: Daptomycin. Effective against most Gram-negative bacteria.

Figure 10.1 describes the principles of antibiotic stewardship – best practice in antibiotic prescribing regarding the prevention of antimicrobial resistance (see Chapter 11).

11 Antimicrobial resistance

Figure 11.1 UK 5-year antimicrobial resistance strategy (DH/DEFRA, 2013): seven key areas for action and key quotes

1 Improving infection prevention and control practices.
'As infections do not respect borders, infection control needs to be addressed nationally and internationally.'

2 Optimising prescribing practices.
'... we equally need to ensure use of the right drug, right dose at the right time and for the right duration to limit unnecessary antibiotic exposure.'

3 Improving professional education, training and public engagement.
'Patients frequently believe, incorrectly, that antibiotics will help them recover from all respiratory tract infections faster... patient consultations can be difficult when patients expect antibiotics for self-limiting infections.'

4 Developing new drugs, treatments and diagnostics.
'The discovery of new drugs takes time (about 10–15 years)...human and veterinary rapid diagnostics are urgently needed to help differentiate between bacterial and viral infections, as well as to enable fast identification of highly resistant strains.'

5 Better access to surveillance data.
'Better sharing of local, regional and national information and data on emerging issues in human and animal health, together with use of early warning systems, is needed to trigger appropriate containment measures to limit the spread of resistant organisms.'

6 Better identification and prioritisation of AMR needs to focus activity and influence our understanding of AMR.

7 Strengthened international collaboration.
'AMR is a global problem and needs concerted global action to tackle it.'

Figure 11.2 Reasons for the development and spread of antibiotic resistance

Reasons for the development of antibiotic resistance in healthcare

Prescribing factors

- Treatment of conditions where antibiotics are not indicated
- Inadequate dose or duration – infection only partially resolved
- Monotherapy, where combination therapy would have been appropriate (i.e. more than one antibiotic)
- Prophylaxis – not indicated, or duration too long
- Over-the-counter availability of antibiotics and indiscriminate prescribing practices
- Use of antibiotics in veterinary medicine – often administered prophylactically in animals bred for human consumption to protect herds from disease – resistant bacteria can be transferred to humans via the food chain, or resistant pathogens in animals can transfer resistant strains to humans

In healthcare settings

- Greater bed occupancy rates – increased opportunities for cross-infection
- Increased patient: staff ratios
- Breakdown in IP&C practice, i.e. hand hygiene
- Environmental reservoirs

Patient factors

- Patient expectation
- Immunosuppression; intensity and duration of exposure to broad spectrum antibiotics; alteration of the patient's own flora as a result of hospitalisation/antibiotic therapy; severity of illness/co-morbidities
- Travel to countries with higher rates of resistant organisms (see Chapter 29)

Suggested resources

Compassion in world farming: www.ciwf.org.uk

Compassion in World Farming (2011). Case Study of a Health Crisis. How human health is under threat from overuse of antibiotics in intensive livestock farming

Antibiotic Research UK: www.antibioticresearch.org.uk

World Health Organization (WHO): www.who.int/

www.nhs.uk/NHSEngland/ARC/pages/AboutARC.aspx

Infection Prevention and Control at a Glance, First Edition. By Debbie Weston, Alison Burgess and Sue Roberts.

The discovery of penicillin and the development of antimicrobial agents revolutionised the treatment of infections and infectious disease, but the increasing global problem of antimicrobial resistance has the potential to transport healthcare back to the pre-antibiotic era. In March 2013, Sally Davies, the Chief Medical Officer for Great Britain and Northern Ireland, declared that 'Antimicrobial resistance is a ticking time bomb not only for the UK but also for the world. We need to work with everyone to ensure the apocalyptic scenario of widespread antimicrobial resistance does not become a reality. This is a threat arguably as important as climate change for the world' (DH, 2011a). She also called for it to be placed on the national risk register and the strategic risk registers for the Department of Health (DH) and the Department for Environment, Food and Rural Affairs (DEFRA). The need for a collaborative international response to tackle the problem was also a priority for discussion by the G8 Science Ministers at the G8 Summit in 2013. Figure 11.1 lists the seven key areas for action from the UK 5-year antimicrobial resistance strategy (DH/DEFRA, 2013).

Definition of antimicrobial resistance

Antimicrobial resistance is the ability of a microorganism to grow in the presence of an 'agent' (chemical or drug) that would normally kill it or inhibit its growth. It is a complex phenomenon, involving the organism, the antimicrobial agent, the environment and the patient, and it gives microorganisms a distinct competitive advantage, perpetuating Darwin's theory of the 'survival of the fittest' (Turnidge and Christiansen, 2005). Antibiotics 'select' for resistance by targeting antibiotic sensitive organisms, 'allowing' the resistant, more dominant organisms to survive. Antibiotic selection pressure can be removed by restricting the use of the antibiotic, either permanently or temporarily, in a particular patient population.

The development of antimicrobial resistance

Within 10 years of the mass production of penicillin in the 1940s, strains of *Staphylococcus aureus*, which was a significant hospital **pathogen** (see Chapter 43), developed resistance to penicillin. Meticillin-resistant *Staphylococcus aureus* (MRSA) was first reported in 1963, a mere three years after the development of meticillin (a semi-synthetic form of penicillin developed to combat the problem of penicillin resistance), and the next five decades saw resistance develop among most microorganisms to the majority of antimicrobial agents.

Mechanisms of resistance

Inherent resistance: Part of the organism's genetic makeup. It is not naturally susceptible to one or more antimicrobial agents.

Acquired resistance: Occurs as a result of spontaneous genetic mutations and / or genetic recombinations. Self-replicating pieces of DNA which exist outside of the bacterial chromosome (plasmids) and mobile DNA segments (transposons) which carry genes for resistance and virulence transfer genetic material from one organism to another. This transfer commonly occurs through conjugation, transduction or transformation.

- **Conjugation:** The major mechanism for the transfer of antibiotic resistance and the exchange of genetic material between a recipient cell and a donor cell from unrelated species of bacteria. DNA is transferred from a donor to a recipient bacterial cell via a specialised structure on the donor cell known as the sex pilus. This makes contact with, and attaches to, the recipient cell, penetrating the cell membrane and allowing the transfer of DNA from one cell to another (Neidhardt, 2004; Willey et al, 2011).
- **Transduction:** DNA can be transferred between bacteria by viruses which infect bacteria, known as bacteriophages. In order for a bacteriophage to infect a bacterial cell, it must randomly collide with a cell which it has a natural affinity to, and then attach and bind to a specific receptor on the bacterial cell wall before injecting its genetic material into the cell membrane.
- **Transformation:** When a bacterial cell is dying and breaking up, closely related species of bacteria are able to 'take up' the DNA and incorporate it into their own chromosome.

Other mechanisms of resistance include:

- **The production of enzymes: Penicillinases / beta-lactamases** are enzymes that cleave or break open the beta-lactam ring, a structural component of penicillins and cephalosporins. Extended spectrum beta-lactamases (ESBLs) are enzymes that confer resistance not only to penicillins and cephalosporins, but also to many other antibiotics. **Carbapenemases** confer resistance to a group of antibiotics known as the carbapenems (see Chapter 29). They are made by a small but growing number of strains of Enterobacteriaceae. Carbapenem resistance poses one of the biggest threats to global public health.
- **Impermeability of the bacterial cell wall:** The protective outer membrane of a Gram-negative bacterial cell wall (see Chapter 3) means that some antibiotics are simply unable to penetrate it. However, the structure of the cell membrane can be altered through chromosomal mutation, which alters the structure of the cell membrane and changes its permeability (Engelkirk and Duben-Engelkirk, 2011).
- **Efflux pumps:** Some bacteria possess an inner membrane protein which acts as an efflux pump, effectively 'pumping' the antibiotic out of the cell. These pumps may be antibiotic-specific, or they may be capable of rejecting multiple classes of antibiotics. Efflux pumps are carried by a number of clinically significant bacteria, including *Campylobacter jejuni* (Chapter 28), *Escherichia coli, Staphylococcus aureus* (Chapter 43), *Pseudomonas aeruginosa, Streptococcus pneumoniae* and *Salmonella typhimurium* (Chapter 42) (Webber and Piddock, 2003)
- **Alteration of target site:** The antibiotic can enter the cell, but structural changes within the cell prevent the antibiotic from attaching or binding to it.
- **Alternative metabolic pathways:** The antibiotic bypasses the site within the bacterial cell at which it would normally be effective (i.e. the aspect of bacterial function which it would normally inhibit).

There are many reasons for the development of antimicrobial resistance; these are described in Figure 11.2.

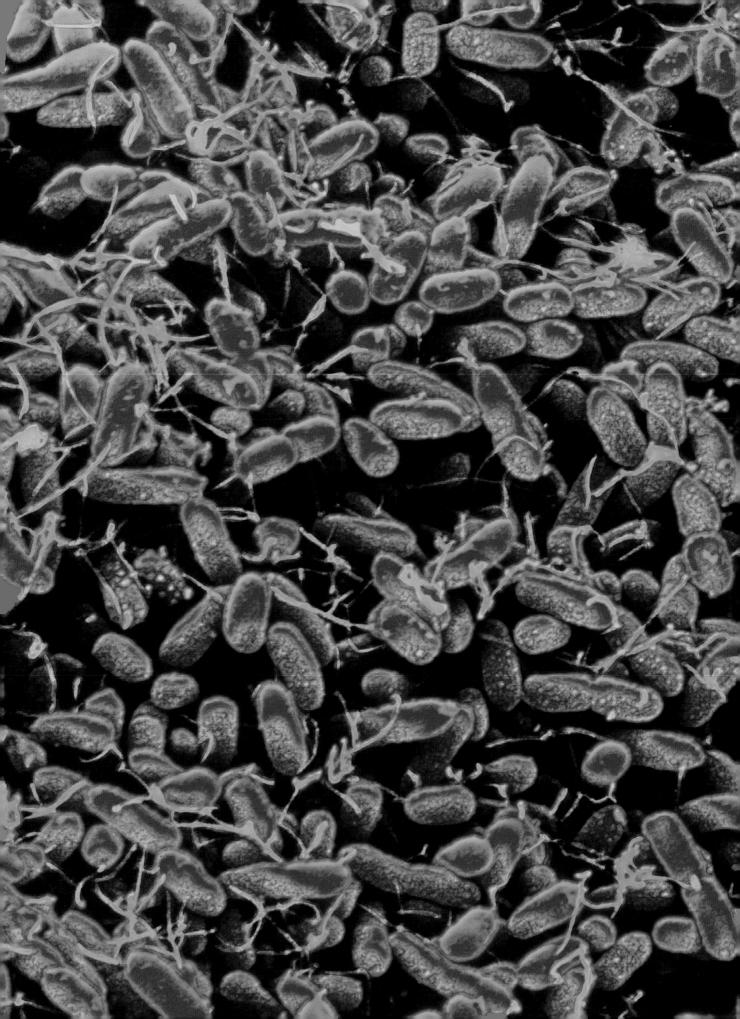

The principles of infection prevention and control

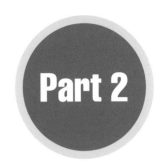

Part 2

Chapters

12 The chain of infection

Figure 12.1 The chain of infection
Source: CDC 2012

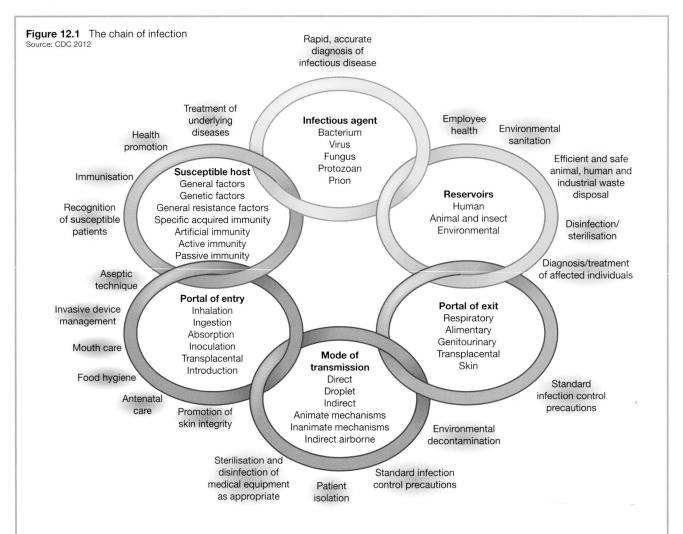

Figure 12.2 Human reservoirs

There are two types of human reservoir: acute cases and carriers.

Acute clinical cases are individuals who are infected with the disease agent and become ill, displaying signs and symptoms. Because they are ill, their contacts may be limited and their normal activities curtailed. They are more likely to be diagnosed and treated.

Carriers are individuals who harbour infectious agents but are not ill and generally have no signs and symptoms of an infectious disease. Carriers do not exhibit signs and symptoms of infection and their activities are not restricted by their illness. As a result they may present more of a risk to others. Carriers may be further subdivided into:

- **Incubatory carriers.** These are individuals that transmit their infection before their own symptoms start. An example is measles (the virus will be shed in nasal and throat secretions 1–2 days before any cold-like symptoms or rash is noticeable).
- **Inapparent infections.** Individuals with inapparent infections never develop the infection themselves but are able to transmit the infection to others. An example is poliomyelitis. Of every 100 individuals infected with poliomyelitis virus only 1 will become paralysed, 4 others will develop mild illness and 95 will exhibit no symptoms at all but will pass the virus in their faeces.
- **Convalescent carriers.** These are individuals that continue to be infectious beyond their recovery phase. Salmonella is an example where individuals may continue to excrete the bacteria in their faeces for several weeks and even up to a year or more. Treatment with antibiotics may prolong the carrier phase.
- **Chronic carriers.** These are individuals that continue their carrier status for a year or more after their recovery. The chronic carrier state is not uncommon with hepatitis B infection and may be lifelong. Approximately 90% of infants infected at birth become chronic carriers of the disease compared to only 1–10% infected after the age of 5.

Source: Adapted from http://health.mo.gov/training/epi/DiseaseProcess.html

Infection Prevention and Control at a Glance, First Edition. By Debbie Weston, Alison Burgess and Sue Roberts.
© 2017 John Wiley & Sons, Ltd. Published 2017 by John Wiley & Sons, Ltd.

Figure 12.3 Animal reservoirs (adapted from PHE, 2013b)

Humans can be subject to diseases that have animal reservoirs. Many of these diseases are transmitted from animal to animal, with humans as incidental hosts. The term zoonosis refers to an infectious disease that is transmissible under natural conditions from vertebrate animals to humans.

Disease	Main reservoirs	Usual mode of transmission to humans
Anthrax	Livestock, wild animals, environment	Direct contact, ingestion
Avian influenza	Poultry, ducks	Direct contact
Brucellosis	Cattle, goats, sheep, pigs	Daily products, milk
Cat scratch fever	Cats	Bite, scratch
Cryptosporidiosis	Cattle, sheep, pets	Water, direct contact
Campylobacter	Poultry, farm animals	Raw meat, milk
Salmonella	Poultry, cattle, sheep, pigs	Foodborne
Hepatitis E	Not yet known	Not yet known
Leptospirosis	Rodents, ruminants	Infected urine, water
Rabies	Dogs, foxes, bats, cats	Animal bite
Ringworm	Cats, dogs, cattle, many animal species	Direct contact
Toxoplasmosis	Cats, ruminants	Ingestion of faecal oocysts, meat
Ebola, Crimean-Congo haemorrhagic fever, Lassa and Marburg viruses	Variously: rodents, ticks, livestock, primates, bats	Direct contact, inoculation, ticks

Source: Department of Health. Used under OGL

Understanding the principles of how infections and infectious disease become established is fundamental to effective infection prevention and control. Infectious disease results from the interaction of an infectious agent, a host and an environment. This process is often referred to as the 'chain of infection', starting with the pathogen (infectious agent) and ending with an infected host. All the links in the chain need to be in place for the infection to occur. Understanding this sequence of events allows appropriate control measures to be implemented to disrupt or 'break' the chain. These are most effective when directed at the links that are most susceptible to intervention. Potential interventions are primarily aimed at controlling or eliminating the agent at source, protecting portals of entry and increasing the host's defences. The chain of infection is made up of six links: pathogen (infectious agent), reservoir, portal of exit, mode of transmission, portal of entry and susceptible host (CDC, 2012) (see Figure 12.1).

Link 1 – The pathogen (infectious agent)

There are five main classes of infectious agents (**pathogens**): bacteria, viruses, fungi, **protozoa** and **prions**.

The factors that determine whether a pathogen will flourish and have the ability to cause an infection are **virulence, invasiveness** and **pathogenicity**.

Link 2 – The reservoir

The reservoir is the natural environment in which the pathogen resides, thrives and reproduces. Reservoirs include humans, animals and the environment. Many common infectious diseases have human reservoirs.

Human reservoirs (see Figure 12.2)

There are two types of human reservoir – acute clinically infected cases and carriers. **Acute clinical cases** who are infected display signs and symptoms of the disease. **Carriers** (colonised individuals) harbour the infectious agent but do not exhibit signs and symptoms of infection and are not ill.

Animal and insect reservoirs (see Figure 12.3)

Animal and insect reservoirs also consist of acute clinically infected cases and carriers. Examples of these are Lyme disease which is transmitted to humans via infected ticks and malaria, West Nile virus and dengue fever which are all transmitted by mosquitoes.

Environmental reservoirs

Plants, soil, water and food may serve as the reservoir for a variety of infectious diseases. Soil is the reservoir for most fungal agents.

Breaking the link

Methods applied for breaking this link are targeted at eliminating or inactivating the infectious agent or preventing it from exiting the reservoir. If effective measures are in place to control the sources of infection there will be fewer opportunities for infection to be transmitted.

Examples of environmental sanitation (inactivation)

• Chlorination of drinking water to provide a clean and safe water supply.
• Efficient and safe disposal of animal, human and industrial waste.
• Protection of food from biological and chemical contaminants, e.g. pasteurisation of milk.
• Measures used to control the risk of *Legionella* (see Chapter 37) from potentially hazardous environments such as cooling towers, pools and spa baths.

Link 3 – Portal of exit

The portal of exit is the route (or routes) by which the pathogen leaves the host or reservoir, generally as excretions, secretions, **skin squames** and droplets. In humans the portal of exit usually corresponds to the site where the pathogen is localised, for example influenza virus exits from the respiratory tract.

Key portals of exit

1 **Respiratory** – coughing, sneezing, and talking. Examples are the common cold (rhinovirus), influenza (see Chapter 35), tuberculosis (see Chapter 44) and childhood diseases such as measles, mumps, rubella (see Chapter 38), pertussis (see Chapter 27), *Haemophilus influenzae* type b (HIB) and pneumococcal disease.

2 **Alimentary** – biting, vomiting, diarrhoea, stool. Examples are enteric diseases and include hepatitis A, salmonella (see Chapter 42), *Shigella*, cholera, *Giardia* and campylobacter (see Chapter 28). An example of a disease transmitted by biting is rabies.

3 **Genitourinary** – sexually transmitted diseases. Examples are syphilis, gonorrhoea, chlamydia and human immunodeficiency virus (HIV) (see Chapter 26). Schistosomiasis and leptospirosis are both spread by urine being released into the environment.

4 **Trans-placental** route from mother to foetus – including the transmission of rubella, HIV, hepatitis B (see Chapter 26) and cytomegalovirus

5 **Skin** – via skin lesions, e.g. varicella causing chickenpox (see Chapter 45), impetigo. Through percutaneous exit, examples are mosquito bites (malaria, West Nile virus) or the sharing of needles (hepatitis B and C, HIV).

Breaking the link
Examples
- Barrier methods, e.g. condoms, use of sheaths for medical equipment.
- Promoting the use of tissues to prevent the spread of influenza and common colds.
- Infection control practices including the use of standard infection control precautions including face masks, as appropriate (see Chapter 16).
- Antenatal care to identify and prevent the transmission of trans-placental infections.

Link 4 – Mode of transmission

An infectious agent may be transmitted from its natural reservoir to a susceptible host in different ways. The two basic modes are **direct** and **indirect:**

Direct transmission

Direct transmission occurs more or less immediately and occurs through direct contact with the infectious agent.
Examples include:
- sexually transmitted diseases, e.g. gonorrhoea
- glandular fever (infectious mononucleosis) caused by the Epstein–Barr virus, commonly called the 'kissing disease'
- tetanus caused by contact with *Clostridium tetani* which lives in soil, house dust and animal and human waste such as manure.

Droplet spread is also considered to be direct transmission. Droplet spread refers to spray with relatively large, short-range aerosols produced by coughing or sneezing. This mode of transmission can infect susceptible individuals up to a metre away. Many respiratory diseases are spread this way, including pertussis.

Indirect transmission

This may occur through an animate or inanimate mechanism.

Animate mechanisms involve vectors. Vectors such as mosquitoes, fleas, ticks and flies may carry an infectious agent in a purely mechanical way. For example, flies may transmit infectious agents such as *Shigella* by walking on faeces and then on to food. Alternatively the vector may support growth or changes in the agent, for example in malaria or Lyme disease. Inanimate mechanisms involve the spread of infectious agents by environmental vehicles or by the air. Anything may act as a vehicle including objects, food, water, milk or biological products. **Food** is a common vehicle for *Salmonella* and *Campylobacter*; **wate**r is commonly implicated in cholera outbreaks; **surgical instruments** and implanted devices may be vehicles of staphylococcal infection.

Indirect airborne transmission occurs when very tiny particles of infectious agents are carried by dust or droplet nuclei suspended in air. Droplet nuclei may remain suspended for long periods of time and may be blown over great distances. Due to their size (1–5 micrometres, which allows them to be inhaled deep into the lungs and retained) they are particularly dangerous. Examples of infectious agents that are spread in this way are *Mycobacterium tuberculosis* and measles.

Link 5 – Portal of entry

A portal of entry is the way in which an infectious agent enters a susceptible host and is usually the same route as the portal of exit from the reservoir (CDC, 2012). Portals of entry by which infectious agents gain access to the human body are:
- inhalation (respiratory tract)
- ingestion (gastrointestinal tract)
- absorption (via mucous membranes, e.g. eyes)
- inoculation (e.g. inoculation injury)
- trans-placental (from the mother to the foetus)
- introduction (e.g. insertion of medical devices that create artificial orifices that are not protected from invasion of pathogens in the same way as natural orifices).

Link 6 – The susceptible host

The final link in the chain of infection is a susceptible host.

Susceptibility is affected by:

General factors that may increase an individual's susceptibility to infection by affecting host defences include:
- extremes of age – the very young due to an immature or suppressed immune system, and the elderly due to degenerative changes and a declining immune response
- malnutrition/dehydration
- alcoholism
- immobility
- underlying chronic disease, e.g. diabetes, asthma
- Medication, e.g. antibiotics, which disrupt the normal flora, and steroids / chemotherapy which suppress the immune response
- genetic factors.

General resistance factors that defend against infection include the skin, mucous membranes, gastric acidity and cilia in the respiratory tract, the cough reflex, and non-specific immune response (see Chapter 6).

Breaking the link

Methods applied to breaking this link focus on supporting and promoting the natural host defences by health promotion, immunisation and medical treatment.

Breaking the chain of infection in healthcare environments

A healthcare environment exposes patients to infection risks not encountered elsewhere. Most healthcare associated infections are caused by opportunistic pathogens that are introduced to susceptible sites as a result of invasive procedures. Key features of healthcare environments and practice promote the integrity of the chain of infection providing significant challenges for healthcare staff.

Common challenges of healthcare environments include:
- high use of antimicrobial agents
- comparatively high prevalence of antimicrobial resistant organisms (survive in favour of sensitive strains), many of which have the ability to spread easily
- patients at the extremes of age
- patients with community and healthcare acquired infections
- patients cared for in relatively close proximity
- high use of invasive devices / procedures
- patients who are frequently immobile
- patients who are undernourished, for a variety of reasons.

Methods used in healthcare to prevent and control infection essentially rely on effective infection prevention and control, including:
- early identification of potentially infectious patients by rapid and accurate diagnosis
- prompt treatment and management of infectious patients
- identification of patients who are 'at risk' of acquiring an infection
- isolation of suspected / confirmed infectious patients (see Chapter 21)
- application of standard infection control precautions including high standards of hand hygiene (see Chapter 14)
- optimising nutrition / hydration
- ensuring appropriate prescribing of antimicrobials – effective antimicrobial stewardship (see Chapter 10)
- promotion and maintenance of skin integrity
- avoidance of the use of invasive devices, where possible; otherwise prompt removal (see Chapters 20)
- providing a clean environment – appropriate cleaning and decontamination of medical equipment and the healthcare environment (see Chapter 17)
- safe management of sharps (see Chapter 18), linen and clinical waste
- infection prevention and control education and training of healthcare staff
- vaccination against vaccine preventable diseases (see Chapter 13)
- diagnoses and treatment of underlying disease that may make patients susceptible to infection
- protection of ports of entry, e.g. skin disinfection prior to invasive device insertion, keeping wounds covered, routinely applying the principles of aseptic non-touch technique, appropriately (see Chapter 19).

Breaking the chain of infection is crucial not only in preventing individuals from developing infection but also from their becoming the new reservoir and further perpetuating the 'chain of infection' see Figure 12.1.

13 Vaccination

Figure 13.1 A 17-month-old child receiving intramuscular (IM) vaccination

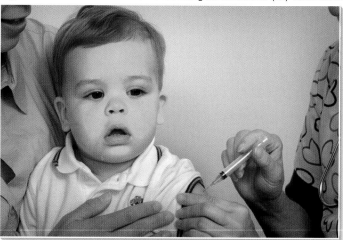

Source: US Centers for Disease Control and Prevention (CDC). CDC/Judy Schmidt. Photographer: James Gathany

Figure 13.2 Key points

- **Immunisation against infectious disease – 'The Green Book'** contains the most up-to-date information on vaccines, administration procedures and specific UK immunisation schedules, for vaccine preventable infectious diseases in the United Kingdom (UK). However, the **on-line version must be used** to ensure information is current as there are frequent updates.
- **Vaccine effectiveness:** Vaccines are not 100% effective. Vaccine failures may be **primary**, whereby individuals fail to make an initial immunological response (for example, 5–10% of children fail to respond to the measles component of MMR), or **secondary**, whereby there is a good initial response to the vaccine but the protection wanes over time (for example the pertussis (whooping cough) vaccine).
- **Vaccine storage:** Vaccines are sensitive biological substances and can lose their effectiveness if too hot or too cold, which can lead to vaccine failures. The maintenance of cold chain compliance (during transport, storage and handling of vaccines) is therefore essential.
- **Training:** All healthcare professionals who administer vaccines must have received *specific training* in immunisation, including recognition and treatment of anaphylaxis, followed by annual updates.
- **Consent:** Consent must be obtained prior to administering a vaccine but may be verbal. For children, consent may be given by a person with parental responsibility.
- **Vaccine information on children/adolescents:** This must be recorded in the **Personal Child Health Record (PCHR – The Red Book)**/ GP Records and Child Health Information System (CHIS).
- **Yellow Card Scheme:** All suspected vaccine-induced adverse drug reactions (ADRs) must be reported via this to the Medicines and Healthcare Products Regulatory Agency (MHRA) or reported via The Black Triangle Scheme for example if a newer drug < 2 years old, or an established drug is used on a new population.
- **Vaccine/immunisation queries:** The local Health Protection Team (**Public Health England**) or Screening and Immunisation Team (SIT) can be contacted for vaccination queries but vaccination errors should be reported to the **Screening and Immunisation Team**.

References:

Mims, Ĉ., Dockrell, H. M., Goering, R. V., Roitt, I., Wakelin, D. and Zuckerman, M. (2004). Medical Microbiology (updated third edition). Spain: Elsevier Mosby.
Public Health England (PHE) (2013). Immunisation Against Infectious Disease. 'The Green Book'. London: PHE.
Newsom, S. W. B. (2009). Infections and Their Control. A Historical Perspective. London: Sage Publications Ltd.
Wilson, J. (2008). Clinical Microbiology. An Introduction for Healthcare Professionals. London: Balliere Tindall Elsevier.

Infection Prevention and Control at a Glance, First Edition. By Debbie Weston, Alison Burgess and Sue Roberts.

Introduction / background

The discovery of **vaccination** as a means of preventing disease is one of the greatest achievements in modern medicine and is the *most effective* public health intervention in the world, after clean water, for saving lives and promoting good health (PHE, 2013c) (Figure 13.1). The first recorded attempts to vaccinate were by the Chinese in the tenth century (Newsom, 2009a). Other significant events included the pioneering work of Edward Jenner, an English doctor, who in 1796 discovered that **inoculating** a person with cowpox made them immune to smallpox, a disease that was killing many people at the time, particularly children (Newsom, 2009a). This work was followed by that of Louis Pasteur, an eminent French scientist who developed a variety of vaccines (to varicella, cholera, diphtheria, anthrax and rabies) during the 1860s to 1890s (PHE, 2013c). The work of both men has been responsible for saving many lives.

The terms vaccination and immunisation are often used interchangeably but there is a subtle difference in definition:

Immunisation is the administration of a vaccine which seeks to make individuals immune from disease. Immunisation means to make someone immune to a disease. Individuals may be vaccinated but because vaccines are not 100% effective, not all individuals will be successfully *immunised*.

Immunisation programmes worldwide vary significantly and because vaccines are given to *healthy* people, and are costly, they are not always given priority, particularly in developing countries. The success of immunisation programmes is influenced by many factors, *not least* the fact that many individuals fear that vaccines are not safe. It is important, therefore, that education forms part of all immunisation programmes.

The aim of vaccination

The aim of vaccination is to prime the adaptive immune system to the **antigens** of a particular microbe so that a first infection induces a *secondary response* (Mims et al, 2004f) (see Chapter 9). Vaccination has both a *direct* and *indirect* effect as it protects those successfully immunised and results in fewer infected individuals to transmit infection, meaning that those still susceptible are indirectly protected (Mims et al, 2004f). This is known as **herd immunity**.

Active and passive immunity

There are two types of acquired immunity as follows:

Active immunity: This protection is produced by an individual's own immune system, is usually long-lasting and can be acquired either by natural disease or by vaccination (PHE, 2013c).

Passive immunity: Passive immunity is protection provided by the transfer of antibodies from immune individuals, most commonly across the placenta or less often from the transfusion of blood or blood products, including immunoglobulin (PHE, 2013c).

Types of vaccine

The most commonly used types of vaccines are as follows:

Live, attenuated vaccines: These use microorganisms that have had their virulence reduced. They induce a greater immune response because they reproduce many of the features of the infection (Mims et al, 2004f). There is, however, a small possibility that the microorganism may revert to a **virulent** form and cause severe disease in immunocompromised individuals. Examples include measles, mumps, rubella (MMR), bacillus Calmette-Guérin (BCG), and yellow fever vaccines.

Inactivated 'non-live' vaccines: These vaccines use whole microorganisms that are killed before being incorporated into the vaccine. Whilst relatively safe, they require *several doses* to elicit an effective immune response (Mims et al, 2004f). Examples include polio, hepatitis A, pertussis and rabies vaccines.

Subunit vaccines: These use fragments of the microorganism instead of the whole organism, for example the hepatitis B vaccine which uses only the surface proteins of the virus.

Toxoids: These vaccines induce immunity against the toxins produced by the bacteria, as it is the effect of these toxins rather than simply the presence of the microbe itself that is harmful (Mims et al, 2004f). Examples are the diphtheria and tetanus vaccines.

Conjugate vaccines: These vaccines are created by joining polysaccharide antigens to carrier proteins of the same microorganism which makes the organism more easily recognisable by the immune system, for example the *Haemophilus influenzae* type B (HIB) vaccine.

Development of future vaccines

Currently DNA and recombinant vaccines are being developed. These introduce *specific components* of the microorganism's genetic material into the body cells and are likely to produce even more efficient vaccines.

The use of immunoglobulins

Sometimes immunoglobulins (containing antibodies against a *specific* infection) are administered to provide *immediate protection* to a susceptible person at risk of acquiring a particular infection (Wilson, 2008b), for example hepatitis B immunoglobulin administered to a *non-immune* individual following needlestick injury, and varicella zoster (VZIG) to susceptible individuals exposed to chickenpox.

Vaccine safety

Whilst current vaccines are generally considered to be safe, having undergone rigorous quality and safety checks, there is still a *small risk* that serious complications can occur. **It is essential therefore that the risk of infection outweighs any risk associated with vaccination.**

Routine immunisation programme in the United Kingdom

Vaccines should be given as early *as possible in life* so children are protected when *at the highest risk from complications* of the diseases. If given too early, maternal antibodies still present may interfere with the effectiveness of the vaccines by neutralising the vaccine viruses. The length of time that maternal antibodies are present varies according to the disease, hence pertussis vaccine is administered at 2 months, whilst MMR is not administered until 1 year (PHE, 2013c).

The UK immunisation Schedule and most up-to-date information on vaccines can be found in: *Immunisation against infectious disease – 'the Green Book'*, which can be found on the Public Health Website (see Figure 13.2).

14 Hand hygiene

Figure 14.1 Handwashing and alcohol handrub technique

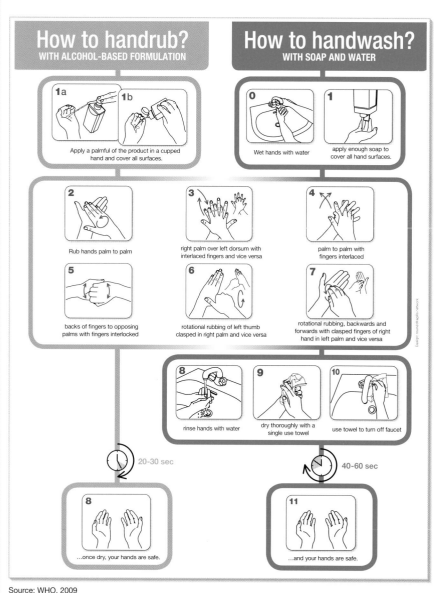

Source: WHO, 2009

Figure 14.2 Benefits of alcohol-based handrub

Alcohol-based handrubs are faster to use, more effective and better tolerated by the skin and have the following immediate advantages:

- elimination of the majority of bacteria and viruses
- the short time required for action (20–30 seconds)
- availability of the product at the point of care
- better skin tolerability compared to other hand hygiene products
- no requirement for any particular infrastructure (washbasin, soap, paper towels)

Source: WHO, 2009

Figure 14.3 Using alcohol handrub – quick and easy

Alcohol-based handrubs take less time to use than traditional handwashing. In an 8-hour shift, an estimated one hour of an ICU nurse's time will be saved by using alcohol handrub (CDC, 2002)

Figure 14.4 Hand care

Expert opinion suggests that skin damage is generally associated with the detergent base of the preparation and/or incorrect handwashing technique (Loveday et al, 2014).

Allergic contact dermatitis due to alcohol handrubs is very uncommon. However, with the increasing use of such products it is likely that true allergic reactions to such products will occasionally be encountered.

Figure 14.9 Code of Practice on the prevention and control of infections and related guidance (Health and Social Care Act 2008)
Source: Department of Health, 2015

The Code of Practice on the prevention and control of infections and related guidance (Health and Social Care Act 2008) requires that registered providers of healthcare have in place:

- a standard Infection prevention and control precautions policy which is evidence based and includes hand hygiene at the point of care
- appropriate management and monitoring arrangements to ensure that relevant staff, contractors and other persons, whose normal duties are directly or indirectly concerned with providing care, receive suitable and sufficient information, and training and supervision in, the measures required to prevent and control the risks of infection.

Figure 14.5 The WHO multimodal Hand Hygiene Improvement strategy

The WHO multimodal Hand Hygiene Improvement strategy and wide range of tools were developed in parallel to the WHO guidelines on hand hygiene in health care to translate recommendations into practice at the bedside. One of the key tools developed was the 5 Moments for hand hygiene in health care.

The concept of the 'My 5 Moments for hand hygiene' aims to:

- foster positive outcome evaluation by linking specific hand hygiene actions to specific infectious outcomes in patients and healthcare workers
- increase the sense of self-efficacy by giving healthcare workers clear advice on how to integrate hand hygiene in the complex task of care. It is practical, simple and easy to remember.
- The concept uses the number 5 like the five digits of the hand, which gives it a 'stickiness factor' (the specific content of a message that renders its impact memorable) (Gladwell, 2000).

'My 5 Moments for hand hygiene' has since been widely adopted worldwide.

Source: WHO, 2009

Figure 14.6 5 Moments for Hand Hygiene

The World Health Organization (WHO) has developed an approach to hand hygiene called the 5 Moments. This approach aims to ensure that hand hygiene is performed:

- at the correct moments
- at the correct location, within the flow of care delivery.

The 5 Moments approach has been adapted by the National Patient Safety Agency (NPSA) for application in the UK context.

The 5 Moments approach to hand hygiene, as adapted by the clean**your**hands campaign, aims to improve hand hygiene across the NHS to ensure that hand hygiene is performed at the right time in the right place (point of care), using the appropriate method soap and water handwashing or alcohol hand rub), using the correct technique (WHO, 2009).

Source: WHO, 2009

Figure 14.7 5 Moments to change the world

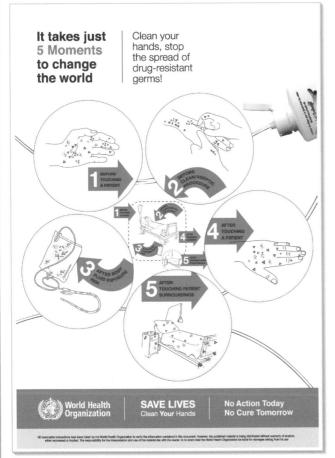

Source: WHO, 2009

Figure 14.8 Your 5 Moments for hand hygiene

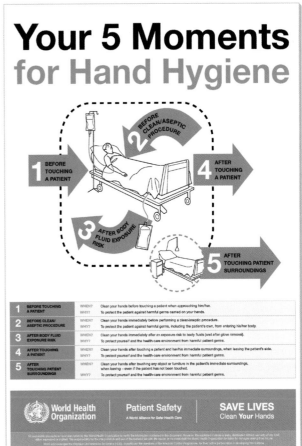

Source: WHO, 2009

Ignaz Semmelweis – the 'father of hand hygiene'

The most important measure in infection prevention and control is hand hygiene and it all began with a Hungarian, Ignaz Philipp Semmelweis, who in 1846 was appointed as a qualified doctor to the Vienna General Hospital – then the largest and most prestigious maternity hospital in the world (Loudon, 2013).

The hospital was divided into two clinics. Doctors, including medical students, worked in one clinic, whilst midwives, training pupil midwives, ran the other. Patients were allocated to the clinics on alternate days regardless of their clinical presentation. Between 1840 and 1846, the maternal mortality rate in the first clinic was 98.4 per 1000 births, whilst the rate in the second clinic was 36.2 per 1000 births. The majority of deaths were due to **puerperal or 'childbed' fever** caused by organisms such as group A streptococcus (GAS) (see Chapter 36). The reasons for this difference were not understood but generally attributed to the poor social and hygiene conditions that prevailed until the arrival of Semmelweis, who postulated that the explanation for the difference was due to the contrasting procedures undertaken by the medical students and the pupil midwives. The medical students would begin each day with the post mortem examination of women who had died of puerperal fever; they would then proceed to the maternity wards to undertake vaginal examinations on the labouring women as part of their training. This was in contrast to the pupil midwives in the second clinic who did not undertake either procedure. Semmelweis believed that the training procedures undertaken in the first clinic resulted in the transfer of what he initially described as 'morbid matter' and subsequently 'decomposing animal organic matter'. In 1847, he introduced a system that required both midwives and medical students to wash their hands in 'chloride of lime', a type of disinfectant, before entering the maternity ward (Newsom, 2009b).

By 1848 the reduction in mortality rates was highly significant; the maternal mortality rate in the first clinic fell to 12.7 per 1000 births, which compared favourably with the rate in the midwife-led clinic of 13.3 per 1000 births (Loudon, 2013). By accident, the process of admission to the two clinics on alternate days had produced the requirements of a controlled trial. The high numbers of births (42 795) and maternal deaths (2977) occurring in the two clinics between 1840 and 1846 meant that chance could be confidently excluded as an explanation of the results demonstrating the differences observed. This was the first evidence that cleansing heavily contaminated hands with an antiseptic agent could effectively reduce healthcare associated infection (HCAI) (Loudon, 2013).

Despite the potential of this breakthrough, Semmelweis experienced significant difficulties convincing his peers and administrators of the benefits of this new approach. He was uninformed of the principles of social marketing and tried to impose a change in practice without engaging the support of those he was trying to influence. In 1843, Oliver Wendell Holmes also concluded independently that puerperal fever was transmitted by the hands of healthcare workers (Rotter, 1999).

Evolution of hand hygiene practice

Despite the seminal work and achievements by Semmelweis and Holmes it took many years for hand hygiene, with an emphasis on handwashing at the time, to become accepted as one of the most important measures for preventing healthcare associated infection. The challenge now in the 21st century is to get alcohol-based handrub accepted as the 'gold standard', given the recently proven benefits over handwashing. Until recently, before the evidence base had been developed and appropriate products were made available, handwashing was considered to be more effective than rinsing with an antiseptic agent and recommendations that antiseptic rinse agents should only be used in emergencies or where sinks were unavailable (Coppage, 1961) were promoted.

During the 1980s the first national hand hygiene guidelines began to be published (Simmonds, 1981; Garner and Favero, 1986). However, it was not until 1995 and 1996 that the CDC / Healthcare Infection Control Practices Advisory Committee (HICPAC) in the USA recommended for the first time that either antimicrobial soap or a **waterless antiseptic agent** should be used for cleansing hands upon leaving the rooms of patients with multi-drug resistant pathogens. By 2002, the revised HICPAC guidelines for hand hygiene in healthcare settings defined alcohol-based *handrubbing*, where available, as the standard of care for hand hygiene practices in healthcare settings, whereas *handwashing* was reserved for particular situations only; this reflected the emerging evidence base and benefits for using alcohol handrubs that had been building during this time (CDC, 2002). A systematic review of publications between 1992 and 2002 on the effectiveness of alcohol-based handrub solutions for hand hygiene demonstrated that alcohol-based handrubs remove organisms more effectively, are quicker to use and cause less skin irritation compared with handwashing with soap or other antiseptic agents and water (see Figures 14.1, 14.2, 14.3 and 14.4).

Multimodal approach to hand hygiene promotion

Pittet et al (2000) published the first landmark study using a multimodal hand hygiene promotion strategy demonstrating significant and sustained, hospital wide, hand hygiene compliance improvement. The improvement was associated with an overall reduction in HCAI prevalence including MRSA. In their seminal work, Pittet et al, describe their experience in Geneva's University Hospitals of the implementation of a strategy based on several essential components. These included the introduction of an alcohol-based handrub, healthcare worker education, hand hygiene audits including performance feedback, prompts, improvement of hand hygiene facilities and an organisation-wide approach to compliance improvement by staff, patients and management. The results of this pivotal study showed remarkable outcomes in terms of a sustained improvement in hand hygiene compliance and HCAI reduction inspiring others to undertake similar studies. In light of its very solid evidence base, this model has been adopted by the First **Global Patient Safety Challenge** to develop the **WHO Hand Hygiene Improvement Strategy** (WHO, 2009).

Figures 14.5, 14.6, 14.7 and 14.8 describe the multimodal approach to hand hygiene and the '**5 Moments for hand hygiene**', which were launched as part of the global Hand Hygiene Improvement strategy.

Resident and transient flora

Bacteria found on the hands can be divided into two categories, namely resident and transient. The **resident flora** consists of microorganisms that reside under the superficial cells of the stratum corneum and can also be found on the surface of the skin; *Staphylococcus epidermidis* is the dominant species. These microorganisms play an important role in protecting the skin from invasion by other harmful species. They are not readily transferable to other people or surfaces and are not easily removed by washing with soap and water. Compared to transient bacteria, resident flora are less likely to be associated with infections but they may cause infections in sterile body cavities, the eyes or non-intact skin. The hands of some healthcare workers may become persistently colonised by pathogenic flora such as *S. aureus* (see Chapter 43), Gram-negative bacilli, or yeast (WHO, 2009).

The **transient flora** consists of microorganisms that do not normally live on the skin but are readily acquired and transferred by touch, either through direct contact with patients or contaminated environmental surfaces.

Transient bacteria are the organisms most frequently associated with HCAI. The transient flora is readily removed by soap and water or antiseptic agents (alcohol-based handrubs, antimicrobial soaps). The transmissibility of transient flora depends on the species present, the number of microorganisms on the surface and the skin moisture content (Marples and Towers, 1979; Patrick et al, 1997).

Hand hygiene compliance

According to the recently published NICE quality standard (QS61), 2014 (https://www.nice.org.uk/guidance/qs61/chapter/Quality-statement-3-Hand-decontamination):

'Effective hand decontamination, even after wearing gloves, results in significant reductions in the carriage of potential pathogens on the hands and decreases the incidence of preventable HCAIs leading in turn to a reduction in morbidity and mortality. Hand decontamination is considered to have a high impact on outcomes that are important to patients. Although hand hygiene has improved over recent years, remaining misconceptions about this standard principle of infection control are reported and good practice is still not universal.'

Compliance with recommended hand hygiene procedures has been reported as variable. Mean baseline rates range from 5% to 89% with an overall average of 38.7%, with performance varying according to work intensity and other factors such as the availability of hand hygiene facilities (WHO, 2009). International studies demonstrate that infection rates can be reduced by 10–50% when healthcare workers clean their hands appropriately and effectively.

Hand hygiene and multi-drug resistant organisms

It is now widely accepted that there is convincing evidence that improved hand hygiene through multimodal implementation strategies can reduce HCAI. In addition, several studies have shown a sustained decrease in the incidence of multi-drug resistant bacteria isolates and patient colonisation following the implementation of hand hygiene improvement strategies (Gordon et al, 2005; Girou et al, 2006; Trick et al, 2007). Failure to perform appropriate hand hygiene is considered to be the leading cause of HCAI and the spread of multi-resistant organisms, and has been recognised as a significant contributor to outbreaks.

Transmission of healthcare associated pathogens

Transmission of healthcare associated pathogens takes place through direct and indirect contact, droplets, air and a common vehicle. Transmission via contaminated healthcare workers' hands is the most common route in most settings and according to the World Health Organization requires five sequential steps:

1 organisms are present on the patient's skin, or have been shed onto inanimate objects immediately surrounding the patient

2 organisms must be transferred to the hands of the healthcare worker

3 organisms must be capable of surviving at least several minutes on the healthcare worker's hands

4 handwashing or hand antisepsis by the healthcare worker must be inadequate or omitted entirely, or the agent used for hand hygiene inappropriate, and

5 the contaminated hand or hands of the caregiver must come into direct contact with another patient or with an inanimate object that will come into direct contact with the patient. (WHO, 2009)

Healthcare associated pathogens can be recovered not only from infected wounds but also from frequently colonised areas of normal, intact skin. Nearly 10^6 **skin squames** containing viable microorganisms are shed daily from normal skin, contaminating the immediate environment with patient's flora including patient gowns, bed linen, medical equipment and bedside furniture (Bonten et al, 1996; Riggs et al, 2007).

Following contact with patients or a contaminated environment, microorganisms can survive on hands for varying lengths of time (2–60 minutes). Healthcare workers' hands become progressively colonised with commensal flora as well as potential pathogens during patient care – a linear increase. In the absence of hand hygiene, the longer the duration of care, the higher the degree of hand contamination. Contaminated hands have been associated with endemic HCAIs (Foca et al, 2000; Sartor et al, 2000) and outbreaks of infection (Boyce et al, 1990; Zawacki et al, 2004).

In general, the effective use of alcohol-based handrubs or handwashing with soap and water will remove transient microorganisms and render the hands socially clean. The additional benefit of the effective use of alcohol handrub is that it will also substantially reduce resident microorganisms. This level of decontamination is sufficient for general social contact and most clinical care activities (WHO, 2009).

epic3: National Evidence-Based Guidelines for Preventing Healthcare Associated Infections in NHS Hospitals in England were revised and published in 2014 (Loveday et al, 2014). Based on the best critically appraised evidence available they provide standard principles for preventing healthcare associated infections in hospital and other acute settings including hand hygiene. The guidance is available at http://www.his.org.uk/files/3113/8693/4808/epic3_National_Evidence-Based_Guidelines_for_Preventing_HCAI_in_NHSE.pdf

Figure 14.9 describes the *Code of Practice* requirements (see Chapter 1) in relation to hand hygiene (DH, 2015).

15 Surgical hand preparation

Figure 15.1 Skin reactions using different hand hygiene products

Skin irritation and dermatitis are more frequently observed after surgical hand scrub with chlorhexidine than after use of an alcohol-based handrub.

Overall, skin dermatitis is more frequently associated with hand antisepsis using a medicated soap than with an alcohol-based handrub.

Source: WHO, 2009

Figure 15.2 Surgical hand preparation

Key steps

- Keep nails short and pay attention to them when washing your hands – most microbes on hands come from beneath the fingernails.
- Do not wear artificial nails or nail polish.
- Remove all jewellery (rings, watches, bracelets) before entering the operating theatre.
- Wash hands and arms with a non-medicated soap before entering the operating theatre area or if hands are visibly soiled.
- Clean subungual areas with a nail file. Nailbrushes should not be used as they may damage the skin and encourage shedding of cells. If used, nailbrushes must be sterile, once only (single use). Reusable autoclavable nail brushes are on the market.

Source: WHO, 2009

Figure 15.3 Intraoperative phase – hand decontamination

The operating team should wash their hands prior to the first operation of the list using an aqueous antiseptic surgical solution, with a single-use brush or pick for nails, and ensure that hands are visibly clean.

Before subsequent operations, hands should be washed using either an alcoholic handrub or an antiseptic surgical solution. If hands are soiled then they should be washed again with an antiseptic surgical solution.

Source: NICE, 2008

Figure 15.4 Method for hand decontamination with an antiseptic soap

Procedural steps

- Start timing. Scrub each side of each finger, between the fingers, and the back and front of the hand for 2 minutes.
- Proceed to scrub the arms, keeping the hand higher than the arm at all times. This helps to avoid recontamination of the hands by water from the elbows and prevents bacteria-laden soap and water from contaminating the hands.
- Wash each side of the arm from wrist to the elbow for 1 minute.
- Repeat the process on the other hand and arm, keeping hands above elbows at all times. If the hand touches anything at any time, the scrub must be lengthened by 1 minute for the area that has been contaminated.
- Rinse hands and arms by passing them through the water in one direction only, from fingertips to elbow. Do not move the arm back and forth through the water.
- Proceed to the operating theatre holding hands above elbows.
- At all times during the scrub procedure, care should be taken not to splash water onto surgical attire.
- Once in the operating theatre, hands and arms should be dried using a sterile towel and aseptic technique before donning gown and gloves.

Source: WHO, 2009

Joseph Lister (1827–1912) first demonstrated the effect of disinfection on the reduction of surgical site infection (Maki, 1976). Since the 19th century surgical hand preparation (disinfection) has been recommended as a key measure to reduce the risk of surgical site infection and represents one of the most important ritual acts in healthcare. Despite the indirect evidence for surgical hand preparation its requirement has never been proven by a randomised controlled trial (Widmer et al, 2010). However, the evidence for surgical hand preparation was recently reviewed within the framework of the World Health Organization *WHO guidelines on hand hygiene in health care*, http://www.who.int/gpsc/5may/tools/9789241597906/en/, and guidance has been included in the National Institute for Health and Clinical Excellence *Surgical site infections: prevention and treatment* (NICE, 2008).

In the days before surgical gloves were available, surgical hand preparation by the surgical team was even more imperative than it is today. During the 19th century, surgical hand preparation consisted of washing the hands with antiseptic (medicated) soap

and warm water, and using a 'scrubbing' brush as a key part of the procedure. In 1894, three steps were suggested.

1 Wash hands with hot water, medicated soap and using a scrubbing brush, brush for **5** minutes.

2 Apply 90% ethanol for 3–5 minutes with a brush.

3 Rinse the hands with an 'antiseptic liquid' (Kampf et al, 2005). In 1939, a similar approach was suggested.

1 An initial 7-minute hand wash with soap, water and the use of a brush, followed by drying with a towel.

2 The second step was the application of 70% ethanol for 3 minutes (Price, 1939).

Over time the duration of the 'scrubbing' time has become much reduced with the appreciation of the damage and increased shedding of bacteria that can be caused. However, the application time of the alcohol-based handrub has remained much the same at 3 minutes (Marchetti et al, 2003). The sequential use of surgical hand scrubs and alcohol handrubs is no longer recommended due to the damaging effects on hands, which also increases the risk of infection. The WHO

Infection Prevention and Control at a Glance, First Edition. By Debbie Weston, Alison Burgess and Sue Roberts.
© 2017 John Wiley & Sons, Ltd. Published 2017 by John Wiley & Sons, Ltd.

now recommends 2–5 minutes if using an aqueous antiseptic surgical solution with advice to follow the manufacturer's guidelines if using an alcohol-based handrub (usually about 3 minutes) (WHO, 2009).

Purpose of surgical hand decontamination

The virulence of the microorganisms, **extent of microbial exposure, and host defence mechanisms** are key factors in the pathogenesis of postoperative infection, so in theory maintaining clean hands throughout the surgical procedure should reduce the incidence of surgical site infection.

The purpose of surgical hand preparation is to minimise the risk that either the **resident flora** that normally colonise the skin or the **transient flora**, acquired by touch, contaminate the surgical wound. In comparison to normal hand hygiene, surgical hand preparation requires more attention as the purpose is to eliminate the transient bacteria and reduce the resident flora as well as inhibit growth of bacteria under the gloved hand for the duration of the procedure. This is to take into account the potential puncture of the surgical glove releasing bacteria into the open wound (Widmer et al, 2010).

Conditions for the rapid multiplication of skin bacteria are ideal inside surgical gloves (warmth, moisture and to some degree, nutrition) and although the skin flora, mainly coagulase-negative staphylococci, is rarely responsible for surgical site infection, in the presence of a foreign body or necrotic tissue **inocula** as low as 100 CFU can initiate such an infection.

Transient bacteria are readily removed by soap and water, but antiseptics are required to eliminate resident organisms residing in the deep crevices and skin follicles. Antiseptics include alcohol or detergent solutions containing chlorhexidine and povidone–iodine. Chlorhexidine has been shown to have a persistent suppressive (residual) effect on bacterial regrowth on the skin. Although alcohol is known to rapidly kill microorganisms, it does not physically remove organic material and therefore should not be used on visibly soiled hands.

Efficacy of aqueous antiseptic surgical solutions (medicated soaps)

The most active agents in order of decreasing activity are chlorhexidine gluconate, iodophors, triclosan and plain soap. Application of chlorhexidine or povidone–iodine results in similar initial reductions in bacterial counts (70–80%), which achieve 99% after repeated application. However, **rapid regrowth occurs after the application of povidone–iodine but not with chlorhexidine**. Despite both in vitro and in vivo studies demonstrating that povidone–iodine is less efficacious than chlorhexidine it remains one of the most widely used products for surgical hand preparation, induces **more allergic reactions** and has comparatively **less residual activity**. At the end of a surgical procedure hands can have more microorganisms when treated with iodophors such as povidone–iodine than before undertaking the surgical hand preparation procedure (WHO, 2009).

Surgical hand preparation with antiseptic surgical solutions or alcohol-based formulations?

Both aqueous antiseptic surgical solutions and **alcohol-based handrub surgical hand formulations** are suitable for the prevention of surgical site infections. It is however, important to note that the antibacterial efficacy of products **containing high concentrations of alcohol far surpasses** that of any antiseptic surgical solution currently available. In addition, the initial reduction of the resident skin flora is so rapid and effective that bacterial regrowth to baseline on the gloved hand takes **more than 6 hours**, negating the need to use an antiseptic surgical solution product with residual activity. **Therefore preference should be given to routine use of alcohol-based handrubs rather than aqueous antiseptic surgical solutions** (WHO, 2009).

Key point

Recommendations for surgical hand preparation

- Remove rings, wrist watch and bracelets prior to performing surgical hand preparation. Artificial nails and nail polish must not be worn in the operating theatre (see Figure 15.2).
- The operating team **should wash their hands prior to the first operation** on the list using **an aqueous antiseptic surgical solution**, with a single-use brush or pick for the nails, and ensure that hands and nails are visibly clean.
- **Before subsequent operations**, hands should be washed using either an alcoholic handrub or an aqueous antiseptic surgical solution, preferably with a product ensuring sustained (residual) activity such as chlorhexidine gluconate (4% w/v). If hands are visibly soiled then they should be washed again with an antiseptic surgical solution. (See http://whqlibdoc.who.int/publications/2009/9789241597906_eng.pdf [page 58].)

1 When performing surgical hand preparation using an **aqueous antiseptic surgical solution,** scrub hands and forearms for the length of time recommended by the manufacturer, typically 2–5minutes (see Figures 15.3 and 15.4).

2 When using an alcohol-based surgical handrub product, (*licensed for this use), follow the manufacturer's instructions for application times. Apply the product to dry hands only. Do not combine surgical hand preparation procedures using **aqueous antiseptic surgical solutions** with alcohol-based handrubs sequentially. (Most commercially available products recommend a 3-minute exposure.)

3 When using an alcohol-based handrub, **use sufficient product** to keep hands and forearms wet with the handrub throughout the surgical hand preparation procedure (Figure 15.5).

4 After application of the alcohol-based handrub as recommended, allow hands and forearms to dry thoroughly before donning sterile gloves. (NICE, 2008; WHO, 2009).

*In Europe alcohol handrubs must meet the requirements of European test standard EN 12791.

Figure 15.5 Surgical hand preparation with an alcohol-based handrub formulation

The handrubbing technique for surgical hand preparation must be performed on perfectly clean, dry hands. On arrival in the operating theatre and after having donned theatre clothing (cap/hat/bonnet and mask), hands must be washed with soap and water. After the operation when removing gloves, hands must be rubbed with an alcohol-based formulation or washed with soap and water if any residual talc or biological fluids are present. (e.g. the glove is punctured) Surgical procedures may be carried out one after the other without the need for handwashing, provided that the handrubbing technique for surgical hand preparation is followed (images 1 to 17).

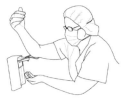
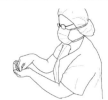
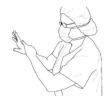
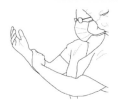

1 Put approximately 5 ml (3 doses) of alcohol-based handrub in the palm of your left hand, using the elbow of your other arm to operate the dispenser

2 Dip the fingertips of your right hand in the handrub to decontaminate under the nails (5 seconds)

3 Images 3 – 7: Smear the handrub on the right forearm up to the elbow. Ensure that the whole skin area is covered by using circular movements around the forearm until the handrub has fully evaporated (10 -15 seconds)

4 See legend for image 3

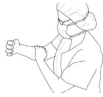
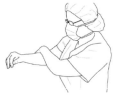
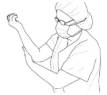
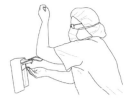

5 See legend for image 3

6 See legend for image 3

7 See legend for image 3

8 Put approximately 5 ml (3 doses) of alcohol-based handrub in the palm of your right hand, using the elbow of your other arm to operate the dispenser

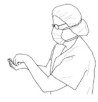

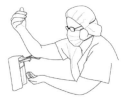
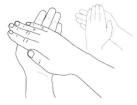

9 Dip the fingertips of your left hand in the handrub to decontaminate under the nails (5 seconds)

10 Smear the handrub on the left forearm up to the elbow. Ensure that the whole skin area is covered by using circular movements around the forearm until the handrub has fully evaporated (10 -15 seconds)

11 Put approximately 5 ml (3 doses) of alcohol-based handrub in the palm of your left hand, using the elbow of your other arm to operate the distributor. Rub both hands at the same time up to the wrists, and ensure that all the steps represented in images 12-17 are followed (20 – 30 seconds)

12 Cover the whole surface of the hands up to the wrist with alcohol-based handrub, rubbing palm against palm with a rotating movement

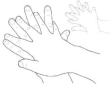
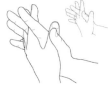
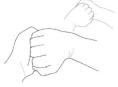
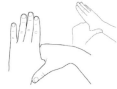

13 Rub the back of the left hand, including the wrist, moving the right palm back and forth, and vice versa

14 Rub palm against palm back and forth with fingers interlinked

15 Rub the back of the fingers by holding them in the palm of the other hand with a sideways back and forth movement

16 Rub the thumb of the left hand by rotating it in the clasped palm of the right hand and vice versa

17 When the hands are dry, sterile surgical clothing and gloves can be donned

Repeat the above-illustrated sequence (average duration, 60 sec) according to the number of times corresponding to the total duration recommended by the manufacturer for surgical hand preparation with an alcohol-based handrub.

Source: WHO, 2009

16 Personal protective equipment

Figure 16.1 Indications for use of PPE – in order of donning, as appropriate

Item	Examples of use
	Plastic apron (as per National Patient Safety Agency (NPSA) colour-coding): Direct contact with patients in isolation side rooms/cohort bays/who are being barrier nursed; venepuncture or cannulation; assisting with washing or bathing; assisting patients with using bedpans or commodes; emptying catheter drainage bags/stoma bags; cleaning or decontaminating equipment; changing soiled or contaminated linen; cleaning ward areas; working in ward kitchens and/or serving patient food
	Full-length disposable gown: Where there is a risk of extensive contamination of the arms and uniform from blood and/or body fluids, or excretions and secretions, i.e. surgery; sterile invasive procedures; childbirth. May also be worn when caring for patients with pandemic/avian influenza
	Coverall: As part of PPE when caring for patients with suspected Ebola virus (see Chapter 33)
	Surgical face mask: A barrier to splashes and droplets, e.g. during surgery; when within 3 metres of a patient with suspected/confirmed *Bordetella pertussis* (see Chapter 27); when undertaking an aerosol-generating procedure on a patient with suspected/confirmed meningococcal meningitis (see Chapter 39)
	FFP3 Respirator: When undertaking aerosol-generating procedures on patients with suspected/confirmed respiratory TB, or when in contact with a patient with suspected or confirmed multi-drug resistant (MDR)-TB (see Chapter 44), pandemic influenza (see Chapter 41) or MERS-CoV
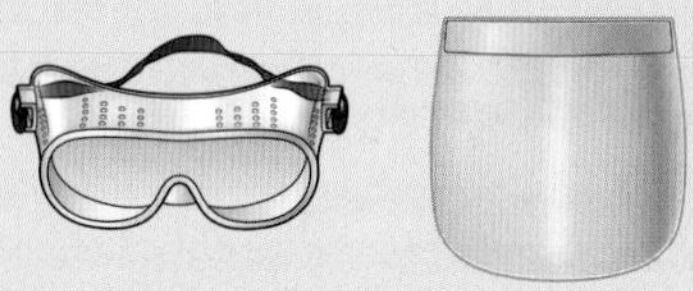	**Goggles/face visor:** During surgery; taking patients on and off haemodialysis; manually cleaning endoscopes or surgical instruments prior to placement in an automated washer disinfector; when undertaking aerosol-generating procedures; any procedure where there is a high risk of blood/body fluid splashes and spray
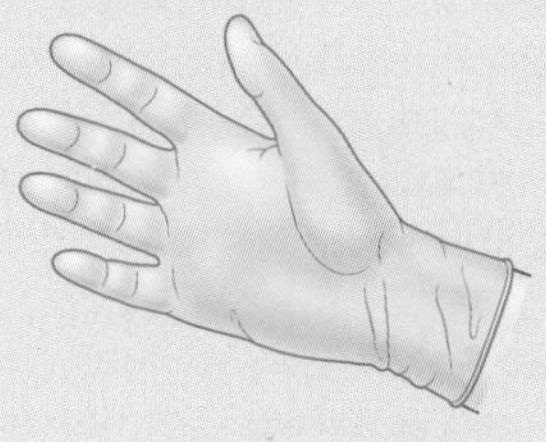	**Gloves:** **Sterile** Surgery and any 'surgical' procedure, e.g. biopsies; insertion of central venous catheters; urinary catheterisation; vaginal examination in obstetric patients and vaginal delivery **Non-sterile** Contact with blood, body fluids, chemicals or infection, e.g. direct contact with patients known to be colonised or infected with microorganisms; cannulation; venepuncture; removal of vascular access devices; vaginal examination in non-obstetric patients; rectal examination; urinary catheter removal; IV drug administration; wound care; nasogastric tube insertion, aspiration and removal; administering suppositories; emptying vomit bowls, urinals and bed pans; changing/handling incontinence pads and nappies; emptying and changing stoma bags; handling or cleaning equipment; handling clinical waste bags; cleaning up blood and body fluid spills; handling soiled bed linen or clothing

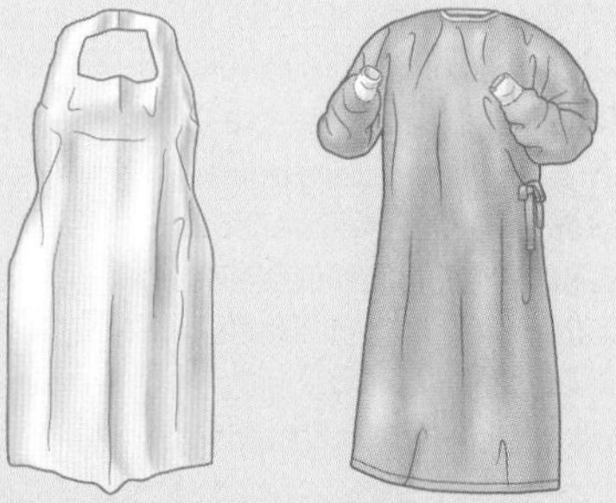

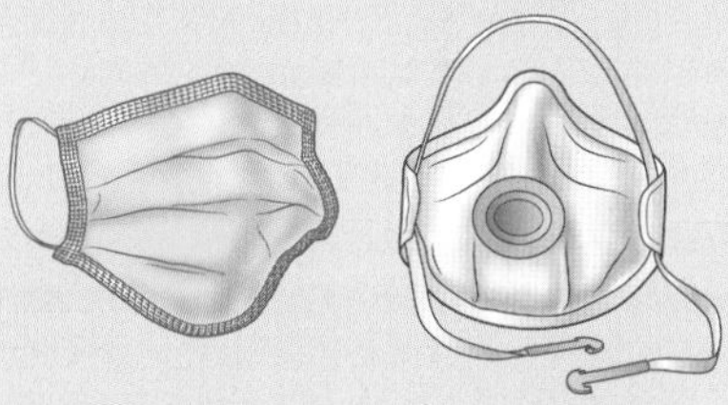

Infection Prevention and Control at a Glance, First Edition. By Debbie Weston, Alison Burgess and Sue Roberts.
© 2017 John Wiley & Sons, Ltd. Published 2017 by John Wiley & Sons, Ltd.

Figure 16.2 PPE – in order of doffing (removal)

Item		How to remove
		Without touching the skin, pinch or grasp one glove at the wrist and pull and peel it away from the hand; the glove will turn inside out (the contaminated outside of the glove will now be on the inside). Then, holding the removed glove in the gloved hand, slide the fingers of the ungloved hand between the glove and the wrist, and roll the glove down the hand and fold it into the first glove
		Grasp the sides of the apron at the top (shoulders), pull to break the ties at the neck, and roll gently downwards
		Using ungloved hands, grasp the sides or headpiece and lift away from the face
		Surgical mask – untie the bottom tie, followed by the top tie, and then lift away from the face **Respirator** – lift the bottom elastic over the top of the head followed by the second elastic, and then lift away from the face

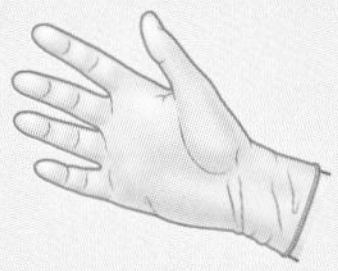

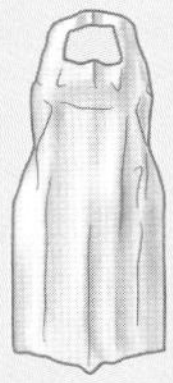

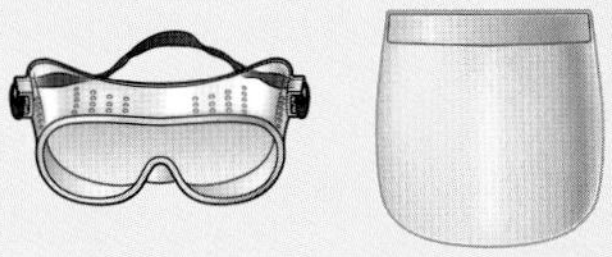

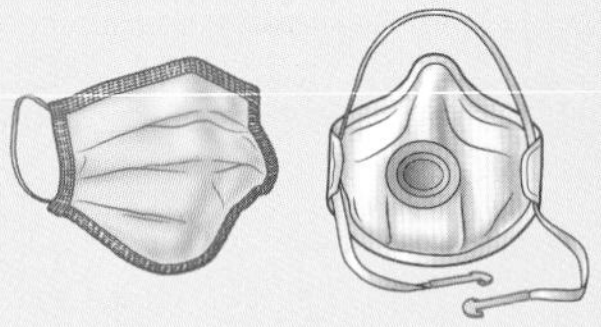

Table 16.1 Surgical face masks and respirators – indications for use

	Surgical face masks	Respirators
Protection against	Blood/body fluids, which can splash or spray as airborne mist during procedures, or if they are expelled violently or hit a surface Respiratory droplets, which are expelled from the nose and mouth and can remain suspended in the air for several minutes. Large droplets fall out of suspension within seconds; smaller droplets evaporate to form droplet nuclei	Droplets and aerosols. Aerosols are small suspensions of solid or liquid particles in gas or air, and can travel long distances depending on the speed with which they are generated and environmental conditions
Indications for use	✓ During surgical procedures ✓ When dealing with spillages of faeces (diarrhoea) or vomit during norovirus outbreaks if there is a risk of splashes ✓ May be worn for contact with patients with seasonal influenza and pertussis if the healthcare worker is within three feet or one metre of a symptomatic patient	✓ Aerosol-generating procedures (AGPs) in healthcare settings include intubation and extubation; sputum induction/chest physiotherapy; suctioning; bronchoscopy ✓ Protection against the inhalation of infectious respiratory particles when: • undertaking AGPs on patients with suspected/confirmed respiratory tuberculosis • in contact with patients with suspected or confirmed multi-drug resistant respiratory tuberculosis (see Chapter 44) • in contact with patients with suspected/confirmed pandemic influenza (see Chapter 41) /Ebola virus (see Chapter 33) and MERS-CoV
Considerations	! Do not filter out microorganisms ! Must be changed when they become wet ! Are not tight-fitting; therefore do not form a protective seal	! Require fit-testing ! Require fit-checking before each use

Personal protective equipment (PPE) is defined as 'all equipment that is intended to be worn or held by a person at work and which protects them against one or more risks to health and safety' (Royal College of Nursing, 2012a). Its use is an integral component of infection prevention and control standard (universal) precautions, used within the healthcare setting to protect healthcare workers from bloodborne **pathogens** and prevent the transmission of microorganisms to both patients and staff. Its use in the workplace is a requirement under the Health and Safety at Work Act 1974, as well as the *Code of Practice* (Health and Social Care Act 2008) (Department of Health, 2015) (see Chapter 1).The epic3 guidelines (Loveday et al, 2014) (https://www.his.org.uk/files/3113/8693/4808/epic3_National_Evidence-Based_Guidelines_for_Preventing_HCAI_in_NHSE.pdf) set out the evidence base for the use of PPE. Figure 16.1 provides examples of when each item of PPE should be worn for various healthcare interventions and also lists the order in which items of PPE should be put on (donned).

Aprons and gowns (Loveday et al, 2014)

Disposable plastic aprons are worn to protect the uniform or clothing if there is a risk of contamination from direct patient contact, the patient's environment, or body fluids / splashes.

They are only clean at the point at which they are put on and must be worn for one procedure or one episode of care only.

Full-length impermeable gowns are required where gross contamination of the uniform / clothing is anticipated.

Gloves (WHO, 2009; RCN 2012b; Loveday et al, 2014)

While gloves provide a barrier between the healthcare worker's skin and contamination from blood, body fluids, secretions and excretions it is essential that healthcare staff understand that:

• The wearing of gloves does *not* negate the need for hand hygiene.
• A pair of *gloved* hands will generally have the same contact with patients and equipment / the environment as a pair *of ungloved* hands.
• The inappropriate use of gloves is potentially just as much of a risk in terms of the transmission of microorganisms / cross-infection as failure to implement effective hand hygiene.
• Gloves do not completely eliminate all risk, as their integrity cannot be guaranteed and they may be punctured or torn by jewellery (rings with stones) or long fingernails.

Face protection: masks, face shields and eye shields / goggles (Coia et al, 2013; Loveday et al, 2014)

The mucous membranes of the eyes, nose and mouth are susceptible portals of entry for microorganisms that are transmitted via sprays or splashes of blood and body fluids, and the inhalation of airborne particles (droplets or aerosols) that can penetrate into the respiratory tract. **Aerosols** are small suspensions of solid or liquid particles in air or gas that can travel short or long distances depending upon the speed with which they are generated (i.e. cough or sneeze) and the environmental conditions (ventilation and air currents). **Droplets** are larger than aerosols and can remain suspended in air for several minutes but are not infectious over long distances (less than 1 metre). Large droplets fall out of suspension within a few seconds and evaporate to form **droplet nuclei**. These can float on air currents and may contain a high microbial load. **Splashes and sprays** are caused by blood and body fluids being expelled violently and / or hitting a surface; blood sprays or splashes may be generated during surgical procedures.

Surgical face masks: These only provide a physical barrier against droplets and splashes that may enter the nose, mouth and respiratory tract. They do not have any filtering capability and do not afford protection against smaller suspended droplets and aerosol particles produced by aerosol-generating procedures or transmissible respiratory infections. They are not considered to be part of respiratory PPE. In addition to being worn for surgery / invasive procedures, they may be worn when caring for patients for infections as described in Figure 16.1.

Respirator filtering face piece (FFP) masks: These provide three different levels of filtering capability (FFP1–3). The FFP3 respirator mask provides the highest level of filtering capability and face fit, reducing exposure to infectious particles by at least a factor of 20 if the respirator is fitted properly. It is the only FFP respirator approved by the Health and Safety Executive (HSE) for protection from infectious aerosols. 'Fit-testing' is an essential requirement of FFP3 use, in order to ensure that the respirator is suitable and a close fit for the shape of the healthcare worker's face, and that there are no gaps under or around the mask through which unfiltered air can enter. Respirators also have to be 'fit-checked' prior to being donned. NHS England has published detailed guidance on the use of FFP3 respirators, including the fit-testing and fit-checking process (http://www.england.nhs.uk/wp-content/uploads/2013/12/guide-ffp3-leaflet-v2.pdf). Respirators must be changed after each use and if the healthcare worker finds breathing difficult and / or it is obviously contaminated. The indications for the wearing of face masks and respirators are described in Table 16.1.

Full face visors or shields: These cover the face, eyes, nose and mouth and provide a high level of protection from splashes and sprays of blood and body fluids. They are most often worn in theatres where there is an increased risk of splashes from body fluids, although they may also be required when caring for a patient with a 'high-risk' infection (see Figure 16.1). The delicate conjunctivae of the eyes can be protected from droplets and splashes by the use of **'goggles'** (wrap-around safety spectacles), full face visors or surgical face masks that incorporate a transparent panel which covers the eyes. Safety spectacles must be fitted over glasses worn for vision, which will *not* afford appropriate protection for the healthcare worker on their own.

Donning and doffing (removing) PPE

There is an order or sequence in which PPE should be donned and removed (Figures 16.1 and 16.2). Ensuring that PPE is removed in the correct order is important not only to minimise the risk of cross-infection but, just as crucially, to minimise the risk of / prevent inadvertent self-contamination of the healthcare worker (see Chapter 33 for the complex PPE donning and removal sequence in relation to Ebola).

17 Environmental cleaning and disinfection

Figure 17.1 Hospital environmental hygiene – epic3

Hospital environmental hygiene	
SP1	The hospital environment must be visibly clean; free from non-essential items and equipment, dust and dirt; and acceptable to patients, visitors and staff. *Class D/GPP*
SP2	Levels of cleaning should be increased in cases of infection and/or colonisation when a suspected or known pathogen can survive in the environment, and environmental contamination may contribute to the spread of infection. *Class D/GPP*
SP3	The use of disinfectants should be considered for cases of infection and/or colonisation when a suspected or known pathogen can survive in the environment, and environmental contamination may contribute to the spread of infection. *Class D/GPP*
SP4	Shared pieces of equipment used in the delivery of patient care must be cleaned and decontaminated after each use with products recommended by the manufacturer. *Class D/GPP*
SP5	All healthcare workers need to be educated about the importance of maintaining a clean and safe care environment for patients. Every healthcare worker needs to know their specific responsibilities for cleaning and decontaminating the clinical environment and the equipment used in patient care. *Class D/GPP*

Source: Loveday et al, 2014

Figure 17.4 An example of cleaning standards – acute NHS Trust

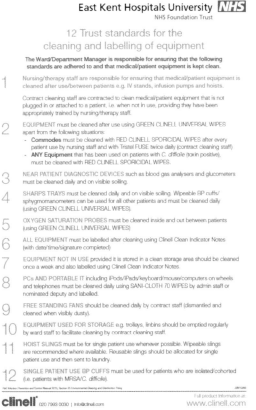

Source: East Kent Hospitals University NHS Foundation Trust and GAMA Healthcare

Figure 17.2 The national specifications for cleanliness in the NHS

The national specifications for cleanliness in the NHS: a framework for setting and measuring performance outcomes (2007) were designed to provide a simple, easy-to-apply methodology within which hospitals in England can assess the effectiveness of their cleaning services, taking account of previous developments such as the 'Matron's charter' and are available at:
http://www.nrls.npsa.nhs.uk/EasySiteWeb/getresource.axd?AssetID=60127&type=full&servicetype=Attachment

Figure 17.3 Indications for cleaning, disinfection and sterilisation

Risk	Application of item	Recommendation
High	• in close contact with a break in the skin or mucous membrane • introduced into sterile body areas	Sterilisation
Intermediate	• in close contact with mucous membranes • contaminated with particularly virulent or readily transmissible organisms • prior to use on immunocompromised patients	Sterilisation or disinfection required Cleaning may be acceptable in some agreed evidence-based situations
Low	• in contact with healthy skin • not in contact with patient	Cleaning

Source: Medical Devices Agency publication, MAC manual (Part 1) 2010

The cleanliness of healthcare premises is an important aspect in the provision of clean safe care (Figures 17.1 and 17.2) (Loveday et al, 2014). Current legislation, regulatory frameworks and quality standards emphasise the importance of cleaning and decontamination to facilitate the prevention and control of infection and maintain public confidence (Health and Social Care Act 2008 – see Chapter 1) (DH, 2015). There is an expectation by the public that the healthcare environment will be clean and the risk of infection controlled.

Pathogens including *Clostridium difficile* (see Chapter 31), meticillin-resistant *Staphylococcus aureus* (MRSA) (see Chapter 43), vancomycin-resistant enterococci (VRE), norovirus (see Chapter

Infection Prevention and Control at a Glance, First Edition. By Debbie Weston, Alison Burgess and Sue Roberts.
© 2017 John Wiley & Sons, Ltd. Published 2017 by John Wiley & Sons, Ltd.

40), and multi-drug resistant (MDR) organisms share the ability to be shed from infected or **colonised** patients, survive on dry surfaces for hours to days and sometimes months, and be difficult to eradicate by cleaning and disinfection. Recent studies indicate that there is a growing body of evidence supporting the theory that contaminated surfaces play an important role in the person-to-person transmission of healthcare associated pathogens, both endemic and epidemic (Otter et al, 2013). Although the main source of healthcare associated pathogens is likely to be the patient's endogenous flora, an estimated 20–40% of HCAI have been attributed to cross-infection via the hands of healthcare workers (Weinstein, 1991) who may have become contaminated from direct contact with the patient or indirectly by touching contaminated surfaces including medical equipment. The degree of patient-to-patient transmission has been found to be directly proportional to the level of environmental contamination.

Weber et al (2013) concluded that contact with the contaminated environment by healthcare personnel is just as likely as direct contact with a patient to lead to contamination of the healthcare provider's hands or gloves that may result in patient-to-patient transmission of healthcare associated pathogens. Admission to a room previously occupied by a patient with MRSA, VRE, Acinetobacter, or *C. difficile* increases the risk for the next patient to acquire the pathogen (Otter et al, 2011). Using a human challenge study, Barker et al (2004) demonstrated that human noroviruses could be consistently transferred via contaminated fingers to surfaces such as toilet seat lids, door handles and telephone receivers and that contaminated fingers could sequentially transfer virus to up to seven clean surfaces.

The continued emergence of antimicrobial resistance in Gram-negative bacteria, in particular, means that there is an urgent need to have in place effective infection prevention and control strategies including effective environmental decontamination if the robustness of the evidence to support this risk increases (Pelag and Hooper, 2010). In 2010, Dancer made a compelling case for not allowing the emphasis on hand hygiene to eclipse the continuing need for robust environmental cleaning, emphasising the need for a multimodal approach to infection prevention, especially given that hand hygiene compliance is rarely 100%.

Decontamination

Decontamination is a combination of processes that removes or destroys contamination so that infectious agents or other contaminants cannot reach a susceptible site in sufficient quantities to initiate infection (Figure 17.3).

Cleaning

Cleaning is the first level of decontamination (HSE, 2015).

The term 'cleaning' is used to describe the physical removal of soil, dirt and dust from surfaces. In healthcare settings this is generally achieved by using a solvent, usually water and detergent, which may be heated; cloths; and mops, with dry mops being used to remove dust from high surfaces. Microfibre cloths and water are sometimes used. Cleaning and / or disinfection of the healthcare environment is usually performed daily to reduce the environmental burden and ensure the patient's environment remains visibly clean. Detergent or disinfectant wipes are commonly used by healthcare staff for the decontamination of medical devices in contact with intact skin. The cleaning process will facilitate the removal of organic matter on which infectious agents thrive. Cleaning may be achieved by either manual or automated methods. The reduction of microbial contamination depends on various factors including the effectiveness of the cleaning process and the amount of bioburden (soil) present. Cleaning will not completely eliminate microorganisms from environmental surfaces and reductions in their number will only be transient. As a rule, cleaning is recommended for items not in direct contact with the patient, and medical equipment in contact with the patient's intact, healthy skin (Figure 17.4).

Enhanced cleaning

'Enhanced cleaning' describes the use of methods in addition to standard cleaning specifications, usually in response to infection prevention and control requirements. These may include increased frequency of cleaning for all or some surfaces such as frequently touched surfaces or the use of additional cleaning equipment or disinfectants. Enhanced cleaning is routinely undertaken for what is frequently referred to as 'terminal cleaning' following the discharge or transfer of a patient colonised or infected with a pathogenic microorganism. Enhanced cleaning can extend to entire wards in the case of a norovirus or *C. difficile* outbreaks, for example (Loveday et al, 2014).

Disinfection

The process of disinfection reduces the number of viable infectious agents but may not necessarily inactivate some microbial agents, such as certain viruses and microbial spores, for example *C. difficile*. This needs to be achieved by chemical or physical means. Chemical disinfection involves the use of a chosen disinfectant, at the specified concentration with good contact between the disinfectant and the surface or medical device for the specified minimum time to disinfect the surface or device being processed (MHRA, 2010).

Blood and body fluid spillages are decontaminated using the process of disinfection, usually using freshly prepared hypochlorite solution containing 10 000 ppm available chlorine (HSE, 2015). Disinfection does not achieve the same reduction in microbial contamination levels as sterilisation – a process used to render an object free from viable infectious agents including viruses and bacterial spores (BS EN 556-1:2001).

Effective cleaning is essential prior to undertaking all subsequent methods of decontamination as these methods have a limited ability to penetrate organic material. Although the introduction of enhanced cleaning and disinfection has been successful both in improving cleaning and reducing healthcare associated infections, studies have shown that this process when undertaken manually is only ever partially effective, relying on the operator to consistently ensure adequate selection, formulation, distribution and contact time of the agents used. Multiple studies have demonstrated that fewer than 50% of hospital ward surfaces are adequately decontaminated when chemical disinfectants are used (Carling et al, 2008). As a result specialist technologies, including automated room disinfection units, have been developed to robustly decontaminate environmental surfaces using either ultraviolet light (UV) or hydrogen peroxide. These technologies supplement but do not replace standard cleaning because surfaces must first be physically cleaned of soil. Although evidence is emerging of their efficacy, from a practical perspective they cannot be used routinely because the room needs to be emptied of people for several hours (Passaretti et al, 2013). Self-disinfecting surfaces, especially copper-coated surfaces, show promise for reducing the bioburden on hospital surfaces and decreasing healthcare associated infections.

18 Sharps

Figure 18.1 When do sharps incidents occur, and what are the risks? (HPA, 2012b; RCN, 2013a)

Sharps injuries occur:
- during use
- after use and before disposal
- between steps in procedures
- during disposal
- while re-sheathing or recapping a needle.

Procedures that have a higher than average risk of causing a sharps injury include intravascular (IV) annulation and venepuncture.

Devices involved in high-risk procedures:
- IV cannulae
- winged steel needles (known as butterfly needles)
- hypodermic needles and syringes
- phlebotomy needles

Figure 18.4 An example of a sharps device incorporating a safety device mechanism. Source: Reproduced with permission of BD Medical

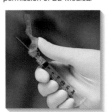

Figure 18.6 epic3 guidelines: Safe use and disposal of sharps (Loveday et al, 2014)

- Sharps must not be passed directly from hand to hand, and handling should be kept to a minimum.
- Needles must not be recapped, bent or disassembled after use.
- Used sharps must be discarded at the point of use by the person generating the waste.
- All sharps containers must:
- conform to current national and international standards
- be positioned safely, away from public areas and out of the reach of children, and at a height that enables safe disposal by all members of staff
- be secured to avoid spillage
- be temporarily closed when not in use
- not be filled above the fill line, and
- be disposed of when the fill line is reached.
- All clinical and non-clinical staff must be educated about the safe use and disposal of sharps and the action to be taken in the event of an injury.
- Use safer sharps devices where assessment indicates that they will provide safe systems of working for healthcare workers.
- Organisations should involve end-users in evaluating safer sharps devices to determine their effectiveness, acceptability to practitioners, impact on patient care and cost benefit prior to widespread introduction.

Figure 18.2 Case study (HSE, 2006)

'A doctor suffered a needlestick injury during her work as a surgeon, which resulted in extended and debilitating treatment for a potential infection of hepatitis C. She was treated with interferon and other antiviral agents for six months. Treatments required constant monitoring of white cell counts and additional medication to stimulate bone marrow. Overall, the sufferer felt tired, nauseous, anaemic and anxious and has suffered from persistent shaking. She took three days off work as a result of the immediate injury, and was unable to carry out surgical work for a further six months while she waited for the results of her blood tests.'

Figure 18.3 What to do if you receive a sharps injury (http://www.hse.gov.uk/healthservices/needlesticks/#know; HSE, 2013)

If you suffer an injury from a sharp that may be contaminated:
- Encourage the wound to gently bleed, ideally holding it under running water.
- Wash the wound using running water and plenty of soap.
- Don't scrub the wound whilst you are washing it.
- Don't suck the wound.
- Dry the wound and cover it with a waterproof plaster or dressing.
- Seek urgent medical advice (for example from your Occupational Health Service or Emergency Department) as effective prophylaxis is available.
- Report the injury to your employer.

Figure 18.5 *The Health and Safety (Sharp Instruments in Healthcare) Regulations 2013* (HSE, 2013)

Main requirements:
Employers need to assess the risk of sharps injuries under the Control of Substances Hazardous to Health (COSHH) regulations. Where risks are identified, the Sharps in Healthcare Regulations require them to take specific risk control measures, as follows:

1. Steps must be taken to avoid the unnecessary use of sharps.
   Where it is not reasonably practicable to avoid the use of sharps, employers are required to:
   - Use safe sharps (incorporating protection mechanisms).
   - Where it is reasonably practicable to do so, prevent the recapping of needles.
   - Place secure containers and instructions for safe disposal of medical sharps close to the work area.

2. Provide information to employees on the risks from injuries, relevant legal duties of employers and employees, good practice in preventing injuries, the benefits and drawbacks of vaccination and the support available to the injured person from their employer. The employer must work with safety representatives in developing and promoting this information.

3. Provide appropriate training to ensure employees know how to work safely. Training must cover the correct use of safer sharps, safe use and disposal of sharps, what to do in the event of an injury and the employer's arrangements for health surveillance.

4. Have arrangements in place in the event of an injury. These include keeping a record of the incident, investigations of the circumstances of an incident and taking action to prevent recurrence. Records should include details of the type of sharp involved, at what stage of the procedure the incident occurred and the severity of the incident.

5. Ensure that injured employees who may have been exposed to a bloodborne virus have immediate access to medical advice, are offered post-exposure prophylaxis or other treatment as advised by a doctor and are offered counselling where appropriate.

6. Review, at suitable periods, the effectiveness of the procedures and control measures.

Infection Prevention and Control at a Glance, First Edition. By Debbie Weston, Alison Burgess and Sue Roberts.
© 2017 John Wiley & Sons, Ltd. Published 2017 by John Wiley & Sons, Ltd.

Sharps injuries are a well-known risk in the health and social care sector and can occur in any setting. Sharps contaminated with an infected patient's blood can transmit more than 20 diseases, including hepatitis B and C and human immunodeficiency virus (HIV) (see Chapter 26). Because of this transmission risk, sharps injuries can cause concern and stress to the many thousands who receive them. Most sharps injuries can be prevented and there are legal requirements on employers to take steps to prevent healthcare staff from being exposed to infectious agents from sharps injuries (HSE, 2013).

What are sharps and what is a sharps injury?

Sharps are needles, blades (such as scalpels) and other medical instruments necessary for undertaking healthcare activities which can cause an injury by cutting or pricking the skin. A sharps injury is an incident that causes a needle, blade or other medical instrument to penetrate the skin. This is sometimes called a **percutaneous** injury or **exposure**.

Who is at risk? (see Figure 18.1)

Workers and others in health and social care are at risk of sharps and exposure incidents. This includes those who directly handle sharps but also workers who may inadvertently be put at risk when sharps are not stored or disposed of correctly. There is a higher risk of infection from a sharps injury involving a hollow-bore needle. Higher risk procedures are listed in Figure 18.1. Clean sharps such as glass ampoules can also represent a risk of injury and steps should be taken to prevent such injuries.

What is the risk?

The main risk from a sharps injury is the potential exposure to infections such as bloodborne viruses (BBV). This can occur where the injury involves a sharp that is contaminated with blood or a bodily fluid from an affected patient. The bloodborne viruses of most concern are:

• hepatitis B (HBV)
• hepatitis C (HCV)
• human immunodeficiency virus (HIV).

The transmission of infection depends on a number of factors, including the person's natural immune response. Although the number of injuries each year is high, only a small number are known to have caused infections that led to serious illness. However, the effects of the injury and anxiety about its potential consequences, including the adverse side effects of post-exposure prophylaxis, can have a significant personal impact on an injured employee (see Figure 18.2).

The risk of infection will depend on a number of factors, including:

• the **depth** of the injury
• the type of sharp used (**hollow-bore** needles present a higher risk although subcutaneous needles also present a risk)
• whether the device was previously in the **patient's vein or artery**
• how **infectious** the patient is at the time of the injury (RCN, 2013a).

When all these factors are taken into account, the risk of infection by a contaminated needle can be as high as:

• **one in 3** for **hepatitis B**
• **one in 30** for **hepatitis C**
• **one in 300** for **HIV** (HPA, 2012b).

A **mucocutaneous** exposure involves exposure of the mucous membrane of the eyes, the inside of the nose or mouth, or an area of non-intact skin. Exposures and bites also present the same risks, although the risk is lower than from a percutaneous exposure, estimated at 1 in 1000 for HIV (HPA, 2012b). In the UK a small but significant number of healthcare staff including nurses have developed potentially life-threatening diseases as a result of a sharps injury. Since the late 1990s at least 20 healthcare workers have contracted hepatitis C and there have been five documented cases of HIV transmission in the UK (HPA, 2012b). All these transmissions have occurred following **percutaneous** exposure.

What to do if you have a sharps injury
(see Figure 18.3)

The majority of incidents where the transmission of bloodborne viruses occurs are caused by **failure to adhere to standard infection prevention and control precautions**. The guidelines on standard precautions (*Guidance for Clinical Health Care Workers: Protection against infection with blood-borne viruses*) were published by the Department of Health in 1998. Their approach to preventing the transmission of bloodborne viruses is based on the principle that all blood and certain body fluids are potentially infectious and therefore specific procedures should be adopted routinely for all patients where contact is anticipated.

Everyone has a role to play in the prevention of sharps injuries to healthcare workers. From the Chief Executive and Board of Directors, who have overall legal responsibility for the health and safety of their staff, to the individual nurse or healthcare worker – all have a duty to ensure that they protect themselves and others around them by safely using and disposing of sharps equipment (HSE, 2013).

Health and Safety (Sharp Instruments in Healthcare) Regulations 2013 (see Figures 18.4, 18.5 and 18.6)

All employers are required under existing health and safety law to ensure that risks from sharps injuries are assessed and appropriate control measures are in place. The most recently published sharps regulations, *The Health and Safety (Sharp Instruments in Healthcare) Regulations 2013,* implement the EU Council Directive 2010/32/ EU[5], building on existing law and providing specific detail on the requirements that must be taken by healthcare employers and their contractors. The Regulations only apply to employers, contractors and workers in the healthcare sector. NHS Trusts/Boards, independent healthcare businesses and other employers whose main activity is the management, organisation and provision of healthcare will be subject to the Regulations. HSE has produced *Health Services Information Sheet 7 - Health and Safety (Sharps Instruments in Healthcare) Regulations 2013* (available at http://www.hse.gov .uk/pubns/hsis7.pdf) to provide guidance on how to comply with the Regulations.

19 Aseptic non-touch technique

Figure 19.1 Aseptic non-touch technique – intravenous drug administration

ANTT IV Drug administration procedure

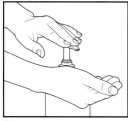

Clean hands

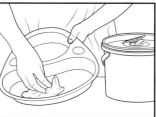

Clean sharps tray with detergent wipes

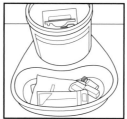

Whilst tray is drying collect equipment and medicines

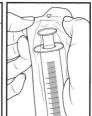

Check expiry dates and packaging

Clean hands

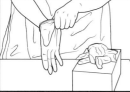

Put on non-sterile gloves

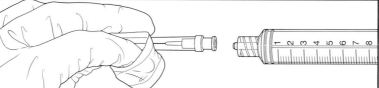

Protecting key-parts, prepare equipment and medicines

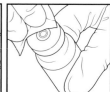

Disinfect vial with chlorhexidine 2%/70% alcohol

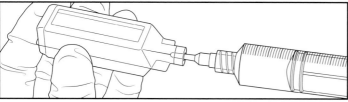

Must draw with needle

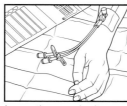

Assess the cannula site (VIP SCORE)

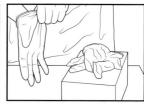

Remove gloves, clean hands, re-apply gloves

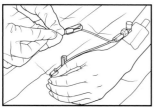

Clean bionnectors with chlorhexidine 2%/70% alcohol
Allow 30 seconds to dry

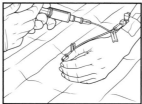

Administer drugs using push pause technique
Flush cannula with 0.9% sodium chloride before and after drug administration
Apply positive pressure as bionnector clamp is closed

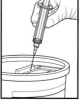

Dispose of all sharps immediately

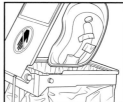

Put waste into clinical waste bin
Remove gloves and dispose in clinical waste bin

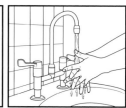

Wash hands

Always:
- Use correct hand hygiene
- Use a non-touch-technique
- Identify and protect the 'key parts'
- Monitor your own and colleagues' practices

Source: Reproduced with permission of East Kent Hospitals University NHS Foundation Trust

Infection Prevention and Control at a Glance, First Edition. By Debbie Weston, Alison Burgess and Sue Roberts.
© 2017 John Wiley & Sons, Ltd. Published 2017 by John Wiley & Sons, Ltd.

In relation to preventing and controlling risks of HCAI, NHS organisations must have in place relevant core policies including 'aseptic technique'. In addition, according to the *Code of Practice on the prevention and control of infections and related guidance* (DH, 2015) the following should be in place.

• Clinical procedures should be carried out in a manner that maintains and promotes the principles of asepsis.

• Education, training and assessment in the aseptic technique should be provided to all persons undertaking such procedures.

• The technique should be standardised across the organisation.

• An audit should be undertaken to monitor compliance with the technique.

Asepsis

Asepsis is commonly referred to as an absence of **pathogenic** microorganisms. Asepsis applies to both medical and surgical procedures. The aim of **medical asepsis** is to minimise the risk of contamination by microorganisms and prevent their transmission by applying standard principles of infection prevention, including decontaminating hands, use of personal protective clothing, maintaining an aseptic area, and not touching susceptible sites or the surface of invasive devices during the procedure. **Surgical asepsis** is considered a more complex process and includes procedures to eliminate microorganisms from an area, thus creating an aseptic environment or what is commonly called a 'sterile field', as practised in operating theatres and for some high-risk invasive procedures such as the insertion of a central venous catheter (Loveday et al, 2014).

Aseptic technique

According to *Mosby's Dictionary of Medicine, Nursing and Health Professions* (2013), the definition of aseptic technique is 'any healthcare procedure in which added precautions, such as the use of sterile gloves and instruments, are used to prevent contamination of a person, object, or area by microorganisms'. This definition fits appropriately with the systems and processes that are generally in place in the operating theatre. Similarly, Loveday et al (2014) describe the aseptic technique as 'a term applied to a set of specific practices and procedures used to assure asepsis and prevent the transfer of potentially pathogenic microorganisms to a susceptible site on the body (e.g. an open wound or insertion site for an invasive medical device) or to sterile equipment/devices. It involves ensuring that susceptible body sites and the sterile parts of the devices in contact with a susceptible site are not contaminated during the procedure'.

Figure 19.2 Aseptic non-touch technique – dressing change

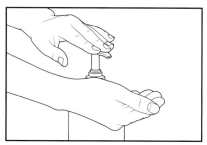

Clean hands

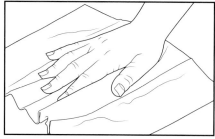

Clean trolley with Clinell universal wipes (green)
and allow to dry
Add a clinical waste bag to side of trolley
(trolley must be used)

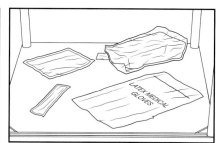

Clean hands, don apron, assemble equipment

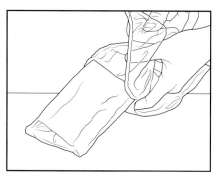

Clean hands
Open dressing pack onto trolley
Clean hands again

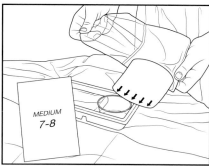

Carefully open required products avoiding
contamination of sterile field/key parts

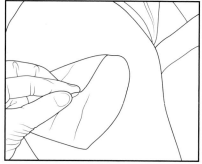

Remove soiled dressing, wearing clean
gloves and dispose into clinical waste bag
Remove gloves

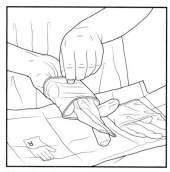

Clean hands and apply sterile gloves

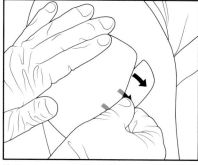

If cleaning is indicated irrigate with
normal saline
Apply appropriate dressing

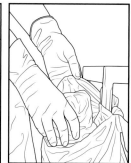

Clear trolley
Dispose of clinical waste,
remove gloves
Clean hands

Always:
- Use correct hand hygiene
- Use a non-touch-technique
- Identify and protect the 'key parts'

Source: Policy for Aseptic Non-Touch Technique (ANTT) Infection Control Manual. Reproduced with permission of East Kent Hospitals University NHS Foundation Trust

Aseptic non-touch technique (ANTT)

Aseptic non-touch technique (ANTT) uses a different approach to aseptic technique. According to Loveday et al (2014), ANTT consists of a framework for the aseptic technique based on the concept of defining key parts and key sites to be protected from contamination. This approach is consistent with the approaches generally used for procedures such as peripheral cannula insertion and dressing changes.

In the past aseptic technique has been performed as a ritualistic procedure normally associated with wound care (Briggs et al, 1996). The evidence base was poor with little consideration given to the technique (Wright, 1989; Gilmour, 1999; Rowley, 2000). This has resulted in variable practice and terminology being used across healthcare settings. Although aseptic technique is considered as an essential element of the prevention of HCAI, and especially important when the body's natural defence mechanisms are compromised, there is currently no evidence either clinically or from a cost effective perspective that any one approach is more clinically or cost effective than another (Loveday, 2014).

Aseptic non-touch technique – a theoretical framework

Aseptic non-touch technique (ANTT) is a relatively new approach utilising a theoretical framework to undertaking aseptic techniques. According to Rowley (2000) this standardised approach has been shown to significantly improve the aseptic technique of healthcare staff by utilising a consistent and rationalised approach.

ANTT operates on the basis, whatever the clinical procedure, of identifying and protecting 'key parts' of equipment which, if touched, either directly or indirectly, could result in cross-infection. It is achieved by ensuring that only sterile equipment and fluids are used and that parts of the components that should remain sterile are not touched or allowed to come into contact with non-sterile surfaces, e.g. the tip of intravenous connectors. In intravenous therapy, the key parts are usually those which come into contact with the liquid infusion, e.g. needles, syringe tips, intravenous line and connections, and exposed central line lumens. The ANTT approach promoted by Rowley et al (2010) has been endorsed by the NICE guideline development group (NICE, 2012) as 'an example of aseptic non touch technique for vascular access device maintenance, which is widely used in acute and community settings and represents a possible framework for establishing guidance on aseptic technique'.

Aseptic non-touch technique is achieved by preventing direct and indirect contact of key parts by a non-touch method. It can be adopted for all aseptic procedures such as intravenous drug administration, urinary catheter care and some aspects of wound care and is applicable in all clinical / non-clinical areas.

Rowley et al have gone on to develop ANTT version 2, an updated theoretical and practice framework expanding on the principles of ANTT version 1, which has been widely adopted in the UK. ANTT version 2 has been developed to reflect current practice and simplify the approach introducing the theory of using micro aseptic fields to protect key parts (Rowley et al, 2010).

The *epic3: National evidence-based guidelines for preventing healthcare-associated infections in NHS hospitals in England* were revised and published in 2014. Based on the best critically appraised evidence available they provide standard principles for preventing healthcare associated infections in hospital and other acute settings including asepsis. The guidance is available at http://www.his.org.uk/files/3113/8693/4808/epic3_ National_Evidence-Based_Guidelines_for_Preventing_ HCAI_in_NHSE.pdf

Figures 19.1 and 19.2 are examples of how the principles of ANTT have been implemented into local procedures in an acute NHS Trust.

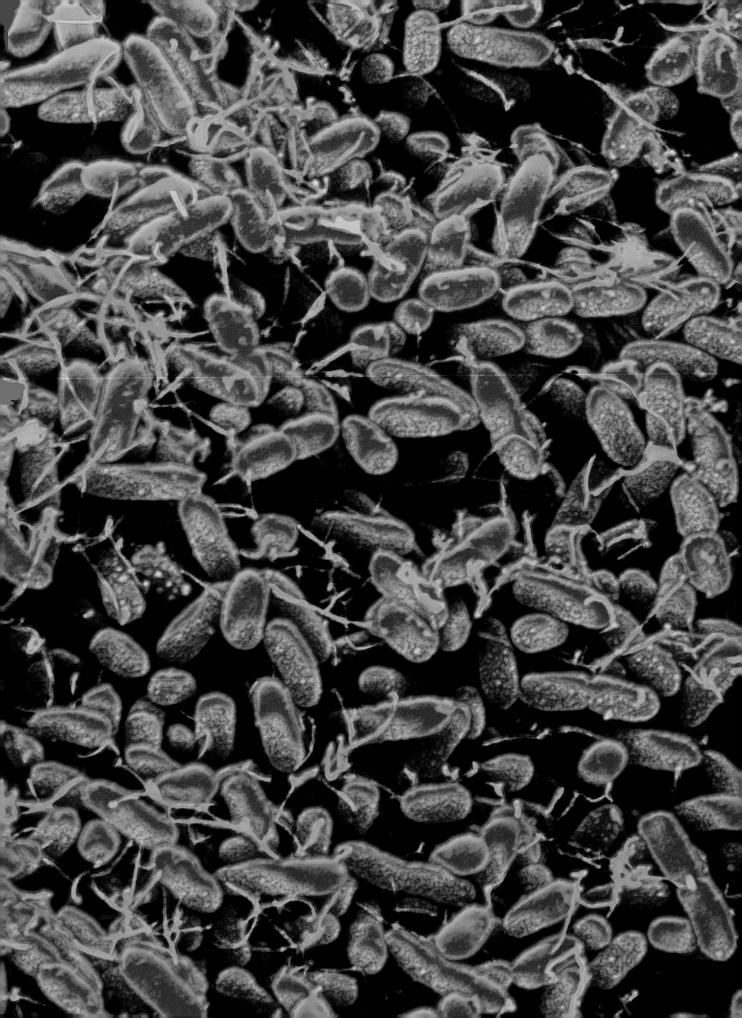

Clinical practice aspects of IP&C

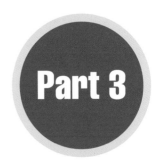

Part 3

Chapters

20 The infection prevention management of intravascular devices

Figure 20.1 Visual infusion phlebitis (VIP) scale

Appearance	Score	Stage
IV site appears healthy	0	No signs of phlebitis Action: OBSERVE CANNULA
One of the following signs is evident: • Slight pain near IV site or • Slight redness near IV site	1	Possibly first signs of phlebitis Action: OBSERVE CANNULA
Two of the following signs are evident: • Pain at IV site • Erythema/redness • Swelling	2	Early state of phlebitis Action: RESITE CANNULA
All of the following signs are evident: • Pain along path of cannula • Erythema/redness around site • Swelling	3	Medium state of phlebitis Action: RESITE CANNULA AND CONSIDER TREATMENT
All of the following signs are evident and extensive: • Pain along path of cannula • Erythema/redness around site • Swelling • Palpable venous cord	4	Advanced stage of phlebitis or start of thrombophlebitis Action: RESITE CANNULA AND CONSIDER TREATMENT
All of the following signs are evident and extensive: • Pain along path of cannula • Erythema/redness around site • Swelling • Palpable venous cord • Pyrexia	5	Advanced stage thrombophlebitis Action: INITIATE TREATMENT/ RESITE CANNULA

Source: Jackson, 1998; Infusion Nurses Society, 2006

Figure 20.2 Peripheral cannula management

The cannula site must also be observed when:

• bolus injections are administered
• IV rates are checked and altered
• solution containers are changed

The incidence of infusion phlebitis varies.
The following best practice points may assist in reducing the incidence of infusion phlebitis and the more serious development of bacteraemia (bloodstream infection):

• Observe cannula site at least daily, record
• Secure cannula with an approved intravenous dressing
• Replace loose, contaminated dressings
• Site cannula away from joints whenever possible
• Aseptic non-touch technique must be followed
• Consider re-siting the cannula every 72–96 hours
• Plan and document continuing care
• Use the smallest gauge cannula suitable for the patient's requirements
• Replace the cannula at the first indication of infusion phlebitis (stage 2 on the VIP score) (RCN, 2010).

Figure 20.3 epic3 Guidelines for preventing infections associated with the use of intravascular access devices

epic3: National evidence-based guidelines for preventing healthcare-associated infections in NHS hospitals in England were revised and published in 2014. Based on the best critically appraised evidence available they provide standard principles for preventing healthcare-associated infections in hospital and other acute settings, including guidelines for preventing infections associated with the use of intravascular access devices.

The guidelines are available at:

http://www.his.org.uk/files/3113/8693/4808/epic3_ National_Evidence-Based_Guidelines_for_Preventing_ HCAI_in_NHSE.pdf

Infection Prevention and Control at a Glance, First Edition. By Debbie Weston, Alison Burgess and Sue Roberts.
© 2017 John Wiley & Sons, Ltd. Published 2017 by John Wiley & Sons, Ltd.

A vascular access device is an indwelling catheter, cannula or other device used to obtain venous or arterial access. Both central and peripheral vascular access devices are available and are used in the management of patients in acute and chronic care settings. Central vascular access catheters (CVCs) are frequently used during clinical care and include peripherally inserted, non-tunnelled and tunnelled, and totally implantable CVCs. The use of these catheters can result in bloodstream infection. Catheter-related bloodstream infections (CR-BSI) associated with the insertion and maintenance of CVCs are potentially among the most serious complications associated with healthcare and are a major cause of morbidity. A prevalence study conducted in 2011 found that 64.2% of bloodstream infections in England were associated with a vascular access device (HPA, 2012a). It has been estimated that treating one case of MRSA bloodstream infection costs £5200 at 2009–10 prices (Plowman et al, 2000). Vascular access devices in general are one of the main causes of healthcare associated infection because they provide a direct route into the bloodstream via the skin. Although CVCs present a greater risk of bloodstream infection than peripheral cannulae, the latter also remain a significant risk to patients because they are by far the most common invasive device used in healthcare (Loveday et al, 2014). **The risk of infection associated with intravascular devices is greatly reduced by complying with all parts of the process for safe insertion and maintenance of the device and prompt removal as soon as it is no longer clinically required.**

The pathogenesis of catheter-related bloodstream infection

The microorganisms that colonise catheter hubs and the skin adjacent to the insertion site are the source of most CR-BSI. Coagulase-negative staphylococci, particularly *Staphylococcus epidermidis*, are the microorganisms most frequently implicated in CR-BSI. CR-BSI is generally caused either by skin microorganisms at the insertion site, which contaminate the catheter during insertion and then subsequently migrate along the cutaneous catheter track, hence the importance of decontaminating the insertion site with 2% chlorhexidine gluconate in 70% isopropyl alcohol prior to inserting intravascular devices and during dressing changes (DH, 2011b; Loveday et al, 2014), or microorganisms from the hands of healthcare workers that contaminate and colonise the catheter hub during care interventions. This point emphasises the importance of effective hand hygiene and the use of 2% chlorhexidine gluconate in 70% isopropyl alcohol to decontaminate ports and the surrounding area prior to administering fluid or injections via the central line or peripheral cannulae (DH, 2011b; Loveday et al, 2014). Less commonly, infusate contamination or seeding (haematogenous spread) from a different site of infection in the body, via the bloodstream, is identified as a cause of CR-BSI.

Biofilms commonly form on devices inserted into the body. The production of biofilm is a strategy utilised for microbial survival with the aim of establishing and spreading infection. Bacteria living within a biofilm, the '*microniche*', are protected from host defence mechanisms and antimicrobials. Central vascular catheters are disposed to biofilm formation as they offer a favourable surface for bacterial attachment. Staphylococci are recognised as the most common bacteria responsible for biofilm-

associated infection, compounded by meticillin-resistant *Staphylococcus aureus* (MRSA) (see Chapter 43). The hallmark of biofilm-embedded microorganisms is their resistance to large doses of traditional antimicrobial agents and as a result treatment outcomes are often unsuccessful, relying on the removal of the device for resolution (Esposito et al, 2013).

Other complications of peripheral cannulae are infrequent and usually minor including cannula blockage, thrombophlebitis, fluid extravasation into the tissues and localised infection. However spinal epidural abscess, although rare, can occur with an incidence of at least 1 in 10 000 hospital admissions. Although most epidural abscesses are a result of epidural anaesthesia or surgery on the spine they can occur following systemic infection or haematogenous spread with the likely involvement of biofilm from an infection at a distant site such as an intravenous line. **Morbidity** and **mortality** associated with this condition are significant and may result in permanent neurological damage if diagnosis and treatment are delayed (Burgess et al, 2005).

Investigating catheter-related bloodstream infection

Catheter-related bloodstream infection involves the presence of systemic infection and evidence implicating the intravascular catheter as its source (i.e. isolation of the same microorganism from blood cultures as that shown to be significantly colonising the intravascular catheter); blood cultures should be taken from a separate peripheral site and the central line when investigating potential infection related to the line (DH, 2011b). In the absence of **systemic** infection, catheter **colonisation** refers to the growth of microorganisms on either the endoluminal or the external catheter surface beneath the skin (Loveday et al, 2014).

Phlebitis scale

Phlebitis is the inflammation of the tunica intima (innermost layer) of the vein. Three types are described: mechanical, chemical and infective (Macklin, 2003). All vascular access sites should be routinely assessed for signs and symptoms of phlebitis. According to Jackson (1998) and Gallant and Schultz (2006), phlebitis should be documented using a standard scale for measuring degree / severity of phlebitis. Each organisation should have guidelines in place regarding the prevention and treatment of phlebitis, including appropriate device and vein selection, dilution of drugs and other pharmacological methods. Any incident of phlebitis, together with the intervention and treatment, should be documented in the patient's notes (RCN, 2010).

All patients with an intravenous (IV) peripheral access device in place must have the site checked at least daily for signs of infusion phlebitis. The subsequent score and action(s) taken (if any) must be documented (see Figure 20.1). Figures 20.2 and 20.3 summarise key points for peripheral cannula management.

Care bundles have been developed in the past by the Department of Health for the insertion and ongoing care of peripheral cannulae and central vascular catheters (2010) and are available at: http://webarchive.nationalarchives. gov.uk/20120118164404/hcai.dh.gov.uk/whatdoido/high-impact-interventions/

21 Isolation and cohort nursing

Figure 21.1 Considerations regarding the 'isolation' of patients

1 The patient

Is the patient going to be '**safe**' in a single room? For example: is the patient confused and apt to wander, **OR** at risk of falls, **OR** at risk of self-harm, **OR** require close observation/monitoring due to their medical condition? The overall safety of the patient has to be taken into consideration, and unless the patient has a communicable disease or is colonised with a highly resistant organism, the risk of cross-infection to other patients (and staff) can be minimised with the strict application of infection prevention and control standard precautions, increased attention to hand hygiene (patients) and additional cleaning (i.e. cleaning of frequent hand touch-points)

Also consider whether or not the patient requires specialist care that can only be given by nursing and medical staff on her/his 'home' ward – it may be detrimental to the patient's medical/surgical treatment to move her/him to another ward for isolation in a single room

Is the patient a hospital inpatient in an acute hospital or a community hospital or in a nursing/residential home? Different healthcare settings will have their own local policies

2 The organism

What is the organism?
Is it antibiotic resistant/multi-antibiotic resistant?
How is it spread?
What is the risk of environmental contamination and cross-infection to other patients and possibly to staff?
What are the implications of cross-infection – could it lead to an outbreak if the patient is not isolated?
Aside from isolation, what other IP&C control measures need to be implemented by staff?
Is there a requirement beyond the wearing of gloves and plastic aprons?
Is additional/enhanced cleaning required?

3 The facilities available

Does the ward design include single rooms for isolation purposes?
Is there a room immediately available or will another patient need to be moved (a risk assessment may need to be undertaken in order to determine isolation priorities)?
Is the room in an observable area or is it located off of the main ward, in an adjacent corridor or annex?
Does the room have en-suite facilities?
Is there a dedicated on-site Isolation/Infectious Ward or 'cohort ward' that the patient could be transferred to?
For patients in community hospitals, there may be no isolation facilities. In nursing / residential homes, the 'isolation room' may be the patient's own bedroom
If the patient cannot be nursed in a single room or a cohort bay, she or he will need to be cared for in the open ward alongside patients who are not known to be colonised or infected. In this instance, the colonised/infected patient should not be in a bed adjacent to a patient with an open wound, or a patient who has invasive devices in situ, as this has greater implications if cross-infection occurs

4 Other

What equipment is needed (i.e. monitors, Dinamap)?
Is there sufficient equipment available for some to be dedicated exclusively to that patient, or will equipment need to be shared?
What are the environmental cleaning/equipment decontamination requirements?
'Isolation' must not impact on the patient's general care and rehabilitation
All risk assessments and exceptions (i.e. where policy cannot be implemented) must be robustly documented and escalated

Figure 21.2 Isolation/cohort nursing – requirements

- Appropriate isolation door sign. Where patients are cohort nursed and there are doors to the bay, signage should be placed on the doors
- Door closed to isolation side room or cohort bay. In the case of isolation side rooms, if it is not safe to close the door, this must be documented in the notes and reviewed daily
- En-suite facilities or dedicated commode. For patients colonised with MRSA in a cohort bay, a bathroom/toilet may be allocated for their use only
- PPE outside the room/bay; for patients who are barrier nursed, a trolley containing PPE is often sited at the foot of the patient's bed
- For patients who are 'barrier nursed' in an open bay alcohol handrub is available outside the side room and at the patient's bedside (NB: availability of alcohol handrub at the bedside needs to be risk-assessed on an individual basis, i.e. risk of deliberate/accidental ingestion)
- Hand washing facilities available within the room/bay
- Domestic and clinical waste bins within the room/bay
- Single patient use tourniquet, blood pressure cuff, pulse oximeter probe and lifting aids (all disposable on discharge). Ideally equipment such as a Dinamap and other monitoring equipment should be dedicated to the isolation side room/cohort bay. If this is not possible, it must be thoroughly decontaminated before being used on another patient
- Disinfectant wipes within the room/bay for the decontamination of surfaces/equipment

Infection Prevention and Control at a Glance, First Edition. By Debbie Weston, Alison Burgess and Sue Roberts.
© 2017 John Wiley & Sons, Ltd. Published 2017 by John Wiley & Sons, Ltd.

Isolation of **colonised** or 'infected' patients in a single room is generally considered to be best practice in preventing and controlling the spread of infection, although it can have adverse psychological effects on patients (Skyman and Sjostrom, 2009; Abad et al, 2010; Barrett, 2010). Where capacity is outweighed by demand, other strategies need to be considered. Whichever method is chosen, it should not be implemented without a **risk assessment** being undertaken, and without the strict application of **infection prevention and control standard precautions.**

Risk assessment considerations
(see Figure 21.1)

The decision as to whether or not a patient who is 'colonised' or 'infected' / 'infectious' is isolated depends upon the nature of that colonisation / infection; some infections pose a significant risk to public health and are notifiable diseases. Although all organisations have local isolation policies, putting them into practice is not necessarily clear cut, and individual patient risk assessments may need to be undertaken in conjunction with the Infection Prevention and Control Team.

Source (standard) isolation

The aim of 'isolating' patients who are known or suspected to be colonised or infected is to isolate the organism, controlling or limiting its route of transmission and reducing the risk of cross-infection to other patients and healthcare staff. Isolation in a single side room, preferably with en-suite facilities, is referred to as source isolation. Although source isolation is commonly sub-categorised into source isolation *with* contact / enteric / droplet or respiratory precautions, these sub-categories are unnecessary, given that they are essentially **standard precautions with added emphasis on hand hygiene (i.e. hand washing when in contact with patients with diarrhoea) or PPE (i.e. surgical face masks or respirator masks when aerosol-generating procedures are undertaken, and / or when caring for patients with suspected MDR-TB) (also see Chapters 14 and 16), where such emphasis is appropriate**. Standard precautions are actually simple to implement; staff just need to understand the basic principles. Although the Centers for Disease Control and Prevention, Atlanta, refer to them in detail (Siegel et al, 2007), the **epic3 Guidelines** (Loveday et al, 2014) make no reference to, or recommendation for, the use of transmission-based precautions sub-categories.

Protective isolation

Patients who are severely immunocompromised through illness / disease are particularly susceptible to infection and may require specialist, protective isolation in order to prevent them from exposure to pathogens. Protective isolation is undertaken within specialist haematology / oncology wards which have purpose- built positive-pressure side rooms where the air pressure within the room is mechanically controlled to ensure that it is higher than the air pressure outside of the room. This prevents 'contaminated' air from entering the room where the patient is nursed. Standard precautions are strictly adhered to, and staff and visitors who are 'unwell' in any way must not have any contact with or visit the patient. Within a general hospital setting, 'protective isolation' is sometimes requested by staff for patients with neutropenic sepsis. However, outside of specialist facilities, this is essentially admission to a side room and the application of standard precautions.

Negative pressure isolation

Air currents can transport bacteria and viruses within buildings and rooms, increasing the risk of infection to other patients and staff. Within standard single (isolation) rooms, there will normally be six air changes an hour; the air changes within the room by passing under the door, or whenever the door or a window is opened, mixing with the air in the corridor. For some infections spread via respiratory droplets, such as multi-drug resistant tuberculosis (see Chapter 44) and pandemic influenza (see Chapter 41), it is important to prevent contaminated air from mixing with 'clean' air. This is achieved by a ventilation system which expels the air from the room and away from other areas, venting it to the outside so that it is not sucked back into the building. The ventilation is balanced so that more air is mechanically extracted *from* the room than is drawn *into* it. This creates a ventilation imbalance, which the ventilation system corrects by pulling air into the room from a gap under the door. Air pressure within the room is controlled and monitored so that if the negative-pressure ventilation system fails, an alarm sounds, alerting staff when the pressure falls. In order to maintain the negative pressure within the room there must be no gaps underneath or around the doors (apart from the deliberate gap underneath the door through which air is drawn in) and it should not be possible to open the windows.

Strict isolation

The isolation of patients with rare infectious diseases such as rabies, viral haemorrhagic fever (see Chapter 33) and pulmonary anthrax will be undertaken in a designated high-level isolation unit (HLIU), of which there is one in England at the Royal Free London NHS Foundation Trust, although in response to the Ebola virus disease outbreak in West Africa during 2014–15 there were plans for additional high-security isolation beds at three other hospitals. The patient is isolated in a negative-pressure patient isolator (Trexler) (flexible film 'tent') within a negative-pressure room. The Trexler isolator provides a physical barrier between the patient and healthcare staff, who have access to the patient via built-in access portholes (DHACDP / HSE, 2015).

Cohort nursing

Cohort nursing is undertaken in situations where there are not enough single rooms to isolate patients. Patients are either cohorted with the same organism, e.g. MRSA colonisation, or if they have the same symptoms, e.g. diarrhoea and vomiting due to norovirus or influenza, and should be cared for by designated staff in a designated area (bay) of the ward wherever possible.

Depending on the organism, and where there are not enough single rooms or enough patients to create a cohort bay, a colonised / infected patient may need to remain in the open bay, with the application of strict IP&C standard precautions.

Figure 21.2 lists everything that needs to be in place in terms of equipment and other precautions where patients are isolated, cohorted or nursed in a bay with other patients.

22 Management of patients with infectious diarrhoea

Figure 22.1 Assessment and management of hospital and community-onset diarrhoea

Diarrhoea within 72 hours of admission to hospital?
- **Bristol Stool Chart types 5 – 7?**
- **Takes the shape of the pot? (see Chapter 8, Figure 8.2)**

Yes

Obtain stool specimen.
Isolate if infectious cause suspected
(i.e. previous history of *C. difficile* infection
(see Chapter 31)
or gastroenteritis/norovirus
(see Chapter 40)

Diarrhoea developed 72 hours post admission?
- **Bristol Stool Chart types 5–7?**
- **Takes the shape of the pot? (see Chapter 8, Figure 8.2)**

Yes

**Does the patient have a history of
C. difficile infection?** (see Chapter 31)

No → Yes → Contact the IP&CT

Is there a simple explanation for the diarrhoea? e.g.:
- Laxatives/aperients/enemas/suppositories in the last 2 weeks
- Constipation with overflow
- Recovery from surgery/paralytic Ileus
- Melaena
- NG/PEG feeding
- Medication (excluding antibiotics) e.g. metformin
- Pre-existing medical condition (i.e. colitis/irritable bowel)

No

Yes →
- Infectious cause highly unlikely
- No indication for specimen collection
- Observe
- Maintain accurate stool chart
- Seek advice if there are any changes

**Is the patient being screened
as per the Sepsis Pathway?**
(see Chapter 25)

Yes → Obtain specimen and wait for result

No → **Has the patient had antibiotics in the last 6 weeks?**

Yes → **Has the patient also had laxatives/enemas?**

No → *C. difficile* or norovirus likely. Follow IP&C policy re stool specimen collection and isolation

Yes → Contact the IP&CT for advice

**Community-onset diarrhoea, patient self-presenting in GP surgery:
Has the patient been discharged from hospital within the last 6 weeks,
AND/OR has the patient been prescribed one or more course of antibiotics in hospital
OR the community, OR does the patient have a history of *C. difficile* infection/carriage?**

Yes → Obtain a stool specimen and seek advice from the local Duty Consultant Medical Microbiologist before prescribing antibiotics

No → **Is the onset < 4 weeks ago and does the patient have:**
- Symptoms severe enough to warrant hospital referral/admission?
- A history of recent foreign travel?
- 'Bloody diarrhoea'?
- A food history that suggests possible 'food poisoning'?
- Contact with domestic pets/animals at a petting farm?
Is the patient a child presenting with acute onset of bloody diarrhoea?

No → Consider reviewing the patient if symptoms do not resolve within 48–72 hours

Yes → Obtain a stool specimen

Infection Prevention and Control at a Glance, First Edition. By Debbie Weston, Alison Burgess and Sue Roberts.
© 2017 John Wiley & Sons, Ltd. Published 2017 by John Wiley & Sons, Ltd.

The word 'diarrhoea' is Greek in origin and means 'flowing through'. It is defined by the World Health Organization (WHO) as '3 or more liquid stools per day, or the passage of more stools than is normal for that person' (www.who.int/topics/diarrhoea/en) and is a symptom of an underlying pathology (RCN, 2013b). The definition commonly used within infection prevention and control is 'stool loose enough to take the shape of a container used to sample it or as Bristol Stool Chart types 5–7' (DH/HPA, 2008). The phrase 'loose stools' on its own should not be used by staff within a healthcare setting, who should ideally refer to a tool such as the Bristol Stool Chart (Lewis and Heaton, 1997) when describing and recording the consistency or type of bowel actions.

The pathogenesis of infectious diarrhoea

The pathogens that cause infectious diarrhoea have to be ingested (consumption of contaminated food or water, or transmitted as invisible contamination via the hands) and can be spread to other individuals via the faecal–oral route (see Chapter 12). The process of bacterial attachment can cause damage to the intestinal microvilli, which affects the ability of the colonic mucosa to absorb nutrients and electrolytes as its absorption capacity is exceeded (Hodges and Gill, 2010). Toxins can cause a severe inflammatory response that directly involves the mucosa, giving rise to **systemic** signs of infection in conjunction with diarrhoea. Viral infections such as rotavirus can cause rapid and extensive epithelial cell death (Hodges and Gill, 2010).

Causes of infectious diarrhoea

- *Clostridium difficile* (see Chapter 31)
- Norovirus (see Chapter 40)
- Rotavirus
- Salmonella (see Chapter 42)
- Campylobacter (see Chapter 28)
- Shigella
- Cryptosporidium
- Giardia
- Enterotoxigenic *E. coli*
- *Vibrio cholerae*
- *Entamoeba histolytica*
- *Staphylococcus aureus* toxin (see Chapter 43)

Assessment (see Figure 22.1)
1. Normal bowel function

Establishing the patient's normal function (frequency and consistency / type) is an essential prerequisite for any patient presenting in a community or hospital setting with 'diarrhoea', or who develops diarrhoea within 72 hours of admission to hospital. It may be readily explained by a coexisting medical condition, whereby episodes of diarrhoea are considered to be normal for the patient.

2. History

Taking a thorough history will help to determine whether or not there may be an infectious cause.

- Onset and duration: less than 4 weeks indicates acute diarrhoea; greater than 4 weeks suggests chronic diarrhoea.
- Frequency, consistency and type.
- Has the patient a previous history of *C. difficile* infection or glutamate dehydrogenase (GHD) antigen carriage? (GHD is an enzyme produced by all strains of *C. difficile*, which may indicate *C. difficile* carriage in the absence of toxin.)
- Are there any associated signs / symptoms such as abdominal pain, vomiting, fever and blood and / or mucus?
- Medical history: inflammatory bowel disease; diverticulitis; irritable bowel syndrome; surgery involving the digestive tract which affects absorption; abdominal or pelvic irradiation secondary to treatment for cancer (radiation colitis).
- History of recent foreign travel ('traveller's diarrhoea', i.e. enterotoxigenic *E. coli*, Giardia, Cryptosporidium and Shigella).
- Medication: antibiotics, laxatives and drugs such as metformin and digoxin can cause diarrhoea.
- Food history: what has the patient had to eat, where and when? Onset of symptoms within 6 hours of eating may be due to 'food poisoning' through ingestion of food contaminated with Bacillus cereus or Staphylococcus aureus toxins. Food allergies / food intolerances can cause diarrhoea.
- Enteral feeding (can cause altered physiological responses as a result of increased water absorption and increased transit time through the colon (Whelan and Schneider, 2011)). The volume / delivery of the feed may also be a factor (Thibault et al, 2013).
- Contact with pets / farm animals: Salmonella infection has been associated with exposure to domestic and wild animals, such as cats, dogs, birds (particularly pigeons), and exotic reptiles kept as pets, such as lizards and terrapins; outbreaks of *E. coli* O157 have been associated with petting farms (HPA, 2009a).

Investigations

If an assessment of the patient's normal bowel function and history indicates a potentially infectious cause, the following investigations are indicated:
- Stool specimen: as much clinical information as possible must be provided on the specimen request form (see Chapter 8).
- Blood tests:
  CRP: C-reactive protein – an acute phase protein made by the liver and found in the blood at very low levels which rise in response to inflammation
  ESR: the rate at which red blood cells separate and fall to the bottom of a test tube of anti-coagulated blood
  White cell count: the number of neutrophils, lymphocytes, eosinophils, monocytes and basophils increases in the presence of infection / inflammation.

Management

Antibiotics may or not be indicated depending on the results of the stool culture.

Anti-diarrhoeal agents such as loperamide should not be administered to patients with infectious diarrhoea. They decrease faecal transit time, meaning that stools remain in the colon for longer, which could potentially increase toxin retention and lead to increased tissue damage to the bowel mucosa (Thielman and Nelson, 2009).

23 Investigation and management of outbreaks

Figure 23.1 Patterns of disease development

Sporadic – A disease that occurs infrequently and irregularly.

Endemic – The constant presence/and or usual prevalence of a disease or infectious agent in a population within a geographical area.

Epidemic – An increase, often sudden, in the number of cases of a disease above what is expected in the population of that area.
NB. This definition also includes 'outbreaks', covering more limited geographical areas.

Pandemic – when an epidemic spreads over several countries or continents, usually affecting a large number of people.

Figure 23.2 Dr John Snow, 1813–1858

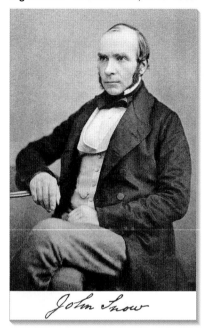

Source: Rsabbatini, https://commons.wikimedia.org/wiki/File%3AJohn_Snow.jpg. Used under CC BY 4.0

Figure 23.3 1854 Broad Street, Soho, cholera outbreak

- **Background:** Cholera was previously thought to be airborne
- **1849:** John Snow published work suggesting that cholera was transmitted by infected water or food
- **1854:** A cholera outbreak occurred with a total of 616 deaths
- John Snow identified the source of the cholera outbreak as a water pump at Broad Street, thus proving his theory
- The pump handle was removed and the outbreak halted

Figure 23.4 Key actions in the management of an outbreak

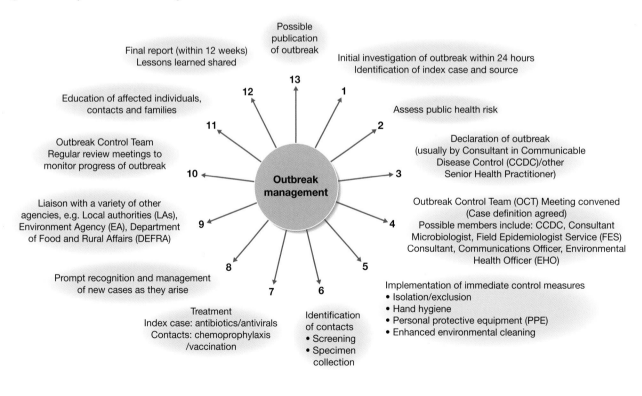

13 Possible publication of outbreak

12 Final report (within 12 weeks) Lessons learned shared

11 Education of affected individuals, contacts and families

10 Outbreak Control Team Regular review meetings to monitor progress of outbreak

9 Liaison with a variety of other agencies, e.g. Local authorities (LAs), Environment Agency (EA), Department of Food and Rural Affairs (DEFRA)

8 Prompt recognition and management of new cases as they arise

7 Treatment
Index case: antibiotics/antivirals
Contacts: chemoprophylaxis /vaccination

6 Identification of contacts
- Screening
- Specimen collection

Outbreak management

1 Initial investigation of outbreak within 24 hours Identification of index case and source

2 Assess public health risk

3 Declaration of outbreak (usually by Consultant in Communicable Disease Control (CCDC)/other Senior Health Practitioner)

4 Outbreak Control Team (OCT) Meeting convened (Case definition agreed)
Possible members include: CCDC, Consultant Microbiologist, Field Epidemiologist Service (FES) Consultant, Communications Officer, Environmental Health Officer (EHO)

5 Implementation of immediate control measures
- Isolation/exclusion
- Hand hygiene
- Personal protective equipment (PPE)
- Enhanced environmental cleaning

Infection Prevention and Control at a Glance, First Edition. By Debbie Weston, Alison Burgess and Sue Roberts.
© 2017 John Wiley & Sons, Ltd. Published 2017 by John Wiley & Sons, Ltd.

Clusters and outbreaks of infection are common in both acute hospital settings and the community, and are caused by a wide variety of different microorganisms. Sometimes the terms 'cluster' and 'outbreak' are used interchangeably but there is an important difference. A 'cluster' refers to a group of people linked by time and place, in whom the causative microorganism causing the infection or colonisation is suspected to be the same. A cluster becomes an 'outbreak' once the specimens are confirmed as being the same by a Public Health England (PHE) reference laboratory. An example of this is when two or more patients on a hospital ward are identified as having *C. difficile* with the same ribotype (see Chapters 9 and 31) (a cluster), but further subtyping of the stool specimens confirms that it is the same strain, thus confirming an outbreak. The internationally recognised patterns of disease development are described in Figure 23.1. The purpose of this chapter is to explain the principles of outbreak recognition and management in general that should be applied whether it occurs in a community or hospital setting.

Definition of an outbreak

Public Health England (2014) defines an outbreak as: 'an incident in which two or more people experiencing a similar illness are linked in time or place, or a greater than expected rate of infection compared with the usual background rate for the place and time where the outbreak has occurred'. However, it may also refer to a *single case* of certain rare diseases such as diphtheria, botulism, rabies, polio and viral haemorrhagic fever, e.g. Ebola (see Chapter 33).

Primary objective in outbreak management

The primary objective in outbreak management is to protect public health by identifying the likely **source** and **mode of transmission** and implementing public health actions, including **infection prevention and control measures** promptly to prevent further spread or recurrence of infection (PHE, 2014a). Understanding the particular characteristics of the causative microorganism is therefore key to identifying these factors.

Recognition of an outbreak

In a hospital, suspicion of a potential or actual outbreak of infection is usually raised by the Infection Prevention and Control Team (IP&CT), and in the community by PHE, through routine surveillance, although vigilant healthcare workers are often the first to alert the IP&CT/PHE to a developing problem. Community outbreaks can be harder to identify than those occurring in hospitals, as affected individuals may be spread out over a wide area. For example, it may take several weeks for the source of a food poisoning outbreak linked to a farm or restaurant to be established as affected individuals may become known over a period of weeks.

Historically important outbreaks

Two of the most famously documented community outbreaks of interest that occurred when **epidemiology** was a new field were the 1854 cholera outbreak in London, discovered by epidemiologist Dr John Snow (see Figures 23.2 and 23.3), and the 1906 typhoid outbreak, in the United States of America (USA) caused by Irish immigrant Mary Mellon, an asymptomatic carrier, known as 'Typhoid Mary' (see Figure 42.3). The former outbreak was halted relatively promptly following identification of the source as a public water pump in Broad Street and removal of the pump handle. The latter continued intermittently over a number of years due to the lack of understanding and cooperation on the part of Mary, who could not believe that she could cause disease in others when she was healthy herself (Newsom, 2009c).

Initial assessment of a suspected outbreak

In both hospital and community settings, it is essential that an initial investigation to clarify the nature of the outbreak begins within 24 hours. This will include establishing the number of infected individuals, date and time of onset of symptoms, likely source and contacts of the index case. An immediate risk assessment must also be undertaken to determine the public health risk, i.e. the risk of transmission of infection to others.

Declaration of an outbreak

The findings of the initial investigation will determine whether an outbreak exists and whether an outbreak control team (OCT) needs to be convened. A press statement may also be prepared, in conjunction with the Communications Team, particularly if media interest is anticipated.

The outbreak control team (OCT)

The purpose of the OCT is to agree a case definition, coordinate activities, undertake a thorough investigation and ensure that control measures are implemented promptly. The first meeting should be held within three days. All agencies and disciplines involved in the investigation and control of the outbreak must be represented at the meeting. It is important that the frequency and format of future meetings is agreed then so that the effectiveness of the outbreak management is continuously reviewed.

Management of an outbreak / immediate implementation of control measures

Prompt implementation of the necessary control measures / PHE interventions is critical in halting the outbreak and will vary according to the microorganism involved. Figure 23.4 describes some of the key actions requiring implementation in an outbreak.

Declaration that the outbreak is over

The OCT will declare the outbreak over when there is no longer a risk to the public health that requires further investigation or management of control measures by an OCT, the number of cases has declined, or the probable source has been identified and withdrawn (PHE, 2014a). A final report will be prepared by PHE/IP&CT within 12 weeks of the formal closure of the outbreak. Lessons learned and recommendations from the outbreak report and debrief process should be disseminated as widely as possible to the relevant staff and may include publication of the outbreak investigation.

Useful information can be obtained from:
Centers for Disease Control and Prevention (CDC): http://www.cdc.gov
National Travel Health Network and Centre (NaTHNaC): http://www.nathnac.org/
World Health Organization (WHO): http://www.who.int/csr/don/en/

24 Prevention and treatment of surgical site infection

Figure 24.1 Epidemiology of surgical site infection

Surgical site infection accounts for about 16% of all healthcare associated infections in England.

The 2011 English national point prevalence survey on healthcare associated infections and antimicrobial use identified the prevalence of healthcare associated infections as 6.4%, a reduction from 8.2% in 2006. Surgical site infection is the third most common.

Most commonly occurring healthcare associated infections in England

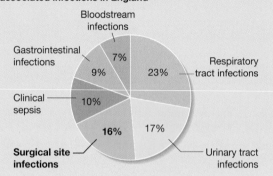

- Bloodstream infections 7%
- Gastrointestinal infections 9%
- Clinical sepsis 10%
- Surgical site infections **16%**
- Respiratory tract infections 23%
- Urinary tract infections 17%

Source: Health Protection Agency, 2012a

Figure 24.3 Cross-section of abdominal wall depicting CDC classifications of surgical site infection

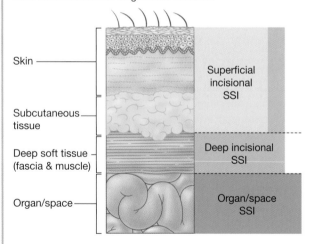

- Skin
- Subcutaneous tissue
- Deep soft tissue (fascia & muscle)
- Organ/space

- Superficial incisional SSI
- Deep incisional SSI
- Organ/space SSI

Figure 24.2 Factors that affect surgical wound healing

Surgical factors
- Presence of suture/foreign body
- Site, duration and complexity of surgery
- Suturing quality
- Pre-existing local or systemic infection
- Prophylactic antibiotics
- Haematoma
- Mechanical stress on wound

Anaesthetic factors
- Tissue perfusion
- Normovolaemia/hypovolaemia
- Perioperative body temperature
- Concentration of inspired oxygen
- Quality of analgesia
- ?Autologous blood transfusion
- ?Epidural anaesthesia and analgesia (through effect on stress-response-induced protein catabolism and immunosuppression)

Patient-related factors
- Diabetes
- Smoking
- Poor nutrition
- Alcoholism
- Chronic renal failure
- Jaundice
- Obesity
- Advanced age
- Poor physical condition

Source: Buggy, 2000

Figure 24.4 Pathogenesis of infection

Microbial contamination of the surgical site is a necessary precursor of SSI. The risk of SSI can be conceptualised according to the following relationship:

$$\frac{\text{Dose of bacterial contamination} \times \text{virulence}}{\text{Resistance of the host patient}} = \text{Risk of surgical site infection}$$

Quantitatively, it has been shown that if a surgical site is contaminated with > 105 microorganisms per gram of tissue, the risk of SSI is markedly increased. However, the dose of contaminating microorganisms required to produce infection may be much lower when foreign material is present at the site (i.e. 100 staphylococci per gram of tissue introduced on silk sutures).

Source: Mangram et al,1999; reproduced with the permission of Cambridge University Press

Figure 24.5 Surgical wound classification

Class I/Clean: an uninfected operative wound in which no inflammation is encountered and the respiratory, alimentary, genital or uninfected urinary tract is not entered. In addition, clean wounds are primarily closed and, if necessary, drained with closed drainage. Operative incisional wounds that follow non-penetrating (blunt) trauma should be included in this category if they meet the criteria.

Class II/Clean-Contaminated: an operative wound in which the respiratory, alimentary, genital or urinary tracts are entered under controlled conditions and without unusual contamination. Specifically, operations involving the biliary tract, appendix, vagina and oropharynx are included in this category, provided no evidence of infection or major break in technique is encountered.

Class III/Contaminated: open, fresh, accidental wounds. In addition, operations with major breaks in sterile technique (e.g. open cardiac massage) or gross spillage from the gastrointestinal tract, and incisions in which acute, non-purulent inflammation is encountered are included in this category.

Class IV/Dirty-Infected: old traumatic wounds with retained devitalised tissue and those that involve existing clinical infection or perforated viscera. This definition suggests that the organisms causing post-operative infection were present in the operative field before the operation.

Source: Mangram et al,1999; reproduced with the permission of Cambridge University Press

Infection Prevention and Control at a Glance, First Edition. By Debbie Weston, Alison Burgess and Sue Roberts.
© 2017 John Wiley & Sons, Ltd. Published 2017 by John Wiley & Sons, Ltd.

Surgical site infection (SSI) is a type of healthcare associated infection (HCAI) in which a wound infection occurs after an invasive (surgical) procedure (NICE, 2008). Surgical site infections are the result of multiple risk factors affecting the patient, the surgical team and the environment which will be covered in this chapter.

Risks of developing SSI

SSI is one of the most common HCAIs (see Figure 24.1) and is a major cause of increased length of hospital stay, morbidity and mortality. It also represents a considerable financial burden for healthcare providers. At least 5% of patients undergoing a surgical procedure develop a surgical site infection (NICE, 2008). A surgical site infection may range from a spontaneously limited wound discharge within 7–10 days of an operation to a life-threatening postoperative complication, such as a sternal infection following heart surgery.

Other associated infection risks

Patients undergoing surgical procedures are also susceptible to other types of healthcare associated infections including postoperative respiratory and urinary tract infections (see Chapters 30 and 32), bacteraemia (including meticillin-resistant *Staphylococcus aureus* (see Chapter 43) and *E. coli*, intravascular cannula-related infections and antibiotic-associated diarrhoea (particularly *Clostridium difficile* – see Chapter 31). Progressive advances in surgery and anaesthesia have resulted in patients who are at greater risk of surgical site infection being considered for surgery and as a result of earlier discharge an increased number of patients are presenting with surgical site infection in primary care. See Figure 24.2 for factors that affect surgical wound healing.

Risk assessment

A risk index comprising data obtained from three factors – **ASA score** (the American Society of Anaesthesiologists physical status classification system), **wound classification** and **duration of operation** – is used routinely to assign a risk score of between 0 and 3 to each operation. Patients with a risk index score of 3 have a higher risk of developing SSI than those with a score of 0. This score is calculated automatically on the basis of data entered and is used to stratify operations and enable rates of SSI to be adjusted by these risk factors (PHE, 2013d).

Definitions of SSI

SSIs are defined by a standard set of clinical criteria according to whether they affect the superficial tissues (skin and subcutaneous layer) of the incision or the deeper tissues (deep incisional or organ space) (Figure 24.3) (PHE, 2013d).

Endogenous and exogenous infection

The majority of surgical site infections are caused by contamination of an incision with microorganisms derived from the patient (**endogenous infection**), being present on their skin (skin flora) or from an opened viscus (internal organ). *Staphylococcus aureus* is the microorganism most commonly cultured from surgical sites. **Exogenous infection** occurs when microorganisms external to the patient contaminate the operative site during the procedure. Sources include surgical instruments, the general theatre environment and the air. Microorganisms from the environment can also contaminate a wound at the time of the incident, for example a traumatic injury occurring as a result of a road traffic incident, or gain access to the wound following surgery, before the skin has sealed. See Figure 24.4 for the pathogenesis of surgical site infection.

Prosthetic-related infections

Rarely, microorganisms from a distant source of infection within the body can cause an SSI by attaching to a prosthesis or other artificial implant within the operative site. This is known as 'haematogenous seeding or spread'. In prosthetic (artificial implant) surgery, the presence of the foreign body, for example a vascular graft after arterial bypass surgery or a prosthetic joint in orthopaedic surgery, increases the risk of SSI significantly. Lower numbers of pathogenic organisms and normally non-pathogenic organisms such as *Staphylococcus epidermidis* (coagulase-negative staphylococcus) may cause an SSI because prosthetic devices provide a nidus for the attachment of the organism. Evidence indicates that prosthesis infections are actually biofilm-correlated infections that are highly resistant to antibiotic treatment and the host immune responses. The application of antibiotic cements and the antibiotic-coated implants partly reduce the risk of prosthetic-related infection due to the slow release of antibiotics from the cements and the formation of a relatively high antibiotic concentration locally (Zhijun et al, 2013).

Classification and measures to reduce the incidence of SSI

Operations on parts of the body that are normally sterile, described as 'clean' surgery, have relatively low rates of SSI, generally less than 2%, compared to operations in 'contaminated' or 'dirty' sites, where rates may exceed 10% (NICE, 2008). See Figure 24.5 for surgical wound classification (clean, clean-contaminated and contaminated). When a viscus, such as the large bowel, is opened, surrounding tissues are likely to be contaminated by a wide range of organisms. For example, after colorectal surgery Enterobacteriaceae and anaerobes are encountered and may act in synergy to cause SSI. Practices to prevent SSI are therefore targeted at minimising the number of microorganisms introduced into the operative site, including:
• removing and reducing the number of microorganisms that normally colonise the skin by encouraging patients to wash prior to surgery and performing antiseptic skin preparation prior to the procedure
• preventing the multiplication of microorganisms at the operative site, for example by using prophylactic antimicrobial therapy
• enhancing the patient's defences against infection, for example by minimising tissue damage and maintaining normothermia
• preventing access of microorganisms into the incision postoperatively by the use of wound dressings.

Evidence-based guidance to support the reduction of SSI

Recognising that most SSIs are preventable by applying measures taken in the pre-, intra-and post-operative phases of care, NICE *Surgical site infection: prevention and treatment* (2008) provides recommendations for the prevention and management of surgical site infections.

The Department of Health (2011c) produced *High Impact Intervention: Care bundle to prevent surgical site infection*, which provides similar guidance to NICE with the exception of recommending 2% chlorhexidine gluconate in 70% isopropyl alcohol for surgical skin antisepsis as opposed to 0.5% chlorhexidine gluconate, based on the work of Darouiche et al (2010).

25 Recognition and management of sepsis

Figure 25.1 Sepsis - risk factors/causes, clinical features, investigations and the 'Sepsis Six'

Box 1 Risk factors for sepsis (NICE, 2016)

- Age < 1 and > 75, or very frail
- Impaired immune systems due to illness / drugs
- Surgery or invasive procedure within the past 6 weeks
- Breaches in skin integrity
- IV drug misuse
- Invasive indwelling devices
- Pregnant women; those who have given birth / had a termination or miscarriage within the past 6 weeks

Box 3 Most common causes of sepsis

- Pneumonia
- Bowel perforation
- UTI
- Severe skin infection

Box 4 Signs of organ dysfunction

- Altered mental state
- Hyperglycaemia (in the absence of diabetes)
- Hypoxia: O_2 saturation < 93% or arterial blood gas (ABG) < 9 kPa
- Urine output < 0.5 ml/kg/h, and/or raised urea and creatinine
- Coagulopathy: international normalised ratio (INR) > 1.5, activated prothrombin time > 60 seconds, or platelets < 100

Box 5 Immediate management – the 'Sepsis Six'

- Administer high-flow oxygen (T)
- Take blood cultures (D)
- Give broad spectrum antibiotics (T)
- Give intravenous fluid challenges (T)
- Measure serum lactate and haemoglobin (D)
- Measure accurate hourly urine output (D)

T = therapeutic intervention
D = diagnostic intervention

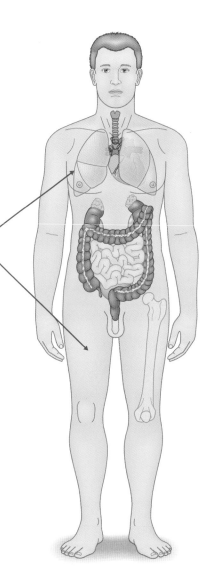

Box 2 Infection as a cause of sepsis

- Pneumonia/lower respiratory tract infection (LRTI)
- Urinary tract infection (UTI) including catheter-associated UTI (CAUTI)
- Intraperitoneal infection
- Biliary tract infection
- Central nervous system (CNS) infection
- Bone and joint infection
- Spinal infection (i.e. discitis)
- Endocarditis
- ENT infection

Box 6 Investigations

- Blood culture
- Blood gases
- Full blood count (FBC)
- Urea and electrolytes
- Clotting screen
- Glucose
- Chest X-ray (CXR)
- ECG
- Cultures – urine, sputum, stool and CSF
- Swabs – wounds, pressure sores, sites of invasive devices, wound drainage sites
- Remove invasive devices and re-site if appropriate

Infection Prevention and Control at a Glance, First Edition. By Debbie Weston, Alison Burgess and Sue Roberts.
© 2017 John Wiley & Sons, Ltd. Published 2017 by John Wiley & Sons, Ltd.

Sepsis is defined as 'a life-threatening organ dysfunction due to a dysregulated host response to infection' (NICE, 2016). The primary cause of death in patients with infections, it is a global problem, affecting 20–30 million people a year (causing more deaths than those from bowel and breast cancer combined), with over 6 million cases occurring in children (neonates and early childhood) and 100 000 during pregnancy and childbirth (maternal sepsis). It is estimated to be responsible for 36 800 deaths in the UK annually, carries a mortality rate of 35–50% (10–15% in children) (NHS England, 2014a; 2014b), which is five times greater than that of myocardial infarction and stroke, and is responsible for 100 000 hospital admissions (College of Emergency Medicine and the UK Sepsis Trust, 2014). 70% of cases originate in the community (NHS England, 2014b).

Approximately 70% of patients with sepsis require care within a critical care environment, and sepsis is the leading cause of death in intensive care units. **Rapid recognition of the deteriorating patient and the implementation of aggressive treatment measures are time critical** as far as sepsis is concerned. A Report by the Parliamentary and Health Service Ombudsman (2013), which summarised the deaths of 10 patients from sepsis, found that although it was not entirely possible to state with any certainty that all 10 patients would have survived if their treatment had been different, systematic failings in the diagnosis and instigation of rapid treatment for these patients meant that any chance of survival was lost. Figure 25.1, Boxes 1, 2 and 3, describe risk factors for, and causes of, sepsis.

The 'normal' immune response: As explained in Chapters 6 and 7, the 'normal' immune response efficiently manages to dispatch pathogens. It is the pathogens' interaction with the host's immune system that gives rise to the clinical features of infection, and although 'help' may be required via the administration of antimicrobial agents and medical intervention, the *regulated* immune response is an efficient defence / **pathogen** eradication mechanism. In cases of sepsis, however, the immune system is overwhelmed and becomes *unregulated,* going into overdrive.

Toxins: The release of toxins (see Chapter 4) triggers the release into the bloodstream of inflammatory mediators such as histamine, serotonin, noradrenaline and plasmakinins, along with tumor necrosis factor (TNF) and interleukin 1 (IL-1), which are released from macrophages. These inflammatory mediators cause the blood vessels to dilate. TNF and IL-1 also cause disturbances in the temperature regulation, giving rise to signs of fever. Macrophages activate the complement system and release other inflammatory **cytokines**, which have an effect on vascular endothelial cell function and integrity. As the blood capillaries become more permeable and fluid leaks out of the general circulation, the blood pressure falls due to the drop in circulating volume, and the patient becomes hypovolaemic. If the patient does not respond to fluid resuscitation at this point and hypotension persists, the physiological manifestations of septic shock, defined as 'persisting hypotension requiring vasopressors to maintain a mean arterial pressure (MAP) of 65 mmHG or more and having a serum lactate of greater than 2mmol/l despite adequate volume resuscitation' (NICE, 2016), become apparent.

The progression of sepsis: The coagulation pathway becomes activated, triggering clotting abnormalities, and DIC may develop. As a result of blood clotting abnormalities, purpuric lesions may develop and manifest as areas of **petechiae** on the skin, as seen in meningococcal septicaemia. Small blood clots develop in the blood vessels which result in poor tissue and organ perfusion and can affect digits or an entire limb. The affected limb will initially appear ice cold, white and bloodless and will eventually become blackened and necrosed as arterial and venous occlusion progresses. Multi-organ dysfunction can swiftly develop with the involvement of the central nervous, respiratory, cardiovascular and renal systems (see Figure 25.1, Box 4). An increasing respiratory rate heralds the onset of impending respiratory failure; impaired cerebral confusion and metabolism attributed to hypotension, **hypoxia** and **acidosis** lead to decreased neurological function and may result in coma; reduced renal perfusion will contribute to renal failure. Although it is estimated that 65 000 people in the UK survive episodes of severe sepsis, many suffer serious, long-term disability (http://www.ncepod.org.uk/pdf/current/SEPSIS/SepsisProtocol.pdf). Figure 25.1, Box 6, lists investigations for sepsis.

The 'Sepsis Six'

Key failings in the management of septic patients, as highlighted by the Parliamentary and Health Service Ombudsman (2013) were:

- failure to act on abnormal vital signs, along with inadequate patient monitoring
- failure to recognise the severity of symptoms and inadequate first line treatment
- delay in escalation.

The 'Sepsis Six' care bundle was developed by the UK Sepsis Trust (http://www.sepsistrust.org) and consists of three diagnostic and three therapeutic medical interventions which, when implemented appropriately, are designed to reduce not only deaths from sepsis, but also length of hospital stay and intensive therapy unit (ITU) bed days (Daniels et al, 2011). The 'Sepsis Six' interventions are listed in Box 5 in Figure 25.1 and can be initiated by any healthcare professional in any setting. Box 6 in Figure 25.1 lists the investigations that need to be undertaken.

All staff have a responsibility / duty of care to patients (see Chapter 1) that requires them to be alert to the possibility of sepsis in *any* patient (particularly those known to have an infection and / or any of the sepsis risk factors listed in Figure 25.1), be competent in recognising the deteriorating patient, and take immediate action to ensure appropriate and timely intervention in order to prevent avoidable deaths.

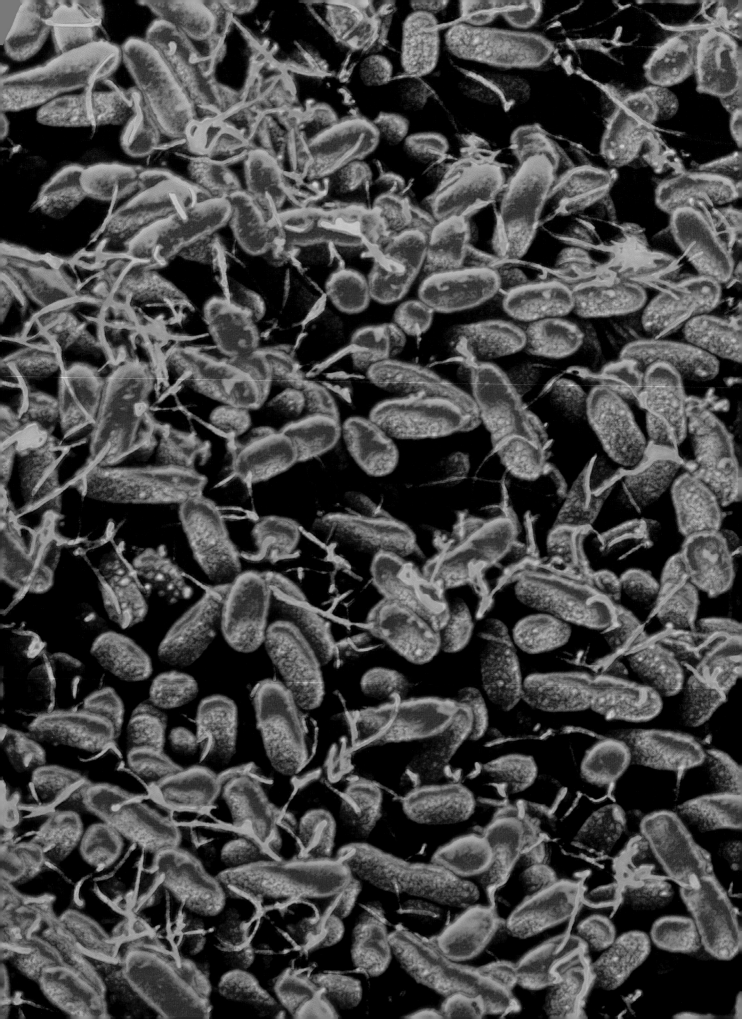

Infections and infectious diseases

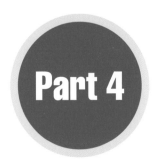

Part 4

Chapters

26 Bloodborne viruses

Figure 26.1 Bloodborne viruses (BBVs): high- and low-risk body fluids

High-risk body fluids	Low-risk body fluids
Blood	Urine
Semen	Faeces
Vaginal secretions	Saliva (*unless bloodstained or exposure occurs during dental work)
Saliva (*only if bloodstained or exposure occurs during dental work)	Vomit
Cerebrospinal fluid (CSF)	
Synovial fluid	
Amniotic fluid	
Pleural fluid	
Pericardial fluid	

Figure 26.2 Exposure to BBVs within the healthcare setting

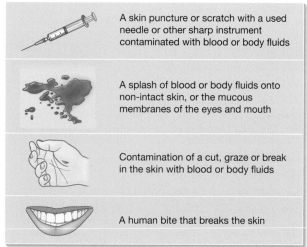

A skin puncture or scratch with a used needle or other sharp instrument contaminated with blood or body fluids

A splash of blood or body fluids onto non-intact skin, or the mucous membranes of the eyes and mouth

Contamination of a cut, graze or break in the skin with blood or body fluids

A human bite that breaks the skin

Table 26.1 Incubation period, transmission and clinical features of HIV, HBV and HCV

	HIV/AIDS	HBV	HCV
Incubation period	**Seroconversion:** within 2–12 weeks of initial infection **Clinical latency:** 9–10 years or longer, although most people in developed countries who are diagnosed promptly and managed effectively will not go on to develop AIDS	45–120 days	6–12 weeks
Transmission risk factors	Unprotected sex – exposure to blood, semen and vaginal and rectal mucosa/secretions Sharing injecting equipment (i.e. needles) Transmission from an HIV-positive mother to baby before or during birth, or through breast feeding	Inoculation from needlestick injuries and blood glucose monitoring (lancer) devices (see Chapter 18) Dialysis patients Acupuncture Tattooing Sexual and perinatal transmission via exposure to high-risk body fluids Sharing toothbrushes, razors and eating utensils that are contaminated with blood Contaminated hospital equipment	Injecting drug users Dialysis patients Men and women with multiple sexual partners and unprotected sex Tattooing and skin piercing Healthcare workers – exposure through poor IP&C practices Recipients of unscreened blood donations prior to 1991 Anyone who may have received blood products such as factor 8, anti-D, and immunoglobulin manufactured before virus inactivation procedures were implemented in 1986
Clinical features	**Seroconversion:** non-specific symptoms that may include a generalised rash, lymphadenopathy, hepatosplenomegaly, fatigue, arthralgia, sore throat, weight loss, diarrhoea, mouth ulcers **AIDS:** opportunistic infections, e.g. recurrent pneumonia, toxoplasmosis, cryptosporidiosis, histoplasmosis, respiratory tuberculosis/other mycobacterial infections, *Pneumocystis jiroveci*, pneumonia, Kaposi's sarcoma	**Pre-jaundice (pre-icteric) phase** (days to weeks after exposure): malaise, anorexia, nausea, mild fever, right-sided upper abdominal discomfort **Jaundice (icteric) phase:** bilirubinuria, enlarged tender liver, jaundice of the skin, mucosa and conjunctivae	Infected individuals may be asymptomatic for 20–50 years – no signs of infection until the liver has become extensively damaged

Infection Prevention and Control at a Glance, First Edition. By Debbie Weston, Alison Burgess and Sue Roberts.
© 2017 John Wiley & Sons, Ltd. Published 2017 by John Wiley & Sons, Ltd.

Table 26.2 CD4 cells and viral load

!	1 billion CD4 cells are produced every day in response to the production of 10 billion HIV particles every day (Ahmad et al, 2010a)
Normal CD4 count	400–1600 cells per mm³ of blood
Damage to the immune system	200–500 cells per mm³ of blood, with the CD4 count estimated to decrease by 45 cells a day, in spite of increased production (thousands of new CD4 cells produced each day) in response to the virus
HIV viral replication	Viral replication can produce > 10 000 new viral copies a day
High viral load	> 100 000 copies per mL of blood
Low viral load	< 10 000 copies per mL of blood
Undetectable viral load	< 50 copies per mL of blood

Table 26.3 HBV blood markers explained

Hepatitis B surface antigen and antibody (HBsAg and anti-HBs)	**HBsAg** – the first marker to be produced and detected; produced in excessive quantities; indicates that the individual is infectious. Detection for longer than 6 months indicates chronic carriage as opposed to acute infection **Anti-HBs** – appears 1–4 months after the onset of symptoms **The disappearance of HBsAg and the appearance of anti-HBs indicate clinical recovery**
Hepatitis B e antigen and HBV-DNA antibody (HBeAg and anti-HBe)	**HBeAg** – indicative of high infectivity, detected with HBV-DNA. Can also appear with, or after, HBsAg **The disappearance of HBeAg, the decline of HBV-DNA and the presence of anti-HBe indicate resolution of viral replication and acute infection**
Hepatitis B core antigen and antibody (HBcAg and anti-HBc)	Core antibodies, present in acute and chronic infection, appear in the bloodstream within weeks of infection occurring. HBcAg stimulates the production of IgG (indicative of chronic infection) and IgM (indicative of acute infection)

Table 26.4 Markers for HBV at different stages of infection

Acute infection and infectiousness	Detection of HBsAg, HBeAg and anti-HBc (IgM)
Chronic infection	Detection of HBeAg for > 6 months; anti-HBc (IgG)
Clinical recovery and immunity	Detection of anti-HBs and anti-HBc

Figure 26.3 The prevention of BBV transmission in the workplace

 Use of personal protective equipment (PPE) based on a risk assessment of the risk of transmission of microorganisms to the patient or carer; the risk of contamination of healthcare practitioners' clothing and skin by patients' blood or body fluids; and suitability of the equipment for proposed use (see Chapter 16)

 Ensure that all staff know the actions to be taken in the event of an inoculation/splash 'injury' or incident

 Protect broken areas of skin, i.e. on the hands, with an occlusive waterproof dressing

 Ensure that all staff know the correct procedure for dealing with blood/body fluid spillages

 Use and dispose of all 'sharps' in accordance with best practice recommendations (see Chapter 18)

Ensure that **all equipment (including instruments)** is decontaminated according to local policy and compliant with national best practice standards (Department of Health, 2013a; 2013b; 2013c)

Bloodborne viruses (BBVs) such as the human immunodeficiency virus (HIV) and hepatitis B (HBV) and C (HCV) pose a significant threat to public health. Many individuals with BBV infection are undiagnosed, and healthcare workers (and those within the emergency services and social services sectors) are exposed to BBVs every day through the nature of their clinical activities and patient–client interactions. Although the risk of BBV transmission is greater from patient to healthcare worker than from healthcare worker to patient, patients can acquire HBV and HCV through healthcare interventions where procedures and policies are not followed. Figure 26.1 lists the body fluids that are high and low risk for BBV exposure. Figure 26.2 describes how percutaneous (exposure through skin puncture) and mucotaneous (exposure via mucous membranes) exposures commonly occur. Table 26.1 lists the incubation period, transmission risk factors and clinical features of each virus.

Human immunodeficiency virus (HIV)
The pathogenesis of infection

HIV is a retrovirus. Retroviruses are *only* transmissible via blood and body fluids, and they are encoded for by an enzyme called reverse transcriptase, which converts viral RNA (see Chapter 5) into a DNA copy that becomes integrated into the DNA of the host cell (Ahmad et al, 2010a). Within the retrovirus family, there are a group of viruses known as lentiviruses ('*lenti*' means 'slow') that cause slow, progressive disease and can persist in a latent state before there are any obvious signs of clinical infection.

The viral envelope is made out of host cell membrane and studded with 72 protein spikes that help the virus bind to and fuse with the CD4 T-helper cells (which aid T-lymphocytes with antibodies and assist in the overall immune response – see Chapter 7). Viral replication is achieved by the work of three proteins contained within the viral capsid:

• reverse transcriptase
• integrase (splices the viral DNA into the gene of the host cell)
• protease (facilitates the assembly and binding of virus particles).

Genes contained within the capsid aid the formation of new virus particles and produce 'copies' of the virus (Collier et al, 2011a).

Within 24–48 hours of 'contact' with the body, intense viral replication takes place within the regional lymph nodes and the bloodstream, and **seroconversion** occurs 2–12 weeks after infection. Although the CD4 count initially increases, damage to the immune system has already occurred and it does not return to baseline values.

Tables 26.2 and 26.3 explain the significance of the CD4 count and the viral load in the development and progression of HIV infection.

Latency and progression to AIDS

Following seroconversion, a long period of clinical latency ensues, lasting 9–10 years or more, and during this time the immune system slowly declines as the proportion of infected CD4 cells increases along with the circulating viral load. Eventually, early signs of symptomatic HIV infection are seen, including malaise, weight loss, fever and night sweats, along with the development of minor **opportunistic** infections, which eventually progress to end-stage AIDS-defining illnesses (see Table 26.1).

Diagnosis

Early detection of HIV, robust monitoring and the prompt instigation of treatment when clinically indicated are central to prolonging life expectancy through halting progression of AIDS, and to reducing the risk to public health. People living with HIV can expect a near-normal life span if they are diagnosed while their CD4 count is still above 350 (Public Health England, 2014b). Of the 107 800 people living with HIV in the UK, it is estimated that 24% are unaware of their diagnosis (Public Health England, 2014b). Combined HIV antigen and antibody testing is the standard in the UK and can be undertaken on a blood sample obtained via venepuncture, or via 'point of care' testing using blood or saliva, which means that HIV can be diagnosed at the earliest opportunity. Combined testing is important because p24 antigen, which is a structural protein and the main component of the viral capsid, is detected in high levels in the blood serum of newly infected individuals during the period between primary infection and seroconversion. However, after seroconversion, antibodies are produced and p24 becomes undetectable (http://www.aidsmap.com).

The British HIV Association recommends that antiretroviral therapy is commenced before the CD4 falls below 200 cells/mm^3 of blood, when there is an increased risk of death due to opportunistic infection or rapid progression to AIDS (British HIV Association, 2012).

Treatment

HIV is treated using highly active antiretroviral therapy (HAART), which includes reverse transcriptase inhibitors such as zidovudine (AZT), lamivudine ($_3$TC), didanosine (ddl) and stavudine (d$_4$T). Protease inhibitors can also be used, such as indinavir, ritonavir and nelfinavir. Drugs may be prescribed in a variety of combinations, and treatment may need to be adjusted or changed due to intolerance of side effects or treatment failure (e.g. drug resistance).

Hepatitis B
The pathogenesis of infection

Hepatitis in general terms means inflammation of the liver and is caused by five different forms of viral hepatitis (A–E). Unlike hepatitis B (HBV) and C (HCV), hepatitis A and D are transmitted via the faecal–oral route (see Chapter 12). Hepatitis E is only seen in individuals with HBV. Like HIV, HBV is both a sexually transmitted and a bloodborne infection. The World Health Organization estimates that HBV kills 780 000 people each year, primarily through the development of liver cancer or cirrhosis (http://www.who.int/mediacentre/factsheets/fs204/en/). Healthy asymptomatic carriers are the primary reservoir of infection. HBV is 50–100 times more infectious than HIV, and can remain viable in dried blood for up to 7 days.

HBV, belonging to the Hepadnaviridae family, is a small-enveloped, double-stranded DNA virus, consisting of an envelope surrounding a core; within the core is the nucleocapsid containing the viral genome. The virus replicates within the liver, attaching itself to hepatocytes (liver cells).

HBV infectivity – antigens and antibodies

HBV antigens and antibodies, known as 'markers' (see Tables 26.3 and 26.4) can be detected in the bloodstream and indicate the course and progress of the infection and the individual's infectivity.

• **Acute (current) infection:**

The detection of hepatitis B surface antigen (**HBsAg**) denotes current infection, and all body fluids should be considered to be highly infectious. **Hepatitis B e antigen (HBeAg)** is the soluble component of the nucleocapsid core and indicative of high infectivity, appearing with, or after, HBsAg. Hepatitis B DNA (**HBV-DNA**) is also detected in the bloodstream. The detection of **IgM** antibody indicates that infection has occurred within the last 6 months, and is also indicative of acute infection.

- **Resolving HBV infection / recovered:**
  Absence of HBsAg; presence of anti-HBs; presence of anti-HBe; HBV-DNA declines.
- **Chronic infection:** Indicated by the persistence of HBsAg in blood serum of > 6 months, and IgG antibody.

Prevention / treatment

The HBV vaccine can be used for pre- or post-exposure prophylaxis for high-risk individuals. Full details, including the vaccination schedule, can be found in the 'Green Book', which is regularly updated (http://www.gov.uk/government/collections/immunisation-against-infectious-disease-the-green-book).

In the event of HBV exposure following an inoculation or contamination incident, specific immunoglobulin (HBIG) is given at the same time as the vaccination, in order to provide immediate (temporary) protection against HBV while the vaccine takes effect. Acute HBV resolves on its own. Chronic HBV carriage, however, requires treatment with peginterferon alfa-2a, or tenofovir or entecavir, in order to reduce the viral load and prevent long-term liver damage.

Hepatitis C
The pathogenesis of infection

HCV, which was first identified in 1989, is the most common form of viral hepatitis in the UK, affecting approximately 214 000 individuals (Public Health England, 2014b). Globally, 130–150 million people are chronically infected with HCV and between 350 000 and 500 000 individuals die from HCV-related illness annually.

HCV is a single-stranded RNA virus, belonging to the genus Hepacivirus, which is a member of the Flaviviridae family (Collier et al, 2011b). Individuals infected with HCV may be asymptomatic for anything from 20 to 50 years. Symptoms only become apparent when there has been extensive damage to the liver, which is caused by the cytopathic effect of the virus on the liver cells and the effect of the immune response. Approximately 15–25% of cases of HCV resolve spontaneously in the acute phase, which is the first 6 months after exposure. However, 70–90% of affected individuals fail to 'clear' HCV during the acute phase and go on to develop chronic HCV. Of these, 5–20% may go on to develop cirrhosis (the development of scarring (fibrosis) and nodules which, over time, affect the normal functioning of the liver and result in liver failure)

(http://www.who.int). HCV-associated cirrhosis is a leading indication for liver transplantation. Chronic HCV carriage is also associated with the development of primary hepatocellular carcinoma in 1–5% of individuals with chronic infection.

Diagnosis

Infection with HCV is indistinguishable from infection with other hepatitis viruses, and diagnosis is dependent upon the detection of HCV-RNA, which can be detected in the blood 1–3 weeks following exposure, and antibody (anti-HBC), which can be detected within 8–9 weeks of exposure.

The viral load is an important indicator regarding treatment: the lower the viral load, the more effective therapy is likely to be.

Treatment

There is no vaccination against HCV. The aim of treatment is to eradicate HCV-RNA in order to prevent progressive fibrosis occurring. The type and duration of treatment is dependent upon the virus subtype and the viral load. Ideally, treatment should begin in the acute stage, although it can be given to individuals with mild chronic hepatitis. Treatment consists of either monotherapy with peginterferon alfa-2a, or combination therapy with alpha-interferon and ribavirin.

The management of BBV-positive patients and the prevention of BBV transmission in the healthcare setting

The application of infection prevention and control standard precautions should, as discussed elsewhere in this book, be applied to **all** patients **all** of the time in **all** settings when dealing with blood and / or body fluids. Patients **do not** need to be nursed in a single room or be placed last on the list for theatre or clinic appointments. However, the operating surgeon / theatre manager should be aware of the patient's BBV status (on a 'need to know' basis). Figure 26.3 describes the key points for the prevention of BBV transmission in healthcare settings.

Healthcare staff undertaking exposure-prone procedures (EPPs)

New healthcare workers who will be undertaking exposure-prone procedures are now required to undergo testing for HIV and HCV and to demonstrate that they are low risk for HBV, prior to commencing employment. EPPs are invasive procedures where there is a risk of injury to the healthcare worker that may exposure the blood and tissues of the patient to the blood of the healthcare worker (i.e. gloved hands in contact with sharp instruments, needletips or fragments of bone / teeth inside a patient's open body cavity, wound or confined anatomical space, where hands or fingertips may not be completely visible at all times).

27 *Bordetella pertussis*

Figure 27.1 Characteristics of *Bordetella pertussis*

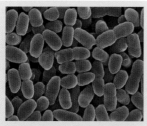

- A small, non-motile, Gram-negative, aerobic coccobacillus of the genus Bordetella
- Grows at an optimal temperature of 35-37°C
- Humans are the only known host
- Bacterial virulence factors include:
  - **Pertussis toxin**
  - Adenylate cyclase toxin
  - Filamentous haemagglutinin
  - Haemolysin

Source: U.S. Centers for Disease Control and Prevention

Figure 27.2 Pathogenesis of *Bordetella pertussis*

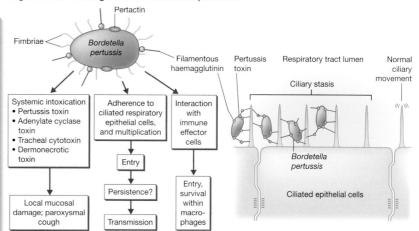

Figure 27.3 Risk factors

Individuals most at risk include:
- Young babies less than 3 months of age – too young to have received their first vaccination
- Infants less than 1 year who have not completed 3 doses of vaccine
- Children and adults who have *not* been vaccinated
- Adults and adolescents whose immunity has diminished (immunity is not life-long)

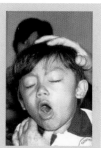

Source: U.S. Centers for Disease Control and Prevention;
photo credit: Michelle Razore

Figure 27.4 Clinical signs and symptoms

Stage 1: Catarrhal (most infectious)
- Usually 7–10 days (range of 4–21 days).
- Coryza (runny nose, sneezing, mild cough, watery eyes).
- Low-grade fever.
- Mild, occasional cough (which gradually becomes more severe).

Stage 2: Paroxysmal (most severe)
- Usually lasts 1–6 weeks but may persist for up to 10 weeks.
- Paroxysms of cough (due to difficulties in expelling mucus).
- Most frequent at night.
- High-pitched 'whoop' at end of paroxysm.
- Cyanosis.
- Vomiting and exhaustion.
- Decreases after 2–3 weeks.

Stage 3: Convalescent
- Usually 7–10 days (range 4–21 days).
- Gradual recovery.
- Less persistent paroyxsmal cough that disappears in 2–3 weeks.
- Cough may flare up again with subsequent respiratory infections.

Source: U.S. Centers for Disease Control and Prevention

Figure 27.5 Correct method for taking a pernasal swab

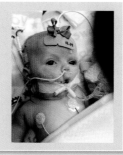

- A flexible ultrafine twisted wire shaft pernasal swab (with nylon rayon swab) is typically used
- Explain the procedure to the patient
- Apply a pair of non-sterile gloves
- Insert the pernasal swab into the nose and gently push along the floor of the nasal cavity towards the posterior wall of the nasopharynx (as this is where the *Bordetella pertussis* bacteria are most likely to be found)
- Gently remove the swab
- Label the swab with correct details, send to the laboratory and record in patient notes
- Remove gloves, dispose of in clinical waste bin and decontaminate hands

Figure 27.6 Infection control precautions

- **Isolation:** Until completion of 5 days of antibiotics
- **Masks:** Surgical face masks are not routinely required but should be worn to reduce the possibility of exposure to large particle droplets during aerosol-generating procedures, e.g. suction
- **Personal protective equipment (PPE):** Gloves and aprons are required for direct contact with secretions
- **Hand hygiene:** Decontaminate hands with alcohol handrub (AHR) unless visibly contaminated when soap and water should be used (refer to Chapter 14 for more information on hand hygiene)
- **Patient hygiene:** Encourage the patient to cover nose and mouth with a tissue when coughing/sneezing
- **Designated equipment:** Recommended
- **Pregnant staff > 32 weeks' gestation:** Must not enter the room
- **Decontamination of isolation room:** The room must be thoroughly cleaned daily according to local Trust Guidelines
- **In the community:** Exclusion from school or nursery until completion of 48 hrs of antibiotics, or 21 days if has not received antibiotics.

Infection Prevention and Control at a Glance, First Edition. By Debbie Weston, Alison Burgess and Sue Roberts.
© 2017 John Wiley & Sons, Ltd. Published 2017 by John Wiley & Sons, Ltd.

Pertussis (whooping cough) is an acute, *highly infectious*, respiratory infection caused by *Bordetella pertussis* bacteria (see Figure 27.1). It was first discovered in 1906 by two scientists named Bordet and Gengou – hence the name *Bordetella*. Pertussis means 'violent cough' (Gladwin and Trattler, 2006d). Pertussis can affect individuals of any age but most commonly affects young babies under 3 months of age. It is a **cyclical** disease with increases seen every 3–4 years. It is one of the **most common vaccine-preventable diseases** among children younger than 5 years of age but despite the widespread use of vaccines the prevalence of pertussis has continued to increase.

Characteristics of *Bordetella pertussis*

Figure 27.2 describes the pathogenesis of *Bordetella pertussis*. The bacteria colonises the lung **ciliated epithelial cells** by binding to the cilia with **adhesins**, so preventing the cilia from moving and clearing secretions. This results in the cough and characteristic 'whoop', although the latter is often absent in adults (Prescott et al, 2005b).

Mode of transmission

Transmission of pertussis occurs primarily via **direct contact** with discharges from the respiratory mucous membranes of an infected person, or via the airborne route. Up to 90% of household contacts will develop the disease and it can be transmitted to others **before** symptoms of the disease develop. Healthcare workers and pregnant women are a frequent and important source of pertussis infection amongst young infants (PHE, 2016).

Risk factors for pertussis

Individuals most at risk include young, unimmunised infants, particularly those prematurely born, < 3 months of age or born to unimmunised mothers. (see Figure 27.3). Pregnant women do *not* appear to be at an increased risk of severe pertussis but the risk relates to the fact that if they become infected in late pregnancy (> 32 weeks) there is potential for transmission of pertussis to the newborn baby (PHE, 2016).

Incubation period and clinical features

The **incubation period** can range from 5 to 21 days but is on average 7–10 days. A case is considered infectious from onset of symptoms until 5 days of appropriate antibiotic treatment has been completed, **or** 21 days from onset of symptoms if the case has not received appropriate antibiotic therapy. **There are three recognised stages of pertussis disease** (see Figure 27.4), and the disease typically lasts 6–10 weeks. Affected individuals are most infectious during the **catarrhal stage**, which is the first 3 weeks after the onset of the cough. Pertussis is a **notifiable disease** in the UK and suspected cases must be reported to Public Health England (see Chapter 2).

Complications

Infants under 3 months (as above) are at the highest risk of developing serious complications being hospitalised, and of dying from the disease. Complications include breathing difficulties (pneumonia, apnoea), seizures and encephalitis, although these are uncommon in children over 1 year of age. In addition, a cough may be severe enough to cause fainting, muscle pain in the ribs (occasionally fractured ribs), a hernia in the groin area or **conjunctival** haemorrhages. Figure 27.3 shows a baby who developed complications.

Diagnosis and treatment

The gold standard diagnostic test is culture from nasopharyngeal swab (NPS)/ nasophayngeal aspirate (NPA) where symptoms < 3 weeks duration in all age groups. The timing of testing is crucial as the sensitivity of the culture is affected not only by patient age but decreases in weeks 1-4.

Polymerase chain reaction (PCR) (See Chapter 9) may also be taken for DNA according to the same criteria.

Oral fluid/saliva tests are usually undertaken for surveillance purposes in children 5- < 17 years with onset of cough > 2 weeks.

Serology (for detection of anti-pertussis toxin [PT] IgG antibody levels) for older children and adults with cough duration > 2 weeks may also be undertaken. All positive isolates should be sent to a PHE Reference Laboratory for confirmation (PHE, 2016).

Treatment

Antibiotics are used to eradicate the organism, lessen the severity of pertussis and reduce the risk of transmission to others, but must be commenced within 21 days of the onset of cough to be most effective. For recommended antimicrobial treatment refer to the Public Health England (PHE, 2016).

Vaccination (see Chapter 13)

Vaccination is without doubt the **most effective** way to prevent pertussis. In the UK the vaccine is currently offered to babies at 2, 3 and 4 months with a fourth dose given as a pre-school booster at 3 years, 4 months. Protection is very high in the first few years after receiving the vaccine or after having the disease but thereafter wanes. The UK vaccination schedule recommends the routine vaccination of pregnant women in between weeks 16–32 as a means of passively protecting infants from birth, through intrauterine transfer of maternal antibodies, until they can be actively protected through vaccination.

Chemoprophylaxis / post-exposure vaccination

The primary purpose of treating cases with **chemoprophylaxis** is to eradicate *B. pertussis* from the nasopharynx and prevent **secondary transmission**. Chemoprophylaxis and post-exposure vaccination are *not* recommended in healthcare settings unless pregnant women or infants are involved. Chemoprophylaxis is only offered to **priority contact groups**, as described in the Guidelines for the Public Health Management of Pertussis in England (2016) followed by vaccination at a later date.

Infection prevention and control

Strict adherence of infection control precautions is essential in a healthcare setting to prevent transmission of pertussis to high-risk individuals (see Figure 27.6).

An outbreak of pertussis in a healthcare setting (> 2 cases) has potentially serious implications. Please refer to Chapter 23 for more information on outbreak management.

28 Campylobacter jejuni

Figure 28.1 Campylobacter bacteria

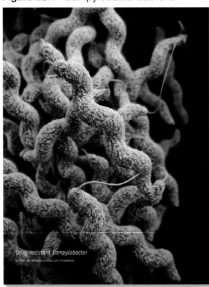

Drug-resistant *Campylobacter*
Centers for Disease Control and Prevention

Source: U.S. Centers for Disease Control and Prevention;
photo credit: James Archer

Figure 28.2 Characteristics of
Campylobacter bacteria

• Spiral or corkscrew appearance

• Gram-negative rods

• Motile

• Unipolar or bipolar flagella

• Toxin-producing

• Non-spore-forming

• Oxidase-positive

• Microaerophilic

• Thermophilic – grows best at 37–42°C

• Fragile bacteria – cannot tolerate
  drying and can be killed by oxygen

Figure 28.3 Chicken

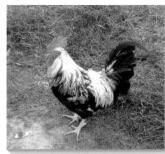

Figure 28.5 Chickens should *not*
be washed!

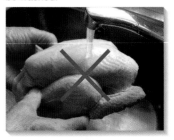

Figure 28.4 Infection prevention and control precautions for hospitalised patients

• Isolation: Until the patient has been free of diarrhoea for a minimum of 48 hours and preferably passed a formed stool
• Personal protective equipment (PPE): Gloves and aprons are required for direct contact with faeces
• **Hand hygiene:** Hand washing should be implemented (refer to Chapter 14 for more information on hand hygiene)
• En suite toilet preferred or designated commode
• Decontamination of isolation room: The room must be thoroughly cleaned daily according to local Trust Guidelines
• As part of general management it is important to ensure that fluids and electrolytes are replaced in dehydrated patients

NB: **Community cases** will be monitored by Public Health England and followed up by an Environmental Health Officer
(EHO) who will try to establish the source and advise individuals/family members on required infection control precautions

Infection Prevention and Control at a Glance, First Edition. By Debbie Weston, Alison Burgess and Sue Roberts.
© 2017 John Wiley & Sons, Ltd. Published 2017 by John Wiley & Sons, Ltd.

The word Campylobacter originates from the Greek word *kampulos*, meaning 'curved', due to its spirally curved rods (see Figure 28.1). It was first discovered in 1963, although not successfully isolated until 1972. Campylobacter bacteria are the most common cause of food poisoning in the UK, affecting an estimated 280 000 people per year. There are at least 12 species causing diarrhoea in humans, *Campylobacter jejuni* and *Campylobacter coli* being by far the most common. Campylobacter accounts for more cases of food poisoning than *E. coli*, Listeria and Salmonella put together.

Campylobacter can also cause disease in domestic animals. *Campylobacter fetus* is a cause of spontaneous abortion in cattle and sheep. Campylobacter commonly lives in the intestines of chickens, although it does not make them ill. Contamination of meat occurs during the slaughtering process. The Food Standards Agency's (FSA) retail survey February 2014–15 (http://www.food.gov.uk) demonstrated that approximately 70% of chickens tested positive for the presence of Campylobacter in varying levels. It takes only a small number of Campylobacter organisms (fewer than 500), to make a person ill. This could result from one drop of juice from a raw chicken. Freezing poultry does not eliminate Campylobacter but will reduce the number of microorganisms. Campylobacter reproduces more readily in the summer months, particularly during 'barbecue season', and is isolated more frequently in infants, young adults, and males.

Characteristics and pathogenesis of Campylobacter jejuni

Figure 28.2 describes the characteristics of Campylobacter bacteria. Most species of Campylobacter produce a toxin (cytolethal distending toxin) and are **pathogenic**. The toxin hinders the cells from dividing and activating the immune system. This helps the bacteria to evade the immune system and survive for a limited time in the cells. *Campylobacter jejuni* causes ulceration and inflamed, bleeding mucosal surfaces in the jejunum, ileum and colon.

Mode of transmission

Infection occurs most commonly by ingestion of contaminated foods, particularly raw or undercooked meats (especially poultry, Figure 28.3), contaminated water and unpasteurised milk, and direct contact with infected animals, particularly farm animals such as cows and chickens, but also household pets. Person to person spread by the faecal–oral route may occur but this is rare, as is transmission from food handlers.

The **incubation** period is 2–5 days, with a range of 1–10 days. The duration of illness is 3 days to 3 weeks.

Clinical signs and symptoms of Campylobacter infection

• Profuse diarrhoea (commonly bloody).
• Fever.
• Cramps.
• Bacteraemia is not uncommon in neonates and debilitated adults rarely nausea and vomiting.

Complications

Campylobacter is usually a self-limiting disease. Complications following Campylobacter infection are relatively rare and occur in approximately 1 in 1000 people but may be severe. Some people may develop arthritis. Others may develop **Guillain–Barré syndrome** that affects the peripheral nervous system, including the spinal and cranial nerves. It begins several weeks after the diarrhoeal illness and is thought to occur as a result of the individual's immune system being triggered to attack its own nerves, resulting in paralysis.

Method of diagnosis

Campylobacter is cultured from a stool specimen on specially selected 'CAMP' agar plates at 42 °C (the normal body temperature of birds).

Treatment

For most people specific treatment is not required and the only advice is for affected individuals to drink more fluids for the duration of the diarrhoea. Recovery generally takes 2–5 days, though it may take up to 10. However, some people, for example those with severe symptoms or weakened immune systems, may require antibiotics and admission to hospital. Azithromycin and fluoroquinalones (e.g. ciprofloxacin) are commonly used but resistance to fluoroquinalones is common.

Infection prevention and control precautions required in a healthcare setting

Infection prevention and control precautions for hospitalised patients are described in Figure 28.4.

Prevention of Campylobacter infection

The Food Standards Agency (2014) recommends that chickens are *not* washed prior to cooking (see Figure 28.5). This will minimise contamination of kitchen surfaces, utensils and other provisions. Provided that chickens are cooked *thoroughly* the risk of Campylobacter infection is very low.
• Hands should be washed before and after handling raw food of animal origin and before touching anything else.
• Separate chopping boards should be used for foods of animal origin.
• Other foods should never be prepared on the same chopping board as that used to prepare the chicken unless it has been thoroughly washed with soap and hot water.
• Following preparation, the cutting board, utensils and kitchen surfaces must be thoroughly washed with soap and water.
• Cook poultry products thoroughly. Make sure the meat is cooked throughout (no longer pink) and any juices run clear.
• Do not drink unpasteurised milk or untreated surface water.

29 Gram-negative carbapenemase-producing organisms, including Enterobacteriaceae

Figure 29.1 The prevention and control of carriage/infection with carbapenemase-producing organisms

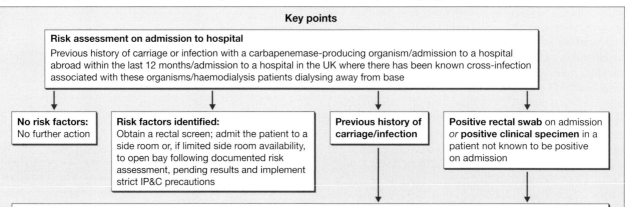

Key points

Risk assessment on admission to hospital
Previous history of carriage or infection with a carbapenemase-producing organism/admission to a hospital abroad within the last 12 months/admission to a hospital in the UK where there has been known cross-infection associated with these organisms/haemodialysis patients dialysing away from base

No risk factors: No further action

Risk factors identified: Obtain a rectal screen; admit the patient to a side room or, if limited side room availability, to open bay following documented risk assessment, pending results and implement strict IP&C precautions

Previous history of carriage/infection

Positive rectal swab on admission *or* **positive clinical specimen** in a patient not known to be positive on admission

Side room with en suite facilities or dedicated commode for the duration of the patient's hospital admission and on all subsequent hospital readmissions; ensure appropriate door signage; explain the need for isolation to patient and relatives. Depending on the organism, its antibiotic resistance pattern and the clinical environment/susceptibility of other patients, the IP&CT may request that 1:1 nursing of the patient is undertaken

All equipment must be single-patient use or dedicated exclusively to that patient for the duration of the patient's admission (i.e. tourniquet, stethoscope, sphygmomanometer, thermometer, lifting aids, monitors). There must be no extraneous items within the room

Hand hygiene: Healthcare workers must decontaminate their hands with alcohol handrub in accordance with the '5 Moments' (see Chapter 14), and wash their hands with liquid soap and water as appropriate; relatives should either wash their hands or decontaminate them with alcohol handrub prior to leaving the room; patients must be assisted with hand hygiene before eating and after using the toilet/commode

Gloves and aprons must be worn for direct patient contact/contact with equipment and removed prior to leaving the room and disposed of as clinical waste (see Chapter 16)

All invasive devices and associated equipment must be inserted and managed with scrupulous attention to IP&C practice

Linen and waste must be managed and disposed of according to local policy

The room and all equipment in it must be cleaned daily using a hypochlorite agent according to local policy. On discharge, the room must undergo a deep/terminal clean according to local policy, and all equipment that is not disposable must be decontaminated according to local policy/manufacturer's instructions. This includes the decontamination of items within the room such as mattresses and pillows and all hard furnishings. Unused wrapped single-use items must be discarded.

Screening: Depending on local policy, repeat rectal screening (weekly until discharge) may or may not be undertaken; as a general rule, once 'positive', patients may be considered to be life-long carriers, and negative rectal screens do not imply clearance. Screening of patient contacts will be required if a carbapenemase-producing/resistant organism is identified from a clinical specimen in an inpatient not previously known to be colonised/infected, and outbreak control measures implemented

Communication: Patients and relatives must be provided with written patient information which includes advice on discharge and advice in the event of the patient's readmission to hospital. The patient's positive status must be recorded on all discharge-related documentation, and the GP informed, along with other healthcare services as appropriate (i.e. community nursing team). If the patient is to be transferred/ admitted to another healthcare provider, the organisation must be informed.

Gram-negative organisms are part of the **commensal** flora (coliforms) of the large bowel, harmlessly colonising the colon and / or the environment in large numbers. However, if introduced into other body sites outside the bowel, they become pathogenic and are common causes of **opportunistic** HCAIs such as urinary tract infections, bloodstream infections (bacteraemia / septicaemia) and intra-abdominal infections. They pose a significant risk to individuals undergoing procedures in healthcare settings and may cause endogenous infections (i.e. they may be spread to other body sites via the patient's own hands) or be transferred to other patients on the hands of healthcare workers and / or via contact with contaminated equipment (see Chapters 14 and 17). **Carbapenemases** are enzymes that destroy carbapenem antibiotics (ertapenem, doripenem, meropenem and imipenem). **Carbapenems are the most medically important class of antimicrobial agents currently available.** They are broad spectrum beta-lactam agents (see Chapter 10), normally reserved for the treatment of serious infections caused by antibiotic-resistant Gram-negative bacteria. Carbapenemases are commonly 'expressed' by Enterobacteriaceae, a large 'family' of Gram-negative bacteria that reside in the bowel as part of the resident bowel flora. Members of the Enterobacteriaceae family that are important causes of healthcare associated and community acquired infections include:

- Salmonella (see Chapter 42)
- *Escherichia coli*
- *Yersinia pestis*
- Klebsiella
- Proteus
- Shigella
- Enterobacter
- Serratia
- Morganella
- Citrobacter.

Classes of carbapenemase

There are several carbapenemase enzymes within the 'A', 'B' and 'D' beta-lactamase classes, and their resistance genes are readily transmissible to other species of bacteria. These enzymes are:
- **NDM** (New Delhi metallo), first reported in 2008 and isolated in a patient repatriated to Sweden from New Delhi, India (Yong et al, 2009)
- **VIM** (Verona imipenemase metallo – endemic in Greece)
- **IMP** (imipenemase metallo – occurs worldwide
- **KPC** (*Klebsiella pneumoniae* carbapenemase, prevalent in the USA since 1999)
- **OXA-48** (widespread amongst *K. pneumoniae* in Turkey, the Middle East and Africa) (Department of Health Advisory Committee on Antimicrobial Resistance and Healthcare Associated Infection/HPA, 2010).

The rapid spread of Gram-negative carbapenemase-producing organisms is a global health problem and a major public health threat.

Risk factors for carriage / infection

- Travel to a country where there is a high incidence of carbapenemase-producing / resistant Enterobacteriaceae.
- Admission to / treatment in a hospital abroad.
- Haemodialysis abroad / away from base (DAFB).

- Treatment in a hospital in the UK where there have been outbreaks of infection (predominantly the North West of England and London) (Public Health England, 2013 e).

Patients who are **colonised** with a carbapenemase-producing organism will be unaware that they are a carrier (unless carriage has previously been detected) because carriage is asymptomatic. If a patient is infected with a carbapenemase-producing or resistant organism their presenting clinical features may be no different from those caused by any other Gram-negative organism. However, antibiotic options are likely to be severely limited, and treatment must only be undertaken under the advice of a microbiologist. Although the risk of infection is greater in hospitalised patients, long-term care facilities, where colonisation of residents is likely, have become increasingly recognised as important reservoirs of antibiotic-resistant organisms in general (Wilson et al, 2015).

Mortality

The mortality rate from infections caused by carbapenem-resistant bacteria ranges from 40 to 70%, depending upon the organism, the site of infection and patient-specific factors, with some bacteria being 'pan-resistant' (i.e. they have no antibiotic sensitivities at all). Isolation of a carbapenem-resistant Enterobacteriaceae from any body site, regardless of whether or not the patient has a clinical infection, is associated with poor outcomes (van Duin et al, 2013).

Prevention and control

In the UK, over the last five years there has been a rapid increase within health and residential care settings in the incidence of sporadic infections, clusters and outbreaks. The implications of the spread of carbapenemase-producing Enterobacteriaceae in the community and in healthcare settings are such that, in 2013, Public Health England launched the *Acute trust toolkit for the early detection, management and control of carbapenemase-producing Enterobacteriaceae*, for implementation during 2014 (PHE, 2013 e). This was followed in 2015 by the publication of a toolkit for non-acute and community care settings (PHE, 2015 b).

Central to preventing and controlling the spread of infections associated with Gram-negative carbapenemase-producing organisms in acute healthcare settings are:
- **risk assessment** of all patients on admission to identify those at risk of carriage and / or patients previously known to be carriers of, or who have had an infection with, a carbapenemase-producing organism
- **rectal screening** of 'at risk' patients (see Chapter 8) in order to detect carriage, and screening of patient contacts
- **isolation** of known carriers / patients with infection for the duration of their hospital admission, and on subsequent readmissions to hospital
- **stringent adherence to infection prevention and control standard precautions, with particular attention to hand hygiene, the use of PPE and cleaning / decontamination of the environment and equipment.**

Figure 29.1 summarises the infection prevention and control management of patients with carriage / infection in a hospital setting. **New guidelines / recommendations on the prevention and control of multi-drug resistant Gram-negative bacteria were published in 2015 by Wilson et al.**

30 Catheter-associated urinary tract infection

Figure 30.1 Indications for catheter removal and insertion

According to the HOUDINI Protocol (Trovillion et al, 2011) a urinary catheter should be removed unless one of the following clinical indicators is present:

Haematuria
Obstruction
Urology surgery
Decubitus ulcer in conjunction with obstruction
Input and output monitoring
Nursing/end of life care
Immobility

NB: The HOUDINI protocol can also be used to ensure that the catheter is inserted appropriately

Figure 30.2 Urinary catheter in situ with balloon inflated

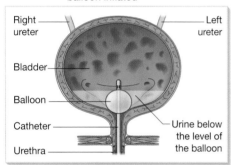

Right ureter
Left ureter
Bladder
Balloon
Catheter
Urethra
Urine below the level of the balloon

Figure 30.3 Points of catheter contamination

Bladder

A Urethral meatus and around catheter

Urethra

C Sample port

B Junction between catheter and connection tube

D Connection to drainage bag and reflux from bag to tubing

E Drainage outlet

Figure 30.4 Features of UTI/CAUTI

UTI in an un-catheterised patient:
• *dysuria*
• frequency of urination
• fever
• *haematuria*

Symptoms indicative of CAUTI:
• new onset/worsening of fever
• rigors
• altered mental status
• malaise or lethargy with no identifiable cause
• flank pain
• costovertebral angle tenderness
• acute haematuria
• pelvic discomfort

In patients where a catheter has been removed:
• *dysuria*
• urgency/frequency of urination
• suprapubic pain or tenderness

In patients with a spinal cord injury:
• a 'sense of unease'
• increased *spasticity*
• *autonomic dysreflexia*

Source: Scottish Intercollegiate Guidelines Network (SIGN), 2012

Figure 30.5 Best practice in the management of urinary catheters and the prevention of CAUTI

• Staff must be trained and competent in the insertion, ongoing management and removal of urinary catheters
• Use a silver-coated urinary catheter to minimise **biofilm** formation and inhibit migration of bacteria along the catheter and into the bladder
• Prevent trauma – use an anaesthetic lubricant gel to facilitate passage of the catheter along the urethra (dilates the urethra, reduces pain and discomfort, increases patient compliance and reduces the risk of infection from traumatic insertion)
• Use an aseptic non-touch technique (ANTT – see Chapter 19) for catheter insertion and when manipulating the drainage system
• Decontaminate hands before and after any contact with the catheter/drainage system (see Chapter 14)
• Ensure that the catheter drainage bag is positioned below the level of the bladder in order to prevent urinary reflux
• Secure the catheter to the thigh or abdomen using a designated adhesive pad/strap in order to prevent 'dragging' of the catheter and trauma
• Use a clean container to empty the catheter; ensure that the drainage tap does not come into contact with the sides of the container
• Ensure that the catheter drainage bag and the tap are not in contact with the floor
• Change the drainage bag every 7 days
• Maintain a closed system, i.e. do not disconnect the catheter from the drainage bag, and use a link drainage bag overnight
• Daily personal hygiene is all that is required for meatal cleansing
• Monitor / record all catheter-related interventions
• Assess the continuing need for the catheter on a daily basis, and remove it as soon as possible
• Catheter protocols and pathways should be used for the insertion of urinary catheters and for the ongoing care of the drainage systems and the patient
• A bladder scanner should be used to assess the residual volume of urine and manage urinary retention
• Patients discharged with a catheter must have a documented plan for its management and removal, including any clinical indications for continuing with catheterisation
• Patients and their relatives/carers should be provided with written information on discharge regarding the need for the catheter, date of review, how to manage the catheter and the drainage system, how to prevent urinary tract infection, and how to access supplies of catheter-related equipment

Source: NICE, 2012; RCN, 2012c; Loveday et al, 2014

Infection Prevention and Control at a Glance, First Edition. By Debbie Weston, Alison Burgess and Sue Roberts.
© 2017 John Wiley & Sons, Ltd. Published 2017 by John Wiley & Sons, Ltd.

'Catheters place patients at significant risk of acquiring a urinary tract infection. The longer a catheter is in place, the greater the danger' (Pratt et al, 2001).

Urinary tract infections (UTIs) account for 17.2% of all healthcare associated infections (HPA, 2012a), and 97% of healthcare associated UTIs are associated with instrumentation such as urinary catheterisation (Hooton, 2010). The method of catheterisation, length of time that the catheter remains in situ, and quality of the ongoing care / catheter management, along with susceptibility of the patient to infection, all influence the development of catheter-associated urinary tract infection (CAUTI). A UTI is defined as being catheter associated if the patient had a urinary catheter in situ at any time during the 7 days preceding the onset of symptoms. The prevalence of catheterised patients in NHS hospitals has been identified as 18.8% (HPA, 2012 a), and catheter-associated urinary tract infections (CAUTIs) are the cause of significant morbidity and mortality. Figure 30.1 lists the indications for catheter removal and insertion.

Pathogenesis of CAUTI
Host defence mechanisms
There are several urinary tract host defences that protect uncatheterised individuals against UTIs (Graham, 2010; Hooton, 2010), such as:
- Urinary flow. Although the urethra is colonised with bacteria, and assuming that there is no known defect of the genitourinary system, the urethra remains closed, protecting the bladder which is sterile except when urine is being voided. The regular emptying of the bladder and the hydrodynamic force of voiding urine flushes away microorganisms.
- Polymorphs on the bladder surface.
- IgA antibody on the bladder wall.
- Exfoliation of bladder epithelial cells.
- Mucin (mucus) layer on the bladder wall – prevents bacterial adherence.
- Urinary pH and osmolality.

In men, the length of the urethra (18–20 cm) offers some protection from the potentially uropathogenic colonic and genital flora that colonise the perineum, making men less susceptible to urinary tract infections. Women on the other hand have a short urethra (4 cm), which is in very close proximity to the perineum, and are more prone to endogenous infections because bacteria can be transiently displaced into the bladder during sexual intercourse, resulting in cystitis (Hooton, 2010; Ray et al, 2010a).

Breaching host defences
A urinary catheter is a 'foreign body'. It forms a bridge between the bladder and the external environment, forcing the urethra to remain open and leaving the normally protected and sterile bladder unprotected, effectively acting as a ladder or gateway for the ascending passage of bacteria. It also interferes with the flushing effect of the urine and the regular and complete emptying of the bladder. The catheter retention balloon prevents complete emptying of the bladder as the catheter drainage holes are sited *above* the level of the balloon, and there is therefore always a small residual volume of urine in the bladder in which bacteria could potentially multiply. The retention balloon can also damage the lining of the bladder if it is under- or over-inflated, irritating the lining of the bladder and interfering with the correct positioning of the bladder tip by resting against the bladder mucosa in an area known as the delicate trigone,

where it can cause the equivalent of a small pressure sore (Robinson, 2001) (see Figure 30.2).

Biofilm formation
Catheters and their associated drainage systems provide an optimal environment for bacteria as they support the growth of bacterial biofilms. Once in situ, the catheter becomes encrusted with proteins and electrolytes from the urine and these serve as a conditioning film that encourages microbial attachment (Trautner and Darouiche, 2004). The bacteria secrete a polysaccharide matrix consisting of sugars and proteins that encases them, affording protection from the effects of antibiotics and host immune defence mechanisms such as phagocytosis. The presence of bacteria such as Proteus, Pseudomonas and Klebsiella encourages formation of a biofilm, parts of which can shear off and seed to other parts of the catheter or the bladder (Jacobsen et al, 2008) or other body sites. When the catheter is removed, biofilm may be visible around the catheter tip as a slimy coating. Encrustation is not always as easily spotted as it may be inside the catheter lumen.

Bacteriuria
Bacterial colonisation of the urine, known as bacteriuria, occurs in 50% of patients who have had a catheter in situ for longer than 7–10 days. The risk of developing bacteriuria increases 5% for each day of catheterisation: 24% of patients with bacteriuria will go onto develop CAUTI, of which 4% may develop a bloodstream infection (Loveday et al, 2014). Although most of the organisms causing CAUTI are derived from the patient's own flora, they can also be acquired exogenously via the hands of healthcare staff, which may be contaminated with antibiotic-resistant organisms. Microorganisms can gain entry to the urinary tract via three main routes (see Figure 30.3).
- Contamination of the distal tip of the catheter on insertion will introduce bacteria into the bladder and colonise the distal urethra.
- Once the catheter has been inserted, bacteria colonising the distal urethra can migrate up and along the outside of the catheter.
- If the catheter drainage bag, sampling port or the junction between the bag and the catheter becomes contaminated, bacteria can migrate up through the lumen of the catheter.

Diagnosing CAUTI
Symptoms indicative of CAUTI are described in Figure 30.4. The prevalence of bacteriuria in catheterised patients means that differentiating between asymptomatic bacteriuria and symptomatic UTI in catheterised patients via urine 'dipsticks' is **not** a reliable indication of whether or not the patient has a CAUTI and should not be undertaken. A clinical specimen of urine (CSU) should only be obtained if the patient has any of the symptoms described in Figure 30.4 (Scottish Intercollegiate Guidelines Network, 2012).

Best practice in the prevention of CAUTI
(see Figure 30.5)
The insertion, ongoing care / management and removal of urinary catheters should conform to best practice guidelines. Figure 30.5 summarises the key best practice points, as per the epic3 Guidelines (Loveday et al, 2014), NICE (2012) and the Royal College of Nursing (2012c).

Clostridium difficile: prevention and control

Figure 31.1 *C. difficile* case and outbreak definitions

To help in identifying and managing incidents of CDI, the following definitions have been recommended (DH/HPA, 2008):

'*C. difficile* infection: one episode of diarrhoea, defined either as stool loose enough to take the shape of the container to sample it or as Bristol Stool Chart types 5–7, that is not attributable to any other cause, including medicines and that occurs at the same time as a positive toxin assay (with or without a positive *C. difficile* culture) and/or endoscopic evidence of pseudomembranous colitis (PMC).

A period of increased incidence (PII) of CDI: two or more new cases (occurring > 48 hours post admission, not relapses) in a 28-day period on a ward.

An outbreak of *C. difficile* infection: two or more cases caused by the same strain related in time and place over a defined period that is based on the date of onset of the first case.'

Typing involves assigning each sample of the bacterium to a recognised type to determine whether there is a common type implying an outbreak.

Figure 31.3 Prevention and control

There are five major factors that have been identified as being necessary to reduce the incidence of infection:
- prudent antibiotic prescribing
- hand hygiene
- environmental decontamination
- isolation/cohort nursing
- use of personal protective equipment (DH/HPA, 2008)

A range of evidence-based measures have been advocated to support hospitals in the reduction of CDI rates including the Department of Health care bundle (DH, 2010).

Management of patients on discharge from hospital

Patients who have recovered from infection are not a risk to others even if they continue to carry the organism in their intestines provided that they observe normal hand hygiene precautions. Having had a diagnosis of infection is not a restriction to a patient returning or being transferred to a care setting (HPA, 2009b).

Figure 31.2 Treatment algorithm

Algorithm 1 - 1st episode of *Clostridium difficile* infection (CDI)

Diarrhoea AND one of the following:
Positive *C. difficile* toxin test **OR**
Results of *C. difficile* toxin test pending **AND** clinical suspicion of CDI

If clinically appropriate discontinue non-*C. difficile* antibiotics to allow normal intestinal flora to be re-established
Suspected cases must be isolated

Symptoms/signs: not severe CDI
None of: WCC >15, acute rising creatinine and/or colitis)
Oral metronidazole 400 mg 8-hourly 10–14 days

DAILY ASSESSMENT

Symptoms improving
Diarrhoea should resolve in 1–2 weeks
Recurrence occurs in ~20% after 1st episode;
50–60% after 2nd episode

Symptoms not improving or worsening
Should not normally be deemed a treatment failure until day 7 of treatment. However, if evidence of severe CDI:WCC >15, acute rising creatinine and/or signs/symptoms of colitis

Switch to oral vancomycin
125 mg 6-hourly 10–14 days

Antimotility agents should not be prescribed in acute CDI

See Algorithm 2 for the management of recurrent *Clostridium difficile* infection - Updated guidance on the management and treatment of *Clostridium difficile* infection including innovative new treatments, e.g. faecal transplants (Public Health England, 2013f)

Symptoms/signs: severe CDI
WCC >15, acute rising creatinine and/or colitis
Oral vancomycin 125 mg 6-hourly 10–14 days.
Consider oral fidaxomicin 200 mg 12-hourly 10–14 days in patients with multiple co-morbidities who are receiving concomitant antibiotics

DAILY ASSESSMENT

Symptoms not improving or worsening
Should not normally be deemed a treatment failure until day 7 of treatment. However, if evidence of severe CDI continues or worsens

Surgery/GI/Micro/ID consultation

AND, depending on degree of ileus/prior treatment
EITHER Vancomycin 125-500 mg PO/NG 6-hourly +/– Metronidazole 500 mg IV 8-hourly x 10 days **OR** Fidaxomicin 200 mg PO 12-hourly
PLUS CONSIDER Intracolonic vancomycin (500 mg in 100–500 ml saline 4–12-hourly) given as retention enema: 18 gauge Foley catheter with 30 ml balloon inserted per rectum; vancomycin instilled; catheter clamped for 60 minutes; deflate and remove (Apisarnthanarak et al., 2002)

Further surgery/GI/micro/ID consultation
Depending on choice of therapy (see above) consider:
1 High dose oral/NG vancomycin (500mg PO 6-hourly)
2 IV Immunoglobulin 400 mg/kg 1 dose, consider repeat

Source: Public Health England, used under OGL 3.0 (PHE, 2013f)

Infection Prevention and Control at a Glance, First Edition. By Debbie Weston, Alison Burgess and Sue Roberts.
© 2017 John Wiley & Sons, Ltd. Published 2017 by John Wiley & Sons, Ltd.

lostridium difficile infection (CDI) is the major infectious cause of diarrhoea acquired in hospitals in the UK and is associated with considerable morbidity and mortality. Between 1990 and 2004, rates of *C. difficile* changed in different age groups in England. Although the greatest increase was seen in the 60–64 age group there were also significant rises in younger people over this period (Department of Health and Health Protection Agency, 2008). Drawing on the *C. difficile* outbreaks at Stoke Mandeville hospital, the University of Leicester NHS Trust and Maidstone and Tunbridge Wells NHS Trust, the Department of Health published *Clostridium difficile infection: How to deal with the problem* (DH/HPA, 2008) to support the delivery of the NHS Operating Framework target to reduce *C. difficile* across the NHS, promote patient safety and ensure that CDI was managed as a 'diagnosis in its own right'. In 2003–04 mandatory surveillance of *C. difficile* in patients over the age of 65 years was introduced as a result of concerns about the increasing incidence. In April 2008 this was extended to all patients over the age of 2 years. In 2007, mandatory quarterly publication of data for *C. difficile* was introduced. The increased focus on *C. difficile* has resulted in significant reductions in cases, decreasing substantially from 55 498 cases in 2007–08 to 13 361 in 2013–14 (Public Health England, 2013f; 2014c). Figure 31.1 provides *C. difficile* case and outbreak definitions.

The organism

C. difficile is an anaerobic, Gram-positive, spore-forming, toxin-producing bacillus (see Chapters 3 and 4). It is part of the normal intestinal flora in humans and is carried by 5% of healthy adults. This carrier status is also known as **colonisation**. Rates of colonisation are considered to be approximately three times higher in inpatients compared to those people treated as outpatients (NICE, 2014a). *C. difficile* exists in both vegetative and spore forms. In the colon it exists as a vegetative cell, whereas outside the colon it survives in spore form. Colonisation of the intestinal tract occurs via the faecal–oral route (see Chapter 12). The accepted model of the pathogenesis of *C. difficile* disease involves disruption to the host defences mediated by the indigenous microflora of the bowel. Healthy adults carry at least 500 recognised bacterial species in the colon. This complex population has an inhibitory effect on incoming, non-indigenous species. *C. difficile* infection occurs in a colonised patient, usually when antibiotic treatment disrupts the colonic microflora, resulting in a proliferation of *C. difficile* with release of toxin A (enterotoxin) and / or toxin B (cytotoxin) leading to mucosal injury and inflammation and signs and symptoms of infection (Weber et al, 2010).

Clinical features

Toxins released by *C. difficile* predominantly cause diarrhoea but may result in a wide spectrum of disease ranging in severity from **mild self-limiting diarrhoea to life-threatening pseudomembranous colitis with toxic megacolon, electrolyte imbalance and even perforation of the bowel, sepsis and death**. Most patients experience abdominal pain with explosive watery foul-smelling diarrhoea; however, in severe cases of infection, diarrhoea may not be a prominent feature. Diarrhoea typically starts within a few days of commencing a course of antibiotics but may occur as a result of taking antibiotics up to two months previously (NICE, 2014). Other symptoms include fever, loss of appetite, nausea and abdominal pain or tenderness. Initial diagnosis can be made on the symptoms and patient history (e.g. having taken antibiotics and / or other risk factors). Examination of the stools of patients with diarrhoea reveals not only the presence of the organism but also, and more importantly for diagnostic purposes, the toxins it produces. Infection refers to patients who exhibit symptoms due to infection and who are also toxin positive (DH, 1994) (see Figure 31.2 for the treatment of *C. difficile*). On average, infection results in an increase of 21 days in the length of hospital stay. Relapses are common, occurring in up to 20% of cases in the first two weeks after treatment has stopped (DH/ Public Health Laboratory service Joint Working Group, 1994). For actions to take on suspicion of a case see: https://www.gov.uk/government/uploads/system/uploads/attachment_data/file/321891/Clostridium_difficile_management_and_treatment.pdf

Cross-infection

Patients with *C. difficile* excrete large numbers of spores in their faeces which contaminate the environment and present a risk of transmission. The spores are highly resistant to drying, chemical disinfectants, alcohol and stomach acid, and can remain in the environment for long periods (up to five months) thereby increasing the likelihood of cross-infection. Spores transferred to other people and ingested can subsequently develop into bacteria that colonise the colon and potentially cause infection. The infection is acquired directly from other infected patients, from healthcare staff (predominantly hands) and from the environment including medical equipment. **The main risk factors for *C. difficile* infection are:**

• Advanced age – the rate of positive *C. difficile* laboratory results in people older than 65 years of age is 20–100 times greater than the rate in people 10–20 years of age.
• Antibiotic treatment within three months (especially those treated with broad spectrum antibiotics which are active against a wide range of bacteria). The use of multiple antimicrobial agents, whether given concurrently or sequentially, is particularly likely to increase the risk of infection. Although none can be excluded, the most commonly implicated antibiotics are: clindamycin; cephalosporins, in particular second and third generation cephalosporins (such as cefuroxime axetil, cefixime, ceftriaxone and cefotaxime); fluoroquinolones (such as ciprofloxacin and norfloxacin); co-amoxiclav; ampicillin and amoxicillin (which may relate mainly to the volume of their use rather than being high risk).
• Underlying morbidity such as abdominal surgery, cancer, chronic renal disease and tube feeding.
• Current use of a proton pump inhibitor (such as omeprazole and lansoprazole) or other acid-suppressive drugs such as H_2-receptor antagonists (NICE, 2014a) other risk factors:
  ◦ Hospitalisation
  ◦ Exposure to cases – as occurs in outbreak situations.
  ◦ Inflammatory bowel disease.
  ◦ Relapses associated with previous infection.

Historically, between 20 and 50% of recurrences have been reinfections and not relapses caused by the same strain of *C. difficile*.

Community- and hospital-acquired pneumonia

Figure 32.1 Risk factors for the development of community- and hospital-acquired pneumonia

- Age (see Chapter 12)
- Life style (i.e. excessive alcohol consumption, smoking, neglect)
- Underlying co-morbidities, i.e. chronic cardiorespiratory diseases (e.g. chronic obstructive pulmonary disease, congestive cardiac failure, bronchiectasis), diabetes mellitus, asplenia, immune compromise
- Impaired cough reflex, i.e. as a result of stroke, neuromuscular diseases (e.g. myasthenia gravis), sedation, presence of a nasogastric tube
- Aspiration of naso- or oropharyngeal secretions or 'foreign' material, such as food, oral fluids, medication and vomit. 45% of all healthy adults may aspirate in their sleep (Kieninger and Lipsett, 2009). Aspiration may occur as a result of altered neurological state (i.e. as a direct result of trauma or anaesthesia, or seizures), impaired swallow reflex/congenital or acquired anatomic abnormalities, gastroesophageal reflux disease
- Previous antibiotic therapy (alteration of commensal flora and colonisation with antibiotic-resistant organisms)
- Restricted mobility due to age, trauma, enforced/prolonged bed rest and surgery
- Surgery involving the head, neck, thorax or upper abdomen
- Intubation/mechanical ventilation
- Exposure to contaminated respiratory therapy equipment (Medicines and Healthcare Products Regulatory Agency, 2004)
- Exposure to contaminated water sources and *Legionella pneumophila* (see Chapter 37)
- Transmission of pathogens on the hands of healthcare staff

Figure 32.2 Clinical features

- Onset over hours to days
- Symptoms of a lower respiratory tract illness (i.e. productive cough), and at least one other respiratory tract symptom such as dyspnoea, pleural pain or tachyapnoea
- Systemic signs of infection, such as temperature ≥ 38°C, sweating/chills/rigors
- Non-specific symptoms such as body aches and headache
- Patients with atypical pneumonia caused by Legionnaires' disease may exhibit confusion, severe headache and diarrhoea (see Chapter 37)

Figure 32.3 The respiratory tract showing pneumonia

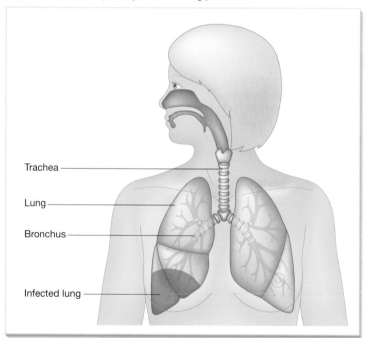

Trachea

Lung

Bronchus

Infected lung

Figure 32.4 Investigations

- C-reactive protein (CRP)
- White cell count
- Full blood count
- Sputum for culture and sensitivity
- Urine for Legionella and pneumococcal antigen
- Blood culture
- Chest x-ray
- Oxygen saturation
- Blood gas

Figure 32.5 Prevention of community-acquired pneumonia

Vaccination in high-risk groups against:

- Influenza (see Chapter 35)
- *Streptococcus pneumoniae*: The pneumococcal vaccine protects against 23 types of pneumococcus which account for approximately 95% of all severe pneumococcal infections. The vaccine is available for adults over the age of 65, and children (> 2 years of age) and adults in the following high risk groups:
  bone marrow transplant; multiple myeloma; asplenic; chronic obstructive pulmonary disease; cystic fibrosis; neuromuscular disease (at risk of aspiration); chronic heart disease; chronic kidney disease; diabetes (tablet or insulin dependent); immunosuppression; cochlear implants; cerebrospinal fluid (CSF) leak following surgery or trauma; on steroids (equivalent to 20 mg/day) for > 1 month (Public Health England, 2013g)
- Lifestyle changes, i.e. smoking cessation
- Good respiratory hygiene/cough etiquette ('catch it, bin it, kill it') to prevent/reduce risk of spread of colds and influenza

Figure 32.6 The pathogenesis of ventilator-associated pneumonia

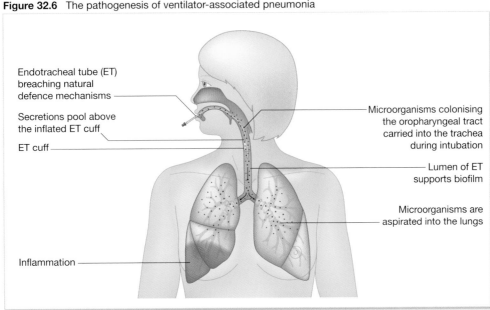

Endotracheal tube (ET) breaching natural defence mechanisms

Secretions pool above the inflated ET cuff

ET cuff

Inflammation

Microorganisms colonising the oropharyngeal tract carried into the trachea during intubation

Lumen of ET supports biofilm

Microorganisms are aspirated into the lungs

Figure 32.7 Prevention of ventilator-associated pneumonia (DH, 2007c)

- Elevation of the head of the bed – the head of the bed is elevated to 30–45° (unless contraindicated)
- Sedation level assessment – unless the patient is awake and comfortable, sedation is reduced/held for assessment at least daily (unless contraindicated)
- Oral hygiene – the mouth is cleaned with chlorhexidine gluconate (≥ 1–2% gel or liquid) 6-hourly (as chlorhexidine can be inactivated by toothpaste, a gap of at least 2 hours should be left between its application and tooth brushing); teeth are brushed 12-hourly with standard toothpaste
- Subglottic aspiration – a tracheal tube (endotracheal or tracheostomy) which has a subglottic secretion drainage port is used if the patient is expected to be intubated for more than 72 hours; secretions are aspirated via the subglottic secretion port 1–2-hourly
- Tracheal tube cuff pressure – cuff pressure is measured 4-hourly, maintained between 20 and 30 cmH$_2$O (or 2 cmH$_2$O above peak inspiratory pressure) and recorded on the ICU chart
- Stress ulcer prophylaxis – stress ulcer prophylaxis is prescribed only to high-risk patients according to locally developed guidelines; prophylaxis is reviewed daily

Figure 32.8 General measures for the prevention of hospital-acquired pneumonia

- Adequate post-operative pain relief to facilitate deep breathing/coughing and mobilisation
- Chest physiotherapy
- Early mobilisation post-operatively
- Hand decontamination in accordance with the '5 Moments' to prevent the exogenous transmission of microorganisms acquired from contact with other patients/the environment
- Compliance with the use of PPE, particularly gloves (see Chapter 16), in order to prevent the spread of pathogens
- Ensure good oral hygiene to prevent colonisation of the orophraynx with pathogens
- In patients who require enteral feeding, keep the patient in the semi-recumbent position while the feed is in progress to prevent aspiration
- Assist patients who have difficulty swallowing with eating, drinking and the swallowing of oral medication to prevent aspiration
- Ensure that nasogastric tubes/enteral feeding tubes are sited correctly to prevent aspiration
- Help preserve gastric acid function and prevent reflux
- Good standards of environmental cleanliness
- Ensure that all respiratory therapy equipment is decontaminated appropriately in between patients according to manufacturer's instructions (i.e. single-use, single-patient use, cleaned, disinfected or sterilised)
- Where nebulisers are single-patient use (as opposed to single-use), the nebuliser must be thoroughly cleaned and dried before re-use, to ensure that no water is left 'standing' in the nebuliser 'acorn', which could then be aerosolised and disseminated
- Change anaesthetic tubing and filters if an anaesthetic machine is used on a patient with a known infection
- Use single-use spirometry mouth pieces
- Vaccination against *Streptococcus pneumoniae* in 'at risk' patient groups (Public Health England, 2013g)
- Staff vaccination against influenza (to prevent patient cross-infection)

Introduction

Pneumonia, a bacterial, viral, fungal or **protozoal** infection of the lung tissue (parenchyma), is the most severe and potentially life-threatening of all community- and hospital-acquired respiratory tract infections. **Community-acquired pneumonia (CAP)** is not associated with care in community or acute healthcare settings (i.e. residential care facilities or hospitals); patients may be diagnosed with CAP on admission, or symptoms may develop within 48 hours of admission. **Hospital-acquired pneumonia (HAP)** has an onset > 48 hours after admission to hospital.

The pathogenesis of pneumonia

During a normal week 14 000 litres of air passes through the respiratory tract (Hoy, 2012) and it is constantly exposed to potential 'insults':

• Gases, vapours and fumes can cause irritation and inflammation.
• Particles: particles greater than 100 μm are not inhaled, whilst those greater than 10 μm are trapped within nasal secretions. However, particles smaller than 5 μm are able to reach the alveoli and can carry up to 100 microorganisms on their surface, depending upon the size of the organism involved (Singh, 2012).

The upper respiratory tract is normally **colonised** with a mixture of commensal flora and pathogenic bacteria but the state of colonisation changes to one of infection when the host's immune defence mechanisms are breached and microorganisms gain access to the lower respiratory tract. These host immune defences are mechanical (i.e. nasal hairs, ciliated epithelium, mucociliary blankets, saliva, the cough and swallow reflex), humoral (i.e. IgA antibody and complement) and cellular (i.e. dendritic cells, alveolar macrophages and phagocytes) (American Thoracic Society and the Infectious Diseases Society of America, 2004) (see Chapters 6 and 7).

Pneumonia can develop as a result of inhalation of a bacterial or viral aerosol, descending infection from the upper respiratory tract to the lower respiratory tract, aspiration of stomach / oropharyngeal contents, or haematogenous spread (seeding) from another site of infection to the lungs via the bloodstream. The organism has to encounter the host and gain entry to the respiratory tract, where it spreads (i.e. from the upper to the lower respiratory tract) and multiplies within the oxygen-rich environment of the lungs. Whether or not entry of the organism results in infection is dependent upon the bacterial or viral load (inoculum), the efficiency of host immune defence mechanisms and host risk factors (see Figure 32.1) and the organism's virulence factors (see Chapters 4 and 5).

Alveolar macrophages are a critical line of defence but if the bacterial / viral load is high, they can be overwhelmed. An inflammatory response is generated within the lung(s), which gives rise to an inflammatory exudate consisting of leukocytes, cytokines and other inflammatory mediators. This exudate 'clogs' the alveoli, impeding gaseous exchange (oxygen and carbon dioxide), and results in breathlessness, increased respiratory rate and sometimes confusion. It also causes damage to the lung parenchyma.

Community-acquired pneumonia

Community-acquired pneumonia (CAP) may be secondary to the development of a bacterial chest infection, a complication of a viral infection such as varicella (see Chapter 45) or influenza (see Chapter 35), or aspiration (see Figure 32.1). Its development depends on the interaction between the host's immune response, the size of the infecting organism and its virulence. It affects between 0.5 and 1% of adults in the UK each year, and is diagnosed in 5–12% of patients presenting in general practice with symptoms of a lower respiratory tract infection (LRTI). Of these, 22–42% will require admission to hospital, and 1.2–10% of hospital admissions will require admission to an intensive therapy unit (ITU) and have a 30% risk of dying (NICE, 2014b). Morbidity and mortality in patients with CAP increase if they are transferred to ITU 24–48 hours post admission (Mandell et al, 2007).

Causes of community-acquired pneumonia

In 50% of cases of CAP, no pathogen is identified (Scottish Intercollegiate Guidelines Network, 2002). However, *Streptococcus pneumoniae* is the most common organism identified from GP specimens, and secondary bacterial infections with *Streptococcus pneumoniae* and *Staphylococcus aureus* are common after influenza. Other causes include:

• *Haemophilus influenzae*
• Influenza (see Chapter 35)
• *Moraxella catarrhalis*
• *Legionella pneumophila* (see Chapter 37)
• Gram-negative bacilli
• *Chlamydophila psittaci*
• *Bordetella pertussis* (see Chapter 27)
• Aspergillus
• Histoplasma
• Cryptococcus.

Assessment of severity of infection

Patients with CAP should be assessed using the **CURB-65** score (Lim et al, 2009), a series of diagnostic indicators that assesses the severity of the pneumonia and informs treatment. One point is allocated for the presence of each of the following criteria:

Confusion (Mental Test score ≤ 8, or delirium)
Urea > 7 mmol
Respiratory rate ≥ 30/minute
Blood pressure (low systolic ≤ 90 mmHg or diastolic ≤ 60 mmHg)
Age ≥ **65**
0 or 1 = low risk (< 3% mortality)
2 = medium risk (3–5% mortality)
3–5 = high risk (> 15% mortality)

Figures 32.2, 32.3, 32.4 and 32.5 describe the clinical features of, and investigations for, pneumonia, and the prevention of community-acquired pneumonia.

Treatment of CAP

'Blind therapy' with amoxicillin and metronidazole is often commenced initially as the number of organisms responsible for causing pneumonia can make the antibiotic treatment of CAP a therapeutic challenge (Donowitz, 2009). In uncomplicated CAP (previously 'healthy' chest and admission to ITU not required), doxycycline or amoxicillin may be prescribed orally. In severe cases, amoxicillin (cefuroxime if penicillin allergic) and clarithromycin may be prescribed in combination.

Hospital-acquired pneumonia

In the 2011 *English National Point Prevalence Survey on Healthcare Associated Infections*, healthcare-associated respiratory tract infections usurped catheter-associated urinary tract infections as the commonest HCAI (HPA, 2012a). In intensive care units, hospital-acquired pneumonia (HAP), which carries a case fatality rate of between 20 and 70%, is strongly associated with endotracheal intubation and mechanical ventilation (ventilator-associated pneumonia (VAP); Masterton et al, 2008; Craven and Chroneou, 2009). The risk of VAP is estimated to be 3% per day during days 1–5 of ventilation, decreasing to 2% during days –5–10, and then 1% each day thereafter (Cook et al, 1998). HAP increases length of stay by approximately eight days and carries a mortality rate of 30–70% (NICE, 2014).

Causative organisms

Pneumonia occurring more than 48 hours after admission to hospital but less than 5 days after admission is generally caused by antibiotic-sensitive organisms (Craven and Chroneou, 2009), whereas pneumonia acquired more than 5 days after admission is more likely to be with a multi-drug resistant organism, acquisition of which is in part due to length of stay. The organisms most commonly encountered are:

- *Staphylococcus aureus*, including MRSA (see Chapter 43)
- *Streptococcus pneumoniae*
- *Haemophilus influenzae*
- *Pseudomonas aeruginosa*
- *Moraxella catarrhalis*
- Acinetobacter species
- Serratia species
- *Klebsiella pneumoniae*
- *Escherichia coli*
- Legionella
- Candida species and *Aspergillus fumigatus* in patients who are immunocompromised or severely **neutropenic**.

The pathogenesis of infection (see Figure 32.6)

The most common cause of hospital-acquired pneumonia is the aspiration of naso- or oropharyngeal secretions. This can occur in patients with impaired cough or swallowing reflexes and through vomiting.

In mechanically ventilated patients, the endotracheal (ET) tube provides a direct route of entry into the normally well-protected respiratory tract. Organisms colonising the oropharynx may be carried into the trachea during intubation, and the process of intubation itself can cause local trauma and inflammation, which increases colonisation of the trachea with resident organisms as well as pathogens (Craven and Chroneou, 2009). In addition, the lumen of the ET tube supports the growth of bacteria which grow within a **biofilm**. Biofilm formation within the ET tube may be a contributing factor in the development of VAP (Craven and Chroneou, 2009). Procedures such as suctioning may dislodge biofilm-encased bacteria, which may be transported to the alveoli (Adair et al, 1999).

Secretions pool above the inflated cuff of the endotracheal tube and often contain Gram-negative bacilli and *S. aureus* which colonise the upper respiratory tract in patients who have been in hospital for longer than five days.

Once the secretions have been aspirated into the lower respiratory tract they cause inflammation and infection in the terminal bronchioles and alveoli in the lung, filling the alveolar spaces with fluid instead of air, preventing gaseous exchange and resulting in consolidation (Dunn, 2005).

The outcome is dependent upon the number and types of organisms that gain entry to the lower respiratory tract and the efficiency of host immune defence mechanisms.

Diagnosis of HAP/VAP – Clinical Pulmonary Infection Score (CPIS) (Masterton et al, 2008)

- Core temperature greater than 38.5 °C.
- Raised or lowered white cell count ($> 10000/mm^3$ or $< 4000/mm^3$).
- Purulent tracheal secretions and / or new or persistent infiltrations on chest x-ray which are otherwise unexplained.
- Worsening gaseous exchange and increased oxygen requirements.
  Figure 32.7 describes the prevention of VAP.

Treatment of HAP

Initial 'blind' therapy pending laboratory confirmation of the causative pathogen is with co-amoxiclav (or clarithromycin if penicillin allergic) and metronidazole (PO or IV depending on whether or not the patient is able to swallow). For patients with severe HAP who are penicillin allergic, IV cefuroxime, with the addition of IV metronidazole if there is suspicion or evidence of aspiration, is the antimicrobial agent of choice. Patients who are prescribed antibiotics by the IV route will be stepped down to an oral prescription as soon as it is possible do so. For severe HAP, oral step-down agents are levofloxacin and metronidazole.

Figure 32.8 describes the prevention of HAP.

33 Ebola virus disease

Figure 33.1 Clinical features and progression of Ebola

Ebola virus may be present: in blood; in body fluids (including urine and semen); on contaminated equipment and instruments; on contaminated surfaces; on contaminated clothing; in waste

The case reproductive rate (the average number of secondary cases arising from one primary case) is 1.5–2.0, compared to 2–3 for influenza and 12–18 for measles. Although it is not particularly 'contagious', the infectious dose (the number of pathogens required to cause infection in a host) is very low at 1–10 virus particles (Leggett et al, 2012; Judson et al, 2015)

Differential diagnosis: differentiating between other infections / infectious diseases which have the same signs and symptoms (i.e. Marburg virus disease; falciparum malaria; typhoid fever; shigellosis; cholera; plague; Q fever), and non-infectious diseases/conditions (i.e. leukaemia; fulminant (sudden severe onset) viral hepatitis; clotting factor deficiencies and platelet disorders) (Patel et al, 2014)

Incubation period: 2–21 days (average 8–10 days). Individuals with fatal disease tend to have severe clinical symptoms early on in the disease process, and generally die between days 6 and 16

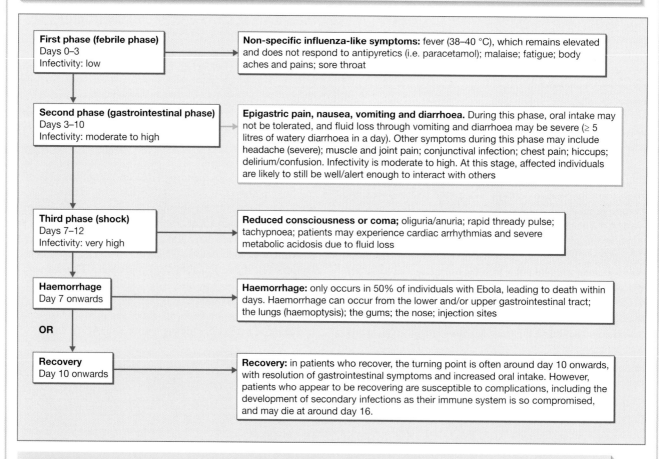

First phase (febrile phase)
Days 0–3
Infectivity: low

Non-specific influenza-like symptoms: fever (38–40 °C), which remains elevated and does not respond to antipyretics (i.e. paracetamol); malaise; fatigue; body aches and pains; sore throat

Second phase (gastrointestinal phase)
Days 3–10
Infectivity: moderate to high

Epigastric pain, nausea, vomiting and diarrhoea. During this phase, oral intake may not be tolerated, and fluid loss through vomiting and diarrhoea may be severe (≥ 5 litres of watery diarrhoea in a day). Other symptoms during this phase may include headache (severe); muscle and joint pain; conjunctival infection; chest pain; hiccups; delirium/confusion. Infectivity is moderate to high. At this stage, affected individuals are likely to still be well/alert enough to interact with others

Third phase (shock)
Days 7–12
Infectivity: very high

Reduced consciousness or coma; oliguria/anuria; rapid thready pulse; tachypnoea; patients may experience cardiac arrhythmias and severe metabolic acidosis due to fluid loss

Haemorrhage
Day 7 onwards

Haemorrhage: only occurs in 50% of individuals with Ebola, leading to death within days. Haemorrhage can occur from the lower and/or upper gastrointestinal tract; the lungs (haemoptysis); the gums; the nose; injection sites

OR

Recovery
Day 10 onwards

Recovery: in patients who recover, the turning point is often around day 10 onwards, with resolution of gastrointestinal symptoms and increased oral intake. However, patients who appear to be recovering are susceptible to complications, including the development of secondary infections as their immune system is so compromised, and may die at around day 16.

Investigations
FBC; U&Es; CRP; blood cultures; glucose; coagulation studies; urine and stool for MC&S; chest x-ray; urgent malaria screen

VHF Screen via the Imported Fever Service if malaria screen is negative, the patient remains pyrexial and no diagnosis has been made (Department of Health Advisory Committee on Dangerous Pathogens /HSE, 2015)

Treatment
Vaccines are in development and trials are underway in West Africa. There has been some success with monoclonal antibodies

Supportive care: fluid replacement for electrolyte disturbances / treatment of hypovolaemic shock; management of haemorrhage, disseminated intravascular coagulation (DIC), septic shock and multi-organ failure

Infection Prevention and Control at a Glance, First Edition. By Debbie Weston, Alison Burgess and Sue Roberts.
© 2017 John Wiley & Sons, Ltd. Published 2017 by John Wiley & Sons, Ltd.

Figure 33.2 Viral Haemorrhagic Fevers Risk Assessment Algorithm (version 6: 15.11.2015).

VHF endemic countries:
Information on VHF endemic countries can be found at
https://www.gov.uk/viral-haemorrhagic-fevers-origins-reservoirs-transmission-and-guidelines or see VHF in Africa map at
https://www.gov.uk/government/uploads/system/uploads/attachment_data/file/365845/VHF_Africa_960_640.png

Additional questions:
- Has the patient travelled to any area where there is a current VHF outbreak? (http://www.promedmail.org/) **OR**
- Has the patient lived or worked in basic rural conditions in an area where Lassa Fever is endemic?
  (https://www.gov.uk/lassa-fever-origins-reservoirs-transmission-and-guidelines) **OR**
- Has the patient visited caves/mines, or had contact with or eaten primates, antelopes or bats in a Marburg/Ebola endemic area?
  (https://www.gov.uk/ebola-and-marburg-haemorrhagic-fevers-outbreaks-and-case-locations) **OR**
- Has the patient travelled in an area where Crimean-Congo Haemorrhagic Fever is endemic
  (http://www.who.int/csr/disease/crimean_congoHF/Global_CCHFRisk_20080918.png?ua=1) **AND**
  sustained a tick bite* or crushed a tick with their bare hands **OR** had close involvement with animal slaughter?
  (*If an obvious alternative diagnosis has been made e.g. tick typhus, then manage locally)

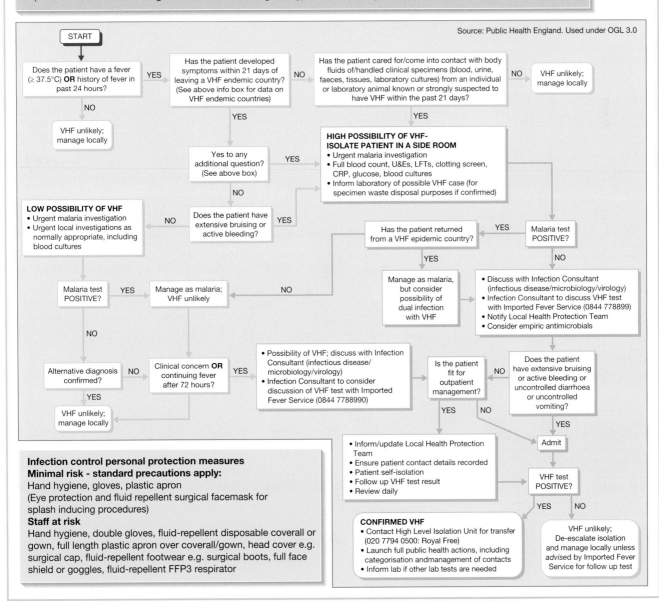

Source: Public Health England. Used under OGL 3.0

Figure 33.3 Order of donning PPE and key points to note (each stage of the donning process must be directed and assisted by a PPE 'buddy')

Healthcare worker must don a set of disposable scrubs; tuck legs of scrubs into socks (if worn); remove all jewellery; tie up/secure hair; cover any minor abrasions (face/hands); wash hands

Gather together and check PPE (for size/integrity): coverall; surgical boots; FFP3 respirator mask; surgical hat/cap; disposable full length plastic apron; full face shield/visor; 2 pairs of examination (non-sterile) gloves

Put on coverall; zip up to the neck; if the coverall has an integral hood, roll the hood down and back on itself so that it does not get in the way.

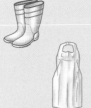

Put on boots and roll the legs of the coverall down over the boots

Put on the full length disposable apron and tie securely. The front of the apron needs to be pulled up and tied at the neck so that it sits at shoulder level

Put on the surgical hat/cap (the purpose of the hat/cap is to help secure the straps of the FFP3 respirator mask)

Put on the FFP3 respirator mask and undertake a fit check

Put on the visor/face shield

Put on inner gloves under the cuffs of the coverall, followed by outer gloves over the cuffs of the coverall

The PPE buddy must check that all PPE has been donned correctly and is secure, checking each item of PPE individually (starting at the head and working down). Before the healthcare worker enters the patient's room, s/he must be reminded that under no circumstances must s/he put her/his hands up to her/his face/head once in the room

Figure 33.4 Order of removal (doffing) of PPE on exiting the isolation room

NB: Each stage of the removal process is verbally directed and controlled by the Safe Undressing Assistant (SUA). It is essential that the healthcare worker does not pre-empt any step in the process and only moves when directed to do so by the SUA. The PPE removal process takes place in a designated area that is divided into Red and Amber zones

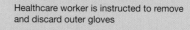

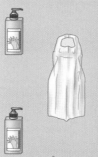

Healthcare worker is instructed to apply alcohol handrub to gloved hands

Healthcare worker is instructed to remove apron by grasping it at the shoulders and pulling it away from the chest so that the neck ties snap, rolling it outwards down the body to waist level to avoid contaminating the coverall, and pulling it at waist level so that the waist ties then snap. The apron is discarded into a burn bin

Healthcare worker is instructed to apply alcohol handrub to gloved hands

Healthcare worker is instructed to remove and discard outer gloves

Healthcare worker is instructed to apply alcohol handrub to gloved hands

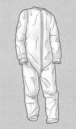

SUA assists with the removal of the coverall and boots; healthcare worker is instructed to:
• tilt head back so the SUA can unzip the coverall from neck downwards, then turn 180° with her/his arms extended out behind them
• stand still while the SUA rolls the coverall away from the healthcare worker's shoulders, down each arm (the healthcare worker will be asked to remove each arm from the sleeves of the coverall, taking care not to come into contact with the SUA), and down the body as far as the tops of the healthcare worker's boots

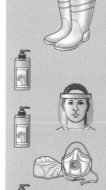

SUA clasps the ankle of the healthcare worker's right boot and requests that they step out of the right boot and put their right foot into the Amber zone. SUA then clasps the ankle of the left boot and requests that the healthcare worker steps out of the left boot and puts their foot into the Amber zone. The SUA places the coverall and boots (removed as one unit) into the burn bin

Healthcare worker is instructed to apply alcohol handrub to gloved hands

Healthcare worker is instructed to remove visor/face shield and discard it in the burn bin

Healthcare worker is instructed to apply alcohol handrub to gloved hands

Healthcare worker is instructed to remove the FFP3 respirator mask, lifting the surgical hat off with it as the straps from the mask are brought over the top of the head

Healthcare worker is instructed to apply alcohol handrub to gloved hands

Healthcare worker is instructed to remove and discard inner gloves

Healthcare worker is instructed to wash her/his hands

Described by the World Health Organization (WHO) as a 'public health emergency of international concern' and 'a crisis for international peace and security', the largest outbreak of Ebola virus disease (EVD) that the world has seen to date is believed to have had its origins in December 2013 in Melliandou, a village in eastern Guinea bordering Liberia and Sierra Leone. 'Patient zero' was a 2-year-old boy who succumbed to a 'mysterious illness characterized by fever, black stools and vomiting' (WHO, 2014) and died two days after the onset of symptoms. Within days family members, mourners and other villagers, including healthcare workers, had become infected and taken the virus into other communities in a geographical area of Africa that had never experienced Ebola before. The outbreak in Guinea hid within towns and villages, unrecognised and undetected, for approximately three months until the WHO was notified on 23 March 2014. By that time, Ebola had crossed borders into Liberia, Sierra Leone and Nigeria, and later spread into Mali and Senegal. At its peak in October 2014, more than 800 new cases in West Africa were being reported per week.

The publicity, climate of fear, and scale of the international response to bring the outbreak in West Africa under control and prevent a global catastrophe have been unprecedented. Although it has always been theoretically possible that Ebola could 'get on a plane and travel anywhere', it has never *really* been considered to pose a *significant* threat to public health outside its natural 'host' areas. However, the sheer *scale* of the 2014 outbreak meant that *all* countries have had to undertake preparedness planning in the event of suspected / confirmed imported cases of Ebola and potential cases arising from secondary transmission.

The West Africa outbreak seeded isolated cases of Ebola in the **United States of America (Dallas)**, **Spain (Madrid), the UK, Germany, France, Norway, Italy** and **Switzerland**.

In **Dallas**, an imported case was seen in a returning traveller from Sierra Leone who was diagnosed with Ebola in the US and subsequently died; two nurses caring for him also contracted Ebola but both recovered. Separately, a repatriated medical aid worker also died. In **Madrid**, a nurse contracted Ebola after caring for two repatriated priests; they died but the nurse recovered. In the **UK**, one nurse was repatriated with confirmed Ebola in August 2014 and recovered. Another became ill shortly after arriving home in Scotland in December 2014. Although she recovered, she suffered severe complications almost ten months later when she developed meningitis as a secondary complication of the original Ebola infection. A third nurse, working as part of the British Military Response Team, contracted Ebola in March 2015 and was repatriated to the UK for care; she too has recovered. The cases seen in **Germany, France, Norway, Italy** and **Switzerland** were repatriated healthcare workers; there were no instances of secondary transmission to healthcare staff caring for them (www.who.int/csr/disease/ebola/en; www.cdc.gov/vhf/ebola).

The WHO declared the outbreak over in January 2016. However, although Ebola no longer poses an international health risk, 'flare-ups' in Guinea and Liberia demonstrate that there is still the potential for Ebola to re-ignite in West Africa.

The Ebola virus

Ebola is a single-stranded, negative-sense, helical, RNA filovirus (Hart, 2007; Bray and Chertow, 2015) which, together with species of arenavirus, bunyavirus and flavivirus, belongs to the family of viruses known as the **viral haemorrhagic fevers (VHFs)** (so called because of the effect that the viruses have on the vascular system) (Department of Health Advisory Committee on Dangerous Pathogens /HSE, 2015). VHFs are severe and life-threatening viral diseases that are endemic in parts of Africa, South America, the Middle East and Eastern Europe. Humans are not the host reservoirs of VHFs; the viruses are **zoonotic** in origin, derived from a wildlife host such as ticks, mosquitos, rodents, bats and primates, and have jumped the species barrier to cause infection in humans.

The fatality rate associated with VHFs ranges from 50 to 90% and they are classed as **Hazard Group 4 Pathogens** – organisms that cause severe disease in humans and spread readily, for which there is no effective treatment or prophylaxis (Department of Health Advisory Committee on Dangerous Pathogens / HSE, 2015).

Although Ebola is the most feared of the VHFs, classifying it as a VHF is, according to Bray and Chertow (2015), something of a misnomer, as only a very small percentage of people with Ebola develop haemorrhage.

It was first discovered in 1976 following two simultaneous outbreaks in the Democratic Republic of Congo (Zaire) and Sudan and was named after the Ebola River that runs through Zaire (Hart, 2007). There are five species:
- **Zaire ebolavirus** – the cause of the majority of outbreaks, including the 2014–2015 West Africa outbreak
- **Sudan ebolavirus**.
- **Bundibugyo ebolavirus** – discovered in the Bundibugyo district in Uganda in 2007).
- **Tai Forest ebolavirus** – emerged in 1994 in the Tai Forest National Park in the Cote d'Ivoire (Ivory Coast), where it caused an outbreak among chimpanzees and infected a scientist who acquired it during a post-mortem on an infected chimp; this is the only known human case of Tai Forest ebolavirus and the only known outbreak of this species among primates
- **Reston ebolavirus** – caused an outbreak among primates in a monkey house in Reston, Virginia, and is the only ebolavirus that is non-pathogenic to humans (www.who.int/csr/disease/ebola/en).

The primary host / reservoir of Ebola virus is not definitively known but is widely believed to be the fruit bat, which is hunted for food and which can infect other species of animal either directly or indirectly (i.e. through contamination of their environment), particularly primates, which has led to a marked reduction in chimpanzee and gorilla populations in known Ebola regions. The family of 'patient zero' are believed to have hunted fruit bats (WHO, 2014).

Contributing factors to the 2014–2015 outbreak (www.who.int/csr/disease/ebola/one-year-report/ebola-report-1-year.pdf; WHO, 2014; Bray and Chertow, 2015)
- Guinea, Liberia and Sierra Leone are among the poorest countries in the world.
- Years of civil war and unrest have resulted in a poor public health infrastructure, including a shortage of healthcare workers (i.e. one to two doctors per 100 000 population). Weak road, transportation and telecommunications systems have severely hindered requests for help / aid, transportation of patients to hospitals / dedicated Ebola treatment centres, and public health information campaigns.
- There is a highly mobile population with movement across uncontrolled borders in search of food and work, and extended families living in different countries. This facilitated the spread of Ebola into densely populated areas.

- As the ecology in the forests has changed as a result of activities by mining and timber companies, fruit bats have moved nearer to villages.
- Infected wild animals are slaughtered for human consumption.
- Cultural beliefs and behavioural practices relating to ancestral funeral and burial rites, include: infected individuals returning to their village of birth to die and be buried next to their ancestors; ceremonial care of bodies after death (burials by military personnel did not observe traditional burial rituals, which led to the dead being hidden in some remote villages); reliance on, and belief in, traditional healers and not conventional medicine.
- Community resistance to outside help due to fear; as the death rate rose, the perception was that hospitals and the 'people in space suits' were to blame.

Health workers 'in the field' are 21–32 times more likely to contract Ebola than the general population, and 418 health workers working in hospitals and Ebola treatment centres in Sierra Leone, Guinea and Liberia died (WHO, 2015a).

The pathogenesis of infection

In an outbreak of Ebola, **the first case of human infection** arises as a result of direct, or indirect, contact with the blood, body fluids, tissues / organs, secretions or excretions of an animal that is infected with, or is a host reservoir of, Ebola virus. The virus enters the human host **via non-intact skin** (i.e. through a scratch, abrasion or macroscopic break) **or via the mucous membranes** of the eyes, nose and mouth as a result of exposure to infected blood and / or body fluids. It attaches to specific receptors on the surface of the cells that it directly infects or targets, such as the endothelial cells lining blood vessels, hepatocytes (cells lining the liver), and white blood cells – primarily monocytes and macrophages – along with dendritic cells (cells that 'present' antigens to T cells, and act as chemical messengers between the two branches of the immune response) (see Chapter 7).

Once it has gained entry, the virus replicates rapidly. The infected macrophages transport the virus to the lymph nodes, where more viral replication takes place, and from there it enters the lymphatic system and the bloodstream. Ebola causes apoptosis ('cell suicide' or programmed cell death) of the infected cells. As the cells break down and die, there is a release of cytokines, chemokines and other inflammatory mediators that generates a massive inflammatory response and adversely affects coagulation pathways. Human to human (H2H) transmission occurs through direct or indirect contact with blood and / or body fluids. Ebola has been detected in the semen of men *after* their clinical recovery (Deen et al, 2015), and it can persist in the aqueous humor (Bray and Chertow, 2015).

Figure 33.1 describes the clinical features and progression of Ebola virus disease.

Individuals at risk of contracting Ebola

During an outbreak, those at most risk of contracting Ebola are healthcare workers, family members in close contact with the patient, and mourners who have direct contact with the deceased during burial rituals (the availability of trained burial teams is a much a priority as healthcare provision).

Within healthcare settings, exposure to Ebola may occur:
- **directly**, through exposure (broken skin or mucous membranes) to blood and / or body fluids during invasive, aerosolising or splash procedures, or percutaneous injury (see Chapter 18)

- **indirectly**, through exposure (broken skin or mucous membranes) to environments, surfaces, equipment or clothing contaminated with splashes or droplets of blood or body fluids (Department of Health Advisory Committee on Dangerous Pathogens /HSE, 2015).

Diagnosis

As the initial clinical features of Ebola are non-specific, there may be a delay in diagnosis, particularly if the disease breaks in a geographical area where Ebola has not previously been seen. In the UK, the Imported Fever Service (IFS) provides a national, single point of contact for advice, risk assessment and diagnostic testing. Testing is undertaken via polymerase chain reaction (PCR) in order to detect viral RNA or antibodies (see Chapter 9) from blood (serum and **EDTA** blood), which is couriered to the Rare and Imported Pathogens Laboratory at Porton Down, Wiltshire.

Treatment

Treatment consists of symptom relief and the management of complications. Clinical trials involving innovative therapies such as monoclonal antibodies (ZMAPP and MIL77) have been underway since 2014, and have had some success, as has the transfusion of convalescent blood / plasma from Ebola survivors. Vaccine trials have been undertaken in Guinea and Sierra Leone; full details are available on the WHO website (http://www.who.int/csr/disease/ebola/en).

The management of Ebola virus disease in the UK

Environmental conditions within the UK do not support the natural reservoirs or vectors of **any** of the VHFs, and therefore the only case (or cases) seen in the UK are:
- deliberately imported (i.e. a healthcare worker infected in Africa is transferred to the UK for treatment)
or
- unwittingly imported (i.e. an individual acquires VHF as a result of travel to / residence in an affected country and has contact with an infected individual or wild animal, potentially giving rise to cases among contacts, including healthcare workers).

Deliberate release (biological warfare) has long been regarded as a possibility.

Revised national guidelines on the Management of Hazard Group 4 viral haemorrhagic fevers and similar human infectious diseases of high consequence were published by the Department of Health and Health and Safety Executive (Advisory Committee on Dangerous Pathogens) in November 2014, and November 2015
(www.gov.uk/government/collections/ebola-virus-disease-clinical-management-and-guidance).

These detail the complex infection control management of patients with suspected and confirmed EVD / VHF presenting within the UK, including risk assessment, testing / screening, all aspects of IP&C, and the transfer / management of positive patients. They are primarily written for the management of people with suspected Ebola within healthcare settings. **Specific guidance documents for the initial infection control management of people within community care settings** (i.e. health centres / GP practices, prison services, immigration / detention centres) are also available at www.gov.uk/government/collections/ebola-virus-disease-clinical-management-and-guidance

The World Health Organization and the Centers for Disease Control and Prevention (Atlanta) websites also have extensive resources on Ebola and the VHFs (www.who.int/csr/disease/ebola/en and www.cdc.gov/vhf/ebola).

Key to the prompt detection and management / treatment of a suspected case and the prevention of secondary cases among healthcare workers are:

Risk assessment

This must be undertaken according to the VHF Risk Assessment Algorithm (see Figure 33.2) for *any* patient presenting with a fever, or history of a fever, within 21 days of returning from **an Ebola / VHF endemic country**_(see www.gov.uk/government/collections/ebola-virus-disease-clinical-management-and-guidance for updated maps and epidemiological data), **and / or** contact with the blood and / or body fluids of an individual, or laboratory animal, known or strongly suspected to have Ebola / VHF.

Risk assessment is a legal obligation (Department of Health Advisory Committee on Dangerous Pathogens/HSE, 2015) and it is essential that the risk assessment is undertaken by a senior member of the medical team (i.e. emergency department consultant or admitting team consultant) and discussed promptly with the IP&CT in order to determine whether or not the criteria for suspecting Ebola / VHF are met.

Isolation in a single room

The patient **must** be isolated in a single room pending confirmation of a negative or positive VHF screen (undertaken via the Imported Fever Service).

There should be a room within the department that is designated specifically for this purpose. Local policy will detail whether or not the patient remains in the department in isolation until Ebola / VHF is confirmed or excluded, or is transferred to another clinical area (i.e. a negative pressure isolation room if there is not one within the emergency department).

PPE (also see Chapter 16)

While the initial risk assessment is undertaken, 'standard precautions and good infection control are paramount to ensure that staff are not put at risk' (Department of Health Advisory Committee on Dangerous Pathogens /HSE, 2015) (i.e. hand hygiene, gloves and a plastic apron). **This risk assessment will determine the level of PPE that staff will then be required to wear.**

Low possibility of VHF / minimal risk
- Hand hygiene, gloves, plastic apron.
- Fluid-repellent surgical face mask and eye protection if **splash-inducing procedures** are to be undertaken.

- FFP3 respirator and eye protection if an **aerosol-generating procedure** is to be undertaken.

High possibility of VHF
There is a **lengthy and complex process** for the donning and removal of the PPE requirements when caring for high-risk patients (local policy may determine that this level of PPE must be worn by staff for the initial risk assessment and the care of low-risk patients due to the level of staff anxiety regarding potential contact with Ebola). This level of PPE consists of:
- a surgical hat
- FFP3 respirator mask
- face visor
- coverall
- double gloves
- full length disposal plastic apron
- surgical boots.

It must be assumed that the patient has Ebola / VHF until it has been excluded (or of course confirmed) by testing, and all IP&C procedures must be implemented and followed to the letter. The incorrect donning of PPE potentially exposes the healthcare worker to contamination while in the isolation room with the patient; **removal therefore carries a significant risk of inadvertent healthcare worker contamination unless staff have received training (although this does not mean that they are competent) and are strictly directed and assisted with each step of the process.** The double glove removal technique in particular must be practised (see http://www.hse.gov.uk/skin/videos/gloves/removegloves.htm).

Figures 33.3 and 33.4 illustrate the complexity of the PPE requirements, which require a PPE 'buddy' and 'Safe Undressing Assistant' (SAU).

Liaison with the Imported Fever Service (IFS)
This will be undertaken by the IP&CT in conjunction with the consultant responsible for the patient's care. If Ebola / VHF is confirmed, arrangements will be made for the patient to be transferred to the nearest high-level isolation unit (HLIU), where s/he will be cared for by a dedicated team of specialist nursing and medical staff in a Trexler isolation unit (see Chapter 21).

Other IP&C precautions
The Department of Health Advisory Committee on Dangerous Pathogens/HSE Guidance provides detailed information on specimen collection, the management and disposal of waste and linen, the management of blood and fluid spillages, and the decontamination of equipment and the environment, and this will be captured at local level in the organisation's policy.

34 Infestation

Figure 34.1 Characteristics of scabies mites
Reference: http://cks.nice.org.uk/scabies

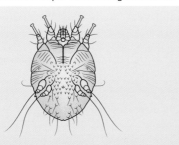

- Size: tiny (may be seen as a tiny speck with the naked eye)
- The female mite is larger at 0.4 mm × 0.3 mm, compared to the male at 0.2 mm × 0.3 mm
- Colour: cream-coloured body
- Covered with bristles and spines on their backs, and four pairs of legs
- Female lays 40–50 eggs in a lifetime
- Six-legged larvae hatch after 3–4 days, transforming into 8-legged nymphs before becoming adults
- Burrows appear as fine, wavy, grey, dark or silvery lines 5 mm long
- Average infestation 10–15 mites

Figure 34.2 Characteristics of head lice
Reference: http://cks.nice.org.uk/head-lice

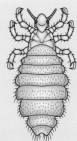

- Size: 2.1–3.3 mm
- Small, flat, wingless. Able to crawl but cannot jump, hop or fly
- Colour: tan, greyish-white in colour
- Six legs
- Eggs are laid as close to the scalp as possible (at the base of the hair shaft) to provide ideal temperature for incubation (> 31 °C)
- Average infestation typically 30 lice per head
- Live for approximately 4 weeks on host
- Die after 2 days away from host without feeding

Figure 34.3 Characteristics of body lice
Reference: www.cdc.gov/parasites/lice/body

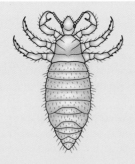

- Size: 2.3–3.6 mm
- Oval in shape
- Colour: tan to greyish white
- Move to skin only at night to feed on blood
- Average infestation: 10–20 lice; in heavy infestations may be many more
- Live for approximately 4 weeks on host
- Die after 5–7 days away from host without feeding
- Known to transmit disease (epidemic typhus, trench fever, epidemic relapsing fever)

Figure 34.4 Characteristics of pubic lice
Reference: http://cks.nice.org.uk/pubic-lice

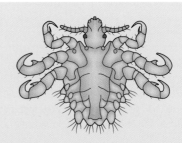

- Size: 1.1–1.8 mm
- Crab-shaped
- Colour: grey or brown in colour
- Feed 10 times a day
- Live for approximately 4 weeks on host
- Can survive 2 days off host without feeding
- Average infestation: 12 lice
- Gorillas are the only other animal affected by pubic lice
- In children, the possibility of sexual abuse should be considered

Infection Prevention and Control at a Glance, First Edition. By Debbie Weston, Alison Burgess and Sue Roberts.
© 2017 John Wiley & Sons, Ltd. Published 2017 by John Wiley & Sons, Ltd.

Figure 34.5 Treatment of scabies

NICE (http://cks.nice.org.uk/scabies) recommends the following treatment:

Permethrin 5% dermal cream (first-line treatment):
Treat whole skin area of body paying particular attention to the scalp, neck, face and ears, and to the webs of the fingers, toes and end of the nails, in addition to the soles of the feet and skin around the buttocks and genitals. Avoid the eyes and around the mouth. Additional treatments may be required for crusted scabies.

Malathion 0.5% *aqueous* liquid (if permethrin inappropriate, for example if the person has an allergy to chrysanthemums). May be used on children over 6 months old.

Treatment of children: For children under 2 months old, specialist advice should be sought from a paediatric dermatologist (NB: scabies is rare in children under 2 years).

Oral ivermectin (named-patient basis only): May be used to treat crusted/Norwegian scabies that does NOT respond to topical treatment alone.

NB: Alcoholic lotions are not recommended as they cause irritation of excoriated skin.

On completion of treatment for both classical and atypical scabies, the individual is considered to be non-infectious.

Figure 34.9 Individual stricken with head and body lice

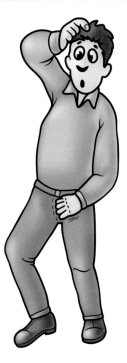

Figure 34.6 Treatment of head lice

NICE (http://cks.nice.org.uk/head-lice) recommends *several treatments*, depending on the preference of the individual or parent as follows:

Dimeticone 4% lotion (Hedrin): This kills the lice by coating them and by blocking their tracheae, so resistance is unlikely to develop. Cure rates of 70% have been reported.

Dimeticone spray 92% (NYDA): This also kills the lice by coating them and blocking the tracheae, so resistance is unlikely to develop. Cure rates of 97% have been reported. However, it is not suitable for use in pregnant or breast-feeding women, or children under 2 years of age.

Wet combing bug buster method: No insecticides are used so resistance is not an issue. The cure rate is thought to be 50–60% provided that a fine-toothed louse detection comb is used.

Isopropyl myristate and cyclomethicone solution (Full Marks Solution): This works by dissolving the wax coating on the louse exoskeleton leading to uncontrolled dehydration and subsequent death so resistance is unlikely to develop. Cure rates of 52–82% have been reported. It is not suitable for people with skin conditions, for use in pregnant or breast-feeding women, or children under 2 years of age.

Malathion 0.5% aqueous liquid: Use is well established, although it has an unpleasant smell, and the prevalence of resistance to insecticides seems to be increasing. It has the advantage of being able to be used on people with asthma and skin conditions, and can be used third-line during pregnancy and wet combing if wet combing and dimeticone are ineffective.

All treatments require more than one treatment session and no treatment can guarantee success. People are advised to check whether treatment has been successful by detection combing on day 2 or day 3 after completing a course of treatment, and again after an interval of 7 days (day 9 or day 10 after treatment). Whilst dry combing takes less time, wet combing is more accurate as the conditioner stops the lice from moving.

NB: Hair should be left to dry naturally, and NOT dried with a hair dryer.

Figure 34.7 Treatment of body lice

No specific treatment is required as they are easily eradicated if clothing is not worn for *at least* 3 days.
Referral to a dermatologist is advised.

Figure 34.8 Treatment of pubic lice

NICE (http://cks.nice.org.uk/pubic-lice) recommends:

Malathion 0.5% aqueous solution: Two applications 7 days apart, *or*
Permethrin 5% dermal cream: Two applications 7 days apart.

For eyelash infestation: Treat with occlusive ophthalmic ointment or topical insecticide.

If acquired via sexual contact: Referral to a genitourinary medicine (GUM) clinic is advised for one week later.

Infestation of the human body with parasites is a common occurrence. Although it is often considered to be nothing more than a nuisance, it can lead to more serious health problems. Body lice in particular can spread serious diseases. It is important therefore that treatment is initiated promptly so that the risk of complications is minimised. This chapter looks at four of the most common causes of infestation: scabies and head, body and pubic lice.

Scabies (Sarcoptes scabei)

Scabies (see Figure 34.1) is a parasitic infestation of the skin caused by the tiny *Sarcoptes scabei* mite. There are an estimated 300 million people with scabies worldwide (WHO, 2015c). Following close contact, the mites burrow into the top layer of the skin within approximately 30 minutes. The adult male mates with the female and, following copulation, dies. The pregnant female mite then enlarges the burrows and starts to lay eggs (http://cks.nice.org.uk/scabies).

There are three main presentations of scabies, the severity and nature of the symptoms being largely dependent upon the immune status and age of the individual.

Classical scabies: This common form is found in healthy individuals with a normal immune system.

Crusted scabies (Norwegian scabies): Although rare, this is *extremely contagious,* occurring in those whose immune systems are severely impaired.

Atypical scabies: This occurs in individuals with an immature or impaired immune response (usually the very young or very old). A greater number of mites are produced than in classical scabies, particularly on the hands, making the person extremely contagious.

Scabies infestations are common in care homes and prisons and sometimes occur in childcare facilities. Scabies is also **endemic** in many developing countries, with **epidemics** frequently occurring where there is poverty, poor sanitation, and overcrowding due to war, mass movement of people and economic crisis (Eberhard et al, 2008).

Mode of transmission

Transmission commonly occurs through prolonged direct contact with infested skin (>15–20 minutes) but may also occur during sexual contact (genital scabies). Transfer from undergarments and bedclothes only occurs if these have been contaminated by an infested individual *immediately* beforehand (Eberhard et al, 2008).

Incubation period

Individuals who have *not* been previously exposed will develop itching –2–6 weeks after infection, which coincides with a widespread eruption of inflammatory papules. Those with previous exposure will develop symptoms 24–48 hours after re-exposure, due to prior sensitisation to the mite, its saliva and faeces (Eberhard et al, 2008).

Clinical signs and symptoms

Classical scabies: The major symptom is a rash with associated burrows that is extremely itchy, especially at night when the person is warm. Common areas of infestation include the wrist, finger webs, forearms, axillary folds, side of chest, waist, lower quadrants of the buttocks and the inside of the legs and ankles (Eberhard et al, 2008).

Crusted scabies: Because there is no allergic response there is no rash or discomfort, and burrows may be difficult to see. Instead there are **hyperkeratotic**, warty crusts, and extensive thickening of the skin. Mites are numerous, and the skin may crumble away. The infestation is sometimes localised to one area of the body such as the scalp, a finger or a toe. Nail hyperkeratosis and discolouration may also occur, in addition to generalised erythema and lymphadenopathy (http://cks.nice.org.uk/scabies).

Atypical scabies: Symptoms are variable. Although scaling or crusting may be present, itching may be very slight or absent, which may lead to a delay in diagnosis.

Complications

These include severe skin conditions, particularly with crusted scabies. Secondary infection occurs as a result of skin damage from scratching or aggravation of existing skin conditions. Acute **glomerulonephritis** may also occur as a result of secondary infection (Eberhard et al, 2008).

Diagnosing scabies

Diagnosis is determined from patient history examination of the affected individual using magnification techniques, and analysis of skin scrapings for crusted scabies. Misdiagnosis of scabies is common because of its similarity to other **pruritic** skin disorders so the diagnosis should always be confirmed by a dermatologist (http://cks.nice.org.uk/scabies).

Treatment

Recommended treatments (as per NICE Guidance) (see Figures 34.5 to 34.9) include:

Permethrin 5% dermal cream (first-line treatment), or **malathion 0.5%** *aqueous* **liquid.** Two treatments one week apart are required as the eggs are more resistant than the mites, although more treatments may be required for crusted scabies. Treatment should be applied to cool dry skin, *not* after a hot bath, and **all** contacts should be treated simultaneously to prevent reinfection. Antibiotics may be required for secondary infection. Antihistamines and calamine lotion may be administered for symptomatic relief. The possibility of underlying immunodeficiency should be investigated for all patients with crusted scabies (http://cks.nice.org.uk/scabies).

Infection control precautions

Isolation / exclusion: is required until 24 hours after completion of first treatment, but is frequently longer for crusted scabies.

Gloves and aprons: Should be worn for the application of topical treatment, with correct disposal in a clinical waste bin.

Environmental cleaning: As per local guidelines.

Laundering: Items such as clothes, towels and bed linen should be machine-washed as per NICE Guidance (http://cks.nice.org.uk/scabies) on the day of the first treatment.

Head, body and pubic lice

Head lice (Pediculus humanus capitis)

Head lice (Figure 34.2) live on the heads of people, most commonly behind the ears and on the back of the neck (http://cks.nice.org.uk/head-lice).

Most people only realise that they have head lice after the itch has developed (due to an allergic reaction to the bites) which can be 2–3 months after the initial infection. The severity of infestation varies from a few lice to thousands.

Body lice (Pediculus humanus)

Body lice (Figure 34.3) are generally easy to see in the seams of an infested person's clothing, particularly around the waist line and under armpits, although occasionally they are seen attached to body hair. Body lice move to the skin at night to feed on the person's blood.

Pubic lice (Phthirus pubis)

Pubic or 'crab lice' (see Figure 34.4) are slightly smaller than other lice and live on coarse body hair, particularly pubic and perianal hair, although they may also be found on axillary hair, the abdomen, chest, and more rarely facial hair, including eyelashes (Eberhard et al, 2008). Eradication from the body is *unlikely* unless treated. Shaving the area does not provide protection from re-infestation because pubic lice need only a *minimal* length of hair on which to lay eggs (Eberhard et al, 2008).

Incubation / life cycle of head, body and pubic lice

All lice have similar life cycles and typically have three different forms:

Nits (lice eggs): These are often the first sign of infestation. They are oval in shape, yellow to white in colour, and difficult to see, frequently being mistaken for dandruff. They are laid at the base of the hair strand and hatch within approximately 7–10 days. The empty nits remain attached to the hair strand as it grows out from the scalp.

Nymphs (immature lice): These are the size of a pinhead when they hatch from the nits, and look like small adults. They mature into adults after three moults, which takes approximately –9–12 days (Eberhard et al, 2008). For pubic lice the nymphal stage is longer at 13–17 days.

Adult lice: These are about the same size as a sesame seed, tan to greyish-white in colour, with hook-like claws on the legs to enable them to hold onto the hair tightly. The female is larger than the male and lays up to eight nits a day. Adults mature after 10 days and live for about 30 days (http://cks.nice.org.uk/head-lice).

Lice risk factors / occurrence

Lice occur worldwide.

Head lice: are more common in preschool and primary school children and their families (http://cks.nice.org.uk/head-lice).

Body lice: are prevalent among populations with poor personal hygiene, especially in cold climates where heavy clothing is worn, bathing infrequent and people cannot change clothes, e.g. refugees (Eberhard et al, 2008).

Pubic lice: are most frequently acquired through sexual contact with an infested person and are common among young adults.

Mode of transmission

Head lice: cannot jump or fly so the rate of transmission is low as infection only occurs when heads come into *direct, prolonged contact* with an infested person.

Body lice: Transmission occurs during direct contact with an infested person or *indirect* contact with their personal belongings, especially clothing and headgear (Eberhard et al, 2008).

Pubic lice: Transmission occurs by close physical contact, which can be from sexual contact or close family contact, such as from infested beard or chest (http://cks.nice.org.uk/head-lice).

Clinical signs and symptoms

Head lice: rarely cause any problem other than an itchy scalp. Individuals with lice sometimes feel a tickling or itching or feeling of something moving in the hair.

Body lice: Small red lumps/bluish spots may occur, although there may not be any symptoms. In some people itching at night may occur and minute dark-brown specks of louse excreta may sometimes be seen on the skin and underwear.

Pubic lice: Similar symptoms to body lice, although the itching is usually intense.

Complications

Head lice: There are no serious complications, although sores can develop due to scratching and becoming infected.

Body lice: can spread epidemic typhus, trench fever, and louse-borne relapsing fever.

Pubic lice: Secondary infections caused by scratching may lead to impetigo or **furunculosis**, and **blepharitis**, **conjunctivitis** or corneal epithelial **keratitis** if the eyelashes are infested (http://cks.nice.org.uk/pubic-lice).

Diagnosis

Head lice: Made if a living, moving louse is found. NB: Lice become dormant when wet, but start to move after two minutes as they dry out.

Body lice: Confirmed by finding adult lice or viable eggs in the seams of the clothing.

Pubic lice: Made by finding a live louse or nits in the pubic region (rarely at other sites), usually with the aid of a magnifying lens (http://cks.nice.org.uk/pubic-lice).

Treatment

Recommended treatments for all forms of lice can be found in the NICE Guidelines, which clearly state the suitability of each, including which treatments are not suitable for key groups of people such as children and pregnant women. All treatments require more than one treatment session to be successful (see Figures 34.5, 34.6, 34.7, 34.8 and 34.9).

Head lice: Treatment should only be commenced if a live head louse is found. The hair should be clean and dry before applying treatment (free from chlorine, conditioner, gels and mousse) and left to dry naturally. All affected household members are treated *simultaneously*.

Body lice: No treatment is required because the lice are easily eradicated if clothing is not worn for *at least* 3 days. Referral to a dermatologist is advised.

Pubic lice: Treatment is as per NICE Guidelines. Eyelash infestation should be treated with an occlusive ophthalmic ointment / topical insecticide. Referral to a genitourinary medicine (GUM) clinic is advised.

Infection prevention and control precautions

Head lice: Isolation / exclusion from school is *not* required, except on paediatric wards when close contact between children may transmit the lice.

Body lice: Isolation is required only until the clothing and bedding has been removed. People with body lice should *not* be nursed on oncology wards.

Pubic lice: Isolation is not required.

35 Influenza

Figure 35.1 Influenza

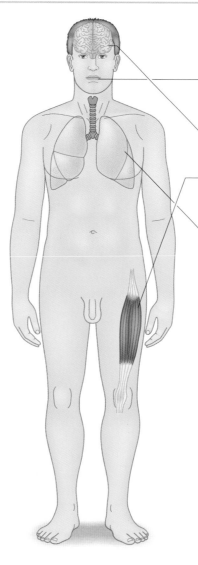

Box 1 At risk individuals eligible for the influenza vaccine. Reference: PHE, 2013h

- People aged 65 and over (including those becoming 65 by 1 March 2015)
- Children aged 2, 3 or 4 (but not 5 years or older) on or before 1 September 2014
- Children aged 6 months or older
- Pregnant women (including women who become pregnant during the flu season)
- Chronic respiratory disease (i.e. asthma, bronchitis, chronic obstructive pulmonary disease)
- Chronic heart disease
- Chronic kidney disease
- Chronic neurological disease (e.g. Parkinson's disease, motor neurone disease)
- Diabetes
- Asplenia, splenic dysfunction
- Immunosuppressed (due to illness/ treatment)
- Residents of long-term care facilities
- Healthcare staff

Box 4 Prevention and treatment Reference: PHE, 2015c

Vaccination campaign – for the public and for healthcare workers

Public health/awareness campaign – good respiratory hygiene
- Cover the mouth when coughing/sneezing
- Use disposable tissues and dispose of them appropriately
- Hand hygiene

Anti-viral agents for the treatment of seasonal influenza in patients at risk of complications, or for the purpose of prophylaxis. **Oseltamivir** (Tamiflu) and **zanimivir** (Relenza) are neuraminidase inhibitors, and block the release of the virus from infected cells. Their early use is recommended in the treatment of proven or suspected seasonal influenza in 'at risk' individuals, and those who are 'considerably unwell', even if they are not in an 'at risk' group.

Oseltamivir – first-line treatment, orally twice daily for 5 days; should commence within 48 hours of onset of symptoms, and may reduce the risk of severe illness up to five days after the onset of symptoms.
Zanimivir – inhaler; twice daily for up to 10 days; prescribed if poor clinical response to oseltamivir.

Box 2 Clinical features

Abrupt onset; incubation period 24–48 hours

Upper respiratory tract
- Initial symptoms of dry cough and pharyngeal pain
- More systemic signs develop within 6–12 hours

Central nervous system
- Fever (intermittently for 4–6 days) and rigors
- Headache

Musculoskeletal
- Myalgia – commonly affecting the long muscles of the back and calves, and may also involve the muscles of the eyes; severity of symptoms related to the height of the fever

Upper and lower respiratory tract
- Signs of both lower and upper respiratory tract infection – respiratory symptoms tend to become dominant by the fourth day of illness
- Recovery generally starts after a week but may take several weeks

Box 3 Complications
References: Sutherland, 2007; Rothberg et al, 2008; Ahmad et al, 2010b

Respiratory tract
- Primary influenza pneumonia
- Secondary bacterial pneumonia ('super-infection')
- Exacerbation of chronic underlying respiratory disease

Cardiovascular system
- Pericarditis
- Myocarditis
- Exacerbation of chronic underlying cardiac disease

Central nervous system
- Encephalopathy
- Aseptic meningitis
- Transverse myelitis
- Guillain–Barré syndrome

Box 5 Infection control management

The isolation of patients admitted to hospital with seasonal influenza, or complications associated with influenza, is not routinely indicated. However, if a single room is available, and the onset of the patient's primary symptoms is within 7 days of admission, isolation may be recommended by the IP&CT to prevent the spread of influenza to susceptible patients. Standard IP&C precautions should be implemented, with particular attention to hand decontamination, cleaning (the environment and equipment), and good respiratory hygiene among patients and staff. Staff should not work if they have symptoms that are suggestive of a respiratory tract infection.

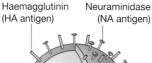

Haemagglutinin (HA antigen)   Neuraminidase (NA antigen)

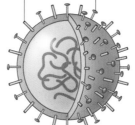

Influenza A virus

Infection Prevention and Control at a Glance, First Edition. By Debbie Weston, Alison Burgess and Sue Roberts.
© 2017 John Wiley & Sons, Ltd. Published 2017 by John Wiley & Sons, Ltd.

The World Health Organization (WHO) estimates that there are 3–5 million severe cases of influenza, globally, each year, and 250 000–500 000 deaths (https://www.who.int). In the UK alone, 10–15 % of the population are affected each year, with 12 000 deaths, predominantly among the elderly and those with pre-existing respiratory disease.

The influenza virus

The influenza virus belongs to the family Orthomyxoviridae (*myxo* is Greek for mucus and refers to the ability of the virus to adhere to mucoproteins on the host respiratory cell; *ortho* = true or regular) (Collier et al, 2011c). Influenza viruses have an amazing ability to change their genetic make-up and essentially recreate themselves, and they have been described as 'the chameleons of the microbial world' (Department of Health, 2002). There are three serotypes. **Influenza A** viruses are promiscuous and highly unpredictable (WHO, 2005). Although mostly prevalent among humans, they also circulate among many mammalian and avian species and it is this ability to jump the species barrier that makes this serotype the biggest threat in terms of the evolution of new influenza viruses and a potential influenza pandemic (see Chapter 41). **Influenza B** can cause severe disease in the 'at risk' groups, and **influenza C** causes mild disease throughout the year, but neither of these serotypes has been linked to previous pandemics.

The virus is covered with surface projections or spikes that consist of two types of antigen – HA antigen and NA antigen (see Figure 35.1). **HA antigen (haemagglutinin)** plays an important role in initiating infection by enabling the virus to attach to receptor sites on the respiratory cell surface in the host. **NA antigens (neuraminidase)** assist fusion of the viral cell envelope with the surface of the host respiratory cell and aid the release of newly formed virus particles from infected cells, which go on to enter and replicate within other cells (Ahmad et al, 2010b).

Influenza A and antigenic drift and shift

Influenza A consists of eight segments of viral RNA and is the only influenza virus that is broken down into subtypes dependent upon its HA and NA antigens. There are at least 16 different and antigenically distinct HAs (H1 to H16) and 9 NAs (N1 to N9), of which H1, H2, H3, H5 and N1, N2 and N9 are the most medically significant (Collier et al, 2011c).

Influenza viruses are able to mutate and swap genes, undergoing frequent changes which may be due to minor point mutations, deletions and insertions in their surface HA and / or NA antigens (antigenic drift) (Nash et al, 2015), or major (antigenic shift). All 16 HA and 9 NA antigens are present in the avian influenza viruses that circulate among migratory swans, ducks and geese, often asymptomatically (Collier et al, 2011c). The significance of avian influenza A viruses is explained in Chapter 41.

Antigenic drift, caused by a single mutation in the viral RNA, occurs constantly among influenza A viruses and is responsible for annual epidemics, with new strains emerging every year. Generally with antigenic drift there is some kind of serological relationship between new and the old HA and NA antigens, so although the virus is 'drifting' and changing subtly, it does not differ too drastically from previous strains. Some of the population will have immunity to the virus and vaccination is an effective preventative measure in those who have no immunity or are in one of the 'at risk' categories.

Antigenic shift poses much more of a problem. Major changes to gene segments on the surface antigens lead to the creation of a 'new' virus and ultimately give rise to a pandemic. As the population will not have previously been exposed to this virus in any shape or form, no preventative vaccine will have been developed and immunity will be virtually non-existent (i.e. the population will be 'immunologically naïve').

Vaccination

The World Health Organization (WHO) decides on the composition of the annual seasonal flu vaccine based on an analysis of virus strains in the Influenza Reference Laboratories in London, Atlanta, Melbourne and Tokyo. The vaccine, offered to individuals in the 'at risk' categories, consists of two subtypes of an influenza A virus (H1N1 and H3N2), and an influenza B virus. Full details on the annual vaccination programme are published in the UK by Public Health England / Department of Health / NHS England, the Centers for Disease Control and Prevention (Atlanta), and the World Health Organization. These plans also include strategies for increasing vaccine uptake among healthcare workers, who have a duty of care towards their patients.

The vaccine matches the circulating strains as closely as possible. However, antigenic drift can cause problems, as seen during the 2014–2015 influenza season, when surveillance in December 2014 identified that 52% of the circulating A/H3N2 viruses had actually drifted away from the vaccine strain. The drifted A/H3N2 strains became the dominant influenza strains, with a higher proportion of H3N2 in circulation over H1N, and affected vaccine efficacy (European Centre for Disease Prevention and Control, 2014).

The pathogenesis of infection

Influenza is transmitted from person to person by respiratory aerosols and droplets. Depending upon the size of the inhaled virus particles, they are either deposited on the mucous membrane lining the respiratory tract, where they destroy the cilia on the epithelial cells within the noses and sinuses (Collier et al, 2011c), or they directly enter the alveoli (Sutherland, 2007). Viral replication occurs within hours, causing functional and structural damage to the cells and releasing virus particles into the airways which go on to infect neighbouring cells (Ahmad et al, 2010b). The damage to the respiratory epithelium initiates an acute inflammatory response, impairing both mechanical and cellular host responses and giving rise to the classic 'flu-like' symptoms.

Risk factors, clinical features, complications, prevention, treatment, and infection control management

See Figure 35.1.

36 Invasive group A streptococcal disease

Figure 36.1 Invasive group A streptococcal infection

Necrotising fasciitis (NF)

Risk factors:
- Underlying medical condition; **increasing age**; renal disease; peripheral vascular disease; underlying malignancy; malnutrition; obesity; varicella infection (see Chapter 45); anti-inflammatory non-steroidal medication; **abdominal or perineal surgery**; incarcerated hernia; **trauma to the extremities** – burns, lacerations, IV drug abuse, animal and insect bites; blunt trauma

Clinical features:
- Localised erythema at the site of infection – may be mistaken for cellulitis
- Prodromal flu-like illness at the onset (headache, temperature, muscular aches and pain) – NF may be misdiagnosed at this stage
- **Local severe pain that does not support the clinical findings (a defining symptom)** (Hasham et al, 2005)
- **Spreading diffuse erythema** over the next 24–72 hours, which should be a warning sign if antibiotics have been commenced; skin becomes smooth, shiny and intensely swollen
- Pain is replaced by numbness as the nerves within the fascia are destroyed
- Skin begins to darken within the area of erythema, which may be spreading by 3–5 cm/hour
- Skin becomes dusky blue with blistering due to necrosis of the superficial fascia and fat
- Skin becomes gangrenous and starts to slough – a large area of the skin/body may be affected by this stage
- Patient displays signs of extreme system toxicity as organisms and toxins are released into the bloodstream – may lead to multi-organ failure secondary to overwhelming sepsis

Infection prevention and control precautions
- Standard precautions, with particular attention to hand hygiene and PPE as appropriate
- For NF – isolation in a single room until all necrotic tissue has been debrided

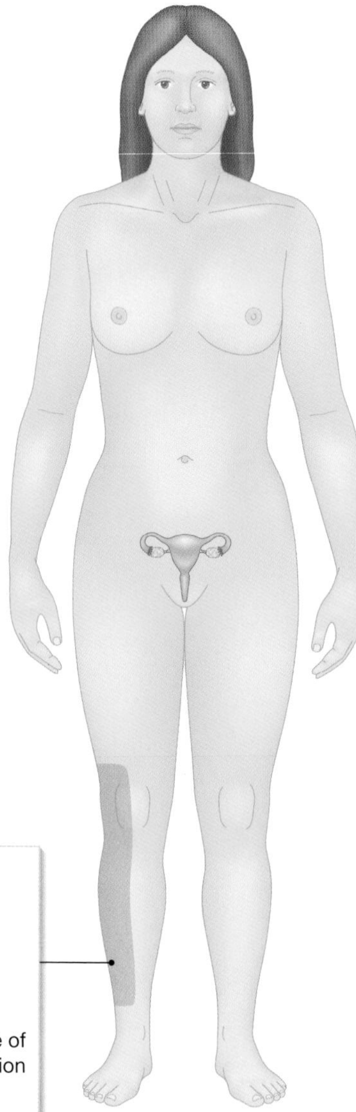

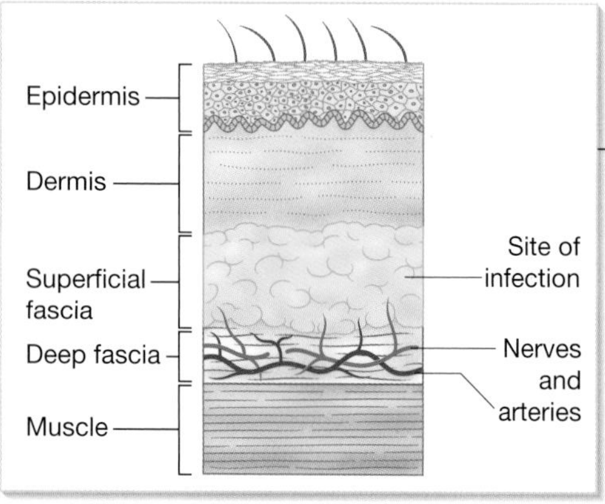

Streptococcal toxic shock syndrome

Risk factors:
- Can affect any age group with or without any underlying medical condition (i.e. 'healthy' individuals)
- Can occur following 'routine' surgery (i.e. hernia repair; vasectomy); childbirth; meningitis; otitis media; urinary and respiratory tract infections; septic arthritis; bacteraemia associated with central venous access devices; blunt trauma

Clinical features:
- May be evidence/history of minor skin or blunt force trauma (pain may be a feature) – increases the risk of NF; or recent illness
- Prodromal flu-like illness in approximately 20% of patients (high fever, chills, muscular aches and pain, vomiting and diarrhoea), along with signs of confusion
- Hypotension/signs of septic shock (see Chapter 25)
- Diffuse erythematous rash

Puerperal sepsis

Risk factors:
- Caesarean section
- Prolonged membrane rupture
- Prolonged labour
- Post-partum haemorrhage
- Retained placental fragments
- Poor nutritional state
- Anaemia

Clinical features (WHO, 2008):
- Fever/rigors (persistent spiking temperature suggests abscess)
- Diarrhoea or vomiting
- Breast engorgement/redness
- Rash (generalised maculopapular rash)
- Abdominal/pelvic pain and tenderness
- Wound infection – spreading cellulitis or discharge
- Offensive vaginal discharge
- Productive cough
- Urinary symptoms
- Delay in uterine involution, heavy lochia
- General – non-specific signs such as lethargy, reduced appetite

GAS Investigations
FBC; U&Es; LFTs; blood cultures; arterial blood gas; renal function; clotting screen; glucose; swabs for culture from any wounds/skin lesions, and sites of invasive devices; specimens from any sites of surgical exploration/debridement

Epidermis

Dermis

Superficial fascia

Deep fascia

Muscle

Site of infection

Nerves and arteries

Infection Prevention and Control at a Glance, First Edition. By Debbie Weston, Alison Burgess and Sue Roberts.
© 2017 John Wiley & Sons, Ltd. Published 2017 by John Wiley & Sons, Ltd.

Group A streptococcus (GAS), also known as *Streptococcus pyogenes*, is one of the most prevalent human pathogens. Historically, it was the cause of 'childbed fever' or **puerperal sepsis** (which remains a leading global cause of maternal death), and it is responsible for a wide range of suppurative infections in the upper respiratory tract, where it is the commonest bacterial cause of sore throats, tonsillitis and scarlet fever, skin infections (such as cellulitis and impetigo), and **invasive life-threatening soft tissue infections**.

Invasive GAS is 'illness associated with the isolation of GAS from a normally sterile body site (i.e. blood; CSF; joint aspirate; pericardial / peritoneal fluids; bone; endometrium; deep tissue or abscess at operation or post-mortem) or associated with necrotising soft tissue infection, or isolated from a non-sterile body site in combination with **necrotising fasciitis** or **streptococcal toxic shock syndrome**' (Steer et al, 2012).

Transmission of GAS can occur within healthcare settings between:
- mother and baby (between 2 and 11% of all severe GAS infections are associated with childbirth)
- patient and close personal contacts
- patient and healthcare worker
- patient and patient
- healthcare worker and patient.

National *Guidelines for prevention and control of group A streptococcal infection in acute healthcare and maternity settings* were published by Steer et al in 2012 (www.his.org.uk/files/5813/7398/0836/Guidelines_for_prevention_and_control_of_group_A_streptococcal_infection_in_acute_healthcare_and_maternity_settings_in_the_UK_a.pdf).

The organism

There are 40 species of streptococci, which are anaerobic, Gram-positive, catalase-negative cocci occurring in pairs or chains. They exist as **commensal** flora in the mucous membranes of the upper respiratory tract and also **colonise** the bowel (enterococci). They are classified according to their ability to cause haemolysis of red blood cells on agar, and their antigenic characteristics (**Lancefield antigens**), which are based upon the C-carbohydrate in the bacterial cell wall.

The cell wall accounts for many of the organism's virulence factors associated with colonisation and evasion of phagocytosis and host immune responses. **Fimbriae** (see Chapter 4) facilitate adherence to host cells and contain **M proteins**, which are strongly anti-phagocytic. **Hyaluronic acid** is a component of the bacterial capsule that is chemically identical to the hyaluronic acid found in connective tissue and 'hides' the organism from the effects of the immune response. **Acids and proteins** facilitate adherence to host tissues and membranes, enabling the bacterium to colonise or invade a portal of entry.

Other proteins aid invasiveness and spread to other areas of the body, killing host cells and initiating an inflammatory response which in turn stimulates the immune response to release cytokines (see Chapter 7), causing shock and tissue injury. **Hyaluronidase**, known as the original 'spreading factor', facilitates the spread of infection along fascial planes, and **haemolysins** (streptolysins O and S) damage cell membranes. **Enzymes** (hyaluronidase, deoxyribonucleases and streptokinase) facilitate the spread of the organism through the tissues (Burton and Duben-Engelkirk, 2004). Ten per cent of GAS produce **superantigen toxins (StrepSAgs)**, which have a profound effect on the immune response (Ryan and Drew, 2010b).

Puerperal sepsis

Puerperal sepsis is any bacterial infection of the genital reproductive tract that commonly occurs after childbirth or miscarriage. The separation of the placenta from the wall of the uterus leaves behind a large raw area of tissue that is a prime breeding ground for GAS, particularly as it has a rich blood supply. This not only encourages bacterial growth but also facilitates their spread into the bloodstream (WHO, 2005). Tears sustained during delivery, including episiotomy, are also a route of entry. Signs and symptoms usually become evident more than 24 hours post delivery, although they can become apparent earlier if there has been prolonged rupture of membranes or prolonged labour without antibiotics. **Risk factors and clinical features are described in Figure 36.1.**

Necrotising fasciitis (NF)

Necrotising fasciitis is a potentially fatal, devastating and rapidly progressive infection of the fascia and deeper subcutaneous tissues. *S. pyogenes* is responsible for 15% of all cases of NF, although it can be polymicrobial. Symptoms may develop over a period of hours to several days. In the 50% of patients without a defined portal of entry, the infection begins deep in the skin, often at the site of a traumatic joint injury, muscular strain or haematoma. **Risk factors and clinical features are described in Figure 36.1.**

Although medical imaging may identify localised swelling of the deep structures and gas in the soft tissues, urgent aggressive and extensive surgical debridement, requiring more than one episode of surgical intervention, is essential. Post-operative dressing changes may need to be undertaken under general anaesthetic, and vacuum-assisted skin closure (VAC) may be required, along with skin grafting and reconstructive surgery. Patients will require intravenous fluid resuscitation, mechanical ventilation and inotropic support in order to manage septic shock. Broad spectrum antibiotic therapy should be initiated at the onset of symptoms, covering Gram-positive cocci, facultative anaerobic Gram-negative rods and anaerobes. Benzylpenicillin and clindamycin are effective against Gram-positive cocci. Flucloxacillin is effective against *Staphylococcus aureus*. Gentamicin is a potent broad spectrum antibiotic in its own right but has a synergistic effect if given in combination with penicillin. Metronidazole is effective against anaerobic bacteria. The antibiotic regimen can be modified once the results of blood and wound cultures are known.

Streptococcal toxic shock syndrome (STSS)

Streptococcal toxic shock syndrome, which first emerged in the 1980s (Ryan and Drew, 2010 b), is any streptococcal infection associated with the sudden onset of shock and multi-organ failure, with or without necrotising fasciitis. Some patients may present only with overwhelming septic shock (see Chapter 25) and die within 24–48 hours of admission. Patients who present with profound septic shock and organ dysfunction should always be carefully examined for a portal of entry, and appropriate cultures taken. As with NF, intensive therapy unit support will be required, along with broad spectrum empirical antibiotic therapy. **Risk factors and clinical features are described in Figure 36.1.**

37 Legionella

Figure 37.1 Legionella

Box 1 Host risk factors for the development of Legionnaires' disease

- Smoking – damage to innate immune response (see Chapter 6)
- Age > 40 years
- Immunocompromised through underlying illness

Of the 286 confirmed and presumptive cases reported in 2013:
- 42 had diabetes
- 59 had underlying heart disease
- 36 had respiratory conditions
- 77 were smokers

Box 2 Index of suspicion and diagnosis

Suspect Legionnaires' disease if:
- Failure to respond to treatment for CAP
- Symptoms of 'pneumonia' are severe enough to require admission to ITU
- Age > 40
- Smoker
- Immunocompromised – underlying illness/disease (Garbino et al, 2004)

Discuss with consultant medical microbiologist – urine for Legionella antigen (rapid detection of Legionella antigen in the urine directs appropriate antibiotic use)

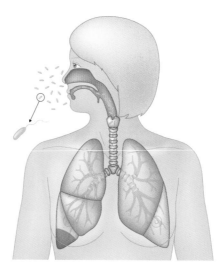

Box 3 Incubation period and clinical features

- Incubation: 2–10 days
- Prodromal illness (lasts hours to days): headache (may be severe), fever with rigors, myalgia, loss of appetite, diarrhoea and abdominal pain
- Cough (develops after the prodrome)
- May complain of pleuritic chest pain and haemoptysis
- Chest x-ray – may be normal in the early stages but changes seen when repeated: patchy infiltrates or multiple areas of consolidation
- Beware differential diagnoses:
  - influenza
  - gastrointestinal infection
  - subarachnoid haemorrhage

Box 4 Treatment/management

Supportive care in ITU may be required for severe cases

Quinolone antibiotics such as levofloxacin, and macrolides such as azithromycin and clarithromycin may be used, sometimes in combination with rifampicin, according to local prescribing guidelines

Box 5 Considerations in the investigation of a confirmed case of Legionnaires' Disease

1. Patient admitted with 'community-acquired pneumonia'
- Establish travel history within the 10–14 days prior to the onset of illness, particularly travel abroad for business or holiday (i.e. type of accommodation; whether there was an air conditioning unit in the room/building; use of leisure facilities/spa; proximity to water cooling tower)
- Consider workplace exposure
- Recreational activities: use of gym/whirlpool/spa bath
- Domestic: home hot and cold water systems
- Have there been any atypical respiratory illnesses within the locality?

The local Environmental Health Team, in conjunction with Public Health England, will undertake water sampling.

2. Patient with 'hospital-acquired pneumonia' who has been an inpatient for more than 10 days
- Location of the patient (ward/bay/single room): if in a bay, which toilet, bathroom shower would s/he have used? Has the patient been on more than one ward? Urgent sampling of water outlets within the patient's environment will need to be undertaken by the Estates Departments
- Has the patient used a spa bath, hydrotherapy pool or respiratory therapy equipment? Investigations will need to be undertaken into how these are decontaminated

If the strain of Legionella isolated from the patient matches those from water sources/outlets either in the community or in the hospital/healthcare environment, outbreak control meetings will be held. The Health and Safety Executive (HSE) will need to be informed, and urgent actions will be implemented in order to safeguard the public and ensure compliance with L8.

Infection Prevention and Control at a Glance, First Edition. By Debbie Weston, Alison Burgess and Sue Roberts.
© 2017 John Wiley & Sons, Ltd. Published 2017 by John Wiley & Sons, Ltd.

Legionella is a water-borne pathogen and a natural inhabitant of natural aquatic environments and artificial / man-made water systems. It was first identified in 1976 following an outbreak of atypical pneumonia among American ex-servicemen attending a reunion of the American Legion at a hotel in Philadelphia, affecting 221 people and killing 34. The culprit was *Legionella pneumophila*, and the infection was named Legionnaires' disease. It is one of the causes of community-acquired pneumonia (CAP) (see Chapter 32), carries a mortality rate of 5–30%, and has caused several notable outbreaks involving the headquarters of the BBC, London (1981), a hospital (Stafford General Hospital, UK, 1985), a city (Murcia, Spain, 2001) and an arts complex (Barrow-in-Furness, UK, 2002). It became a notifiable disease in 2010, and in 2013 there were 284 confirmed cases, of which 191 were attributed to exposure in the community, 88 to travel abroad, and 5 associated with exposure within a healthcare setting (PHE, 2013i).

The organism

Legionella are motile, aerobic, Gram-negative bacilli, of which there are more than 45 species and more than 60 serogroups; 18 of these are **opportunistic** human **pathogens**, and *Legionella pneumophila* serogroup 1 accounts for more than 80% of infections. **Virulence** factors (see Chapter 4) include pili, which promote attachment to the macrophages and epithelial cells, flagella which aid motility and promote invasion, and lipopolysaccharide (LPS), which is an endotoxin. Legionella often grow in a **biofilm** with other aquatic bacteria and may be ingested by free-living amoeba in which they survive and grow as intracellular parasites. They thrive in water temperatures of 20–50 °C, particularly in water that is stagnant or where the water supply is disrupted, but cannot withstand temperatures higher than 60 °C. Environments that support the growth of Legionella include rivers, lakes and ponds; air conditioning systems; domestic hot water systems; air humidifiers; architectural / decorative fountains; whirlpool spa baths; ice making machines; shower heads and respiratory therapy equipment. As well as Legionnaires' disease, Legionella can also cause a milder, non-pneumonia respiratory illness called **Pontiac fever**.

The pathogenesis of infection

Although they are **ubiquitous** organisms, Legionella are opportunistic bacteria and only cause infection in susceptible individuals where the right individual and environmental conditions come together.

- **Virulent** strains of bacteria must be present within an environment that supports their survival and multiplication.
- The infectious dose must be transmitted via a virulent aerosol.
- The aerosol must be inhaled by a susceptible individual.

The bacteria are present in water-borne particles suspended in the air as an aerosol. A water droplet containing a single Legionella bacterium will remain suspended in the air for long periods of time and can travel considerable distances in suitable air conditions, where it can enter the air conditioning and ventilation systems of buildings.

Following inhalation of a contaminated aerosol, the bacterium enters the lung, where it is phagocytosed by alveolar macrophages (see Chapter 6). The bacteria replicate within the macrophages, destroy them and escape, and are re-phagocytosed by other macrophages. This process of re-amplification increases the concentration of bacteria within the lungs, which become flooded with an inflammatory exudate. In spite of this, there is generally little sputum production (Hood and Edwards, 2007). The inflammatory process triggers the release of cytokines and chemokines from the infected macrophages and, in conjunction with the bacteria's virulence factors, triggers a severe immune response.

Figure 37.1 describes host risk factors, the incubation period and clinical features, and the diagnosis and treatment of Legionnaires' disease, along with considerations in the investigation of a confirmed case.

The prevention and control of Legionella

- Compliance with Legionella control is a statutory requirement under The Health and Safety at Work Act (1974), Control of Substances Hazardous to Health (COSHH) Regulations (1988), Public Health (Infectious Diseases) Regulations (1988), and Water Quality Regulations (1989 and 1991).
- *The control of legionella bacteria in water systems: Approved Code of Practice and guidance* (L8) (Health and Safety Executive, 2013) applies to any premises / work activity where water is stored or used, or where there is a means of creating and transmitting water droplets that may be inhaled.
- In June 2014, following the death of a neonate, Public Health England and NHS England issued a Patient Safety Alert (Public Health England/NHS England, 2014), warning of the risk of Legionella infection from birthing pools *filled in advance of labour in home setting*s **and** *where the water temperature is maintained by use of a heater and a pump*. If Legionella is present in the pool pump equipment or the domestic supply, the warm water in the heated pool provides ideal growth conditions, potentially over several weeks.
- **Within healthcare settings**, **basic actions** to reduce the risk of outbreaks of Legionnaires' disease include:
  - the removal of any redundant pipework, which serve as 'dead-legs'
  - the running of *all* water outlets (taps, baths, showers, toilet cistern flushes) daily, particularly in areas such as unoccupied side rooms, or infrequently used bathrooms, examination / treatment rooms)
  - where spa baths are used (e.g. ARJO), disinfecting the bath as per the manufacturer's instructions (i.e. twice daily when not in use, and in between every episode of patient use)
  - disconnecting toilets, showers and baths that are no longer in use
  - using automatic self-purging showers that run for several minutes a day
  - replacing old pipework.

NB: Legionella infection is **not** transmissible between infected individuals, and hospital patients with Legionnaires' disease do not require isolation in a single room.

38 Measles, mumps and rubella

Figure 38.1 Presentation of measles

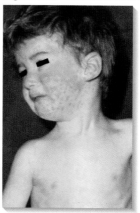

Source: U.S. Centers for Disease Control and Prevention; photo credit: Brian W. J. Mahy

Figure 38.4 Presentation of mumps

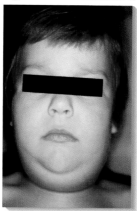

Source: U.S. Centers for Disease Control and Prevention; photo credit: Patricia Smith, Barbara Rice

Figure 38.7 Presentation of rubella

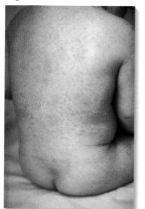

Source: U.S. Centers for Disease Control and Prevention; photo credit: CDC

Figure 38.2 Characteristics of measles

- Measles (*rubeola* means 'red' in Latin)
- Acute viral illness, **highly infectious** disease
- Genus: Morbillivirus
- Family: Paramyxoviridae
- RNA virus – single strand, negative sense
- Enveloped
- Shape: pleomorphic
- Size: 120–250 nm
- Nucleocapsid helical
- Lifelong immunity after infection
- Pathogenesis: The virus enters the body through the respiratory tract or conjunctiva of eyes. The virus then spreads rapidly to the lymph nodes, and throughout the body

Source: Mims et al, 2004g; 2004h; Prescott et al, 2005c

Figure 38.5 Characteristics of mumps

- An acute viral illness
- Genus: Rubulavirus
- Family: Paramyxoviridae
- RNA virus – single strand, negative sense
- Enveloped
- Shape: pleomorphic
- Size: 120–250 nm
- Nucleocapsid helical
- Lifelong immunity
- Pathogenesis: The virus enters the body via the respiratory tract

Source: Mims et al, 2004g; 2004i; Prescott et al, 2005c

Figure 38.8 Characteristics of rubella

- Rubella (from the Latin *rubellus*, meaning 'reddish')
- A mild viral illness
- Genus: Rubivirus
- Family: Togaviridae
- RNA – single strand, positive sense
- Enveloped
- Shape: spherical
- Size: 60–70 nm
- Nucleocapsid icosahedral
- Not as infectious as measles but more infectious than mumps

Source: Mims et al, 2004g; 2004h; Prescott et al, 2005c

Figure 38.3 Measles – clinical features

Prodromal symptoms:
- Fever
- Malaise
- Coryza (inflammation of mucous membranes → cold symptoms)
- Conjunctivitis: red, watery eyes
- Cough
- Rash develops over 3 days – erythematous, *maculopapular*. Starts at the head and spreads to the trunk and limbs
- Koplik's spots (small red spots with bluish centre) may be present on mucous membranes of mouth 1–2 days before rash appears

Figure 38.6 Mumps – clinical features

Prodromal symptoms a few days before the parotid glands swell include:
- Fever of 38°C (100.4°F) or above, headache, malaise, myalgias anorexia, joint pain, nausea, dry mouth, abdominal pain

Then:

- Swelling of the parotid the most common symptom – usually bilateral but may be unilateral

Figure 38.9 Rubella – clinical features

Prodromal symptoms:
- Low-grade fever
- Malaise
- Coryza
- Mild conjunctivitis
- Enlarged lymph nodes often evident behind the ear (may precede rash)
- Rash usually transitory: Irregular *maculopapular*, lasting 3 days

Figure 38.10 Infection prevention and control precautions

In hospital
Isolation with *standard precautions* until no longer infectious (local policies may vary).
Risk assessment of all patients and staff exposed to the case.
For susceptible measles contacts, MMR and/or HNIG may be required. Non-immune staff may need to be excluded (as per PHE guidance).

In the community
Measles/rubella: Exclusion from school/nursery/work until 4 days from the onset of the rash.
Mumps: Exclusion until parotid (salivary) glands have gone down – 5 days from onset of swelling.

Infection Prevention and Control at a Glance, First Edition. By Debbie Weston, Alison Burgess and Sue Roberts.
© 2017 John Wiley & Sons, Ltd. Published 2017 by John Wiley & Sons, Ltd.

Measles, mumps and rubella, whilst often mild diseases in childhood, can nevertheless cause **serious complications** in vulnerable individuals. **Measles**, in particular, one of the most highly communicable infectious diseases, has a high **morbidity** and **mortality** rate in less well developed countries than the UK. **Mumps** can cause unpleasant complications in adults, and **rubella** whilst rare, is well known for the serious complications it causes in the first trimester of pregnancy (PHE, 2013j). The introduction of the MMR vaccine in 1988 initially led to a large reduction in cases of these diseases. Since then, however, there has been an increase in the number of cases due to different factors, not least the fear generated following publication of research undertaken by Andrew Wakefield regarding the suggested risk of autism and bowel disease in association with the MMR vaccination. Although this research was discredited it led to a reduced uptake of the vaccine. All three of these diseases are **notifiable** (see Chapter 2). Further information on national figures can be found on the Public Health England website (www.gov.uk/topic/health-protection/infectious-diseases).

Measles
Mode of transmission, incubation period and clinical features

Measles is spread by airborne or droplet transmission through coughing and sneezing or close personal contact with infected nasal or throat secretions (i.e. more than 15 minutes in direct contact with someone infected) (PHE, 2013j).

The incubation period of measles ranges from 7 to 18 days but is on average 10–12 days after exposure. The affected individual is infectious from 4 days before the onset of the rash to 4 days after (PHE, 2013j). Figures 38.1, 38.2 and 38.3 describe the clinical appearance of measles, the characteristics of the measles virus and clinical features.

Complications

The most common complications of measles are as follows: ear infections (otitis media) 7–9%, pneumonia 1–6%, severe diarrhoea and dehydration 8% and, less commonly, convulsions (1 in 100 cases). A rare complication is **encephalitis** (1 in 1000 cases), and very rare is **subacute sclerosing panencephalitis**. Death occurs in 1 in 5000 cases (high in children < 1, lower in children between the ages of 1 and 9, and higher in teenagers and adults). Complications are more common and more severe in malnourished, chronically ill and immunocompromised children (PHE, 2013j).

Mumps
Mode of transmission, incubation period and clinical features

Mumps is spread through direct contact with respiratory secretions or saliva or through fomites. The incubation period ranges from 14 to 25 days after exposure but is on average 17 days. The affected individual is infectious from up to a week before to 5 days after the onset of the swelling. In approximately 1 in 3 cases, mumps does not cause any noticeable symptoms.

Figures 38.4, 38.5 and 38.6 describe the presentation of mumps, characteristics of the virus and clinical features.

Complications

Mumps is rarely fatal but it frequently affects the nervous system and complications may include viral meningitis, and encephalitis. Post puberty, 25% of men will develop orchitis (swelling of the testes) and deafness (bilateral or unilateral). **Nephritis** and cardiac abnormalities may also develop.

Rubella ('German measles')
Mode of transmission, incubation period and clinical features

Rubella is spread by airborne or droplet transmission. It is less contagious than measles but more so than mumps (Mims et al, 2004g). The incubation period ranges from 14 to 21 days, but is on average 14–17 days after exposure. Affected individuals are infectious for one week before symptoms appear to 4 days after the onset of the rash. Figures 38.7, 38.8 and 38.9 describe the presentation of rubella, characteristics of the virus and clinical features.

Complications

Complications include **thrombocytopenia** (estimated at 1 in 3000 infections) (PHE, 2013j) and post-infectious **encephalitis** (1 in 6000 cases). Adults may occasionally develop arthritis (which rarely becomes chronic) and **arthralgia**. Infection in pregnancy is particularly dangerous and may result in foetal loss or congenital rubella syndrome with one or more of the following: cataracts, deafness, cardiac abnormalities, retardation of intra-uterine growth, and inflammatory lesions of brain, liver, lungs and bone marrow (PHE, 2013j). **Infection in the first 8–10 weeks of pregnancy will lead to damage in 90% of surviving infants.**

Diagnosing measles, mumps and rubella

Diagnosis is made on clinical signs and symptoms. Oral fluid (saliva) testing is undertaken by Public Health England for every clinically suspected case of measles, mumps or rubella (as a means of surveillance) and sent to a PHE reference laboratory. Blood serum for IgM will also demonstrate IgM antibodies (see Chapter 7) and current infection.

Risk factors

Those most at risk of becoming infected with measles, mumps and rubella include unvaccinated individuals who have not received the MMR vaccine, or those who are partially vaccinated, infants too young to have received the first MMR, specific communities who choose not to be vaccinated, unvaccinated individuals living in undeveloped countries, unvaccinated pregnant women, and immuno-compromised individuals.

Treatment

There is no antiviral treatment available for these diseases. Most individuals recover with rest, and supportive treatment (hydration and antipyretics). Secondary infection may be treated with antibiotics. Following risk assessment, MMR vaccine may be offered as prophylaxis to measles contacts (within 72 hrs), and for future protection of unvaccinated individuals, and offered opportunistically to all unvaccinated contacts, but is contraindicated in pregnancy ('live' vaccine). Human normal immunoglobulin (HNIG) may be administered to some susceptible measles contacts e.g. immunocompromised, neonates, pregnant women, but is not given to mumps and rubella contacts as no proven benefit (PHE, 2013).

Prevention

The prevention of measles, mumps and rubella can be achieved by vaccination with the MMR vaccine (see Chapter 13), thus ensuring that a large number of the population are vaccinated which in turn prevents onward transmission to unvaccinated individuals (Herd immunity). Affected individuals should avoid contact with others until they are no longer infectious and receive MMR vaccine as soon as possible when clinically recovered.

Infection prevention and control

The recommended infection prevention and control precautions are described in Figure 38.10

39 Meningococcal disease

Figure 39.1 Meningococcal disease

Risk factors
- Smoking
- Residence in overcrowded houses/institutions (e.g. halls of residence)
- Travel to parts of the world where meningitis is *endemic*
- Age < 1 year
- Lack of immunity to circulating strains
- Recent influenza infection
- Complement deficiency

Prodromal illness
- Vomiting
- Diarrhoea
- Fever
- Muscle and joint pain
- Lethargy and headache

In newborn babies and infants non-specific symptoms may include:
- Fever
- Vomiting
- Diarrhoea
- Irritability
- Distress when handled
- Refusing feeds

Signs of meningococcal sepsis with/without meningitis
- Pallor
- Tachycardia
- Tachypnoea
- Cyanosis
- Rigors
- Cold extremities
- Altered mental state

Meningitis
- Severe headache
- Neck stiffness and *photophobia*

In babies neck stiffness and photophobia may be absent

Raised intracranial pressure (ICP)
- Headache
- Hypertension
- Tachycardia
- Fluctuating/decreasing level of consciousness
- Unequal, dilated or poorly reactive pupils
- *Papilloedema* (late sign)
- Bulging fontanelle in babies (late sign)

Non-blanching *petechial* rash
- Red or brown
- Pin prick/flea bites
- Purple blotches or bruises
- Profuse or scanty

Examine entire skin surface, including conjunctivae, palate of mouth, soles of feet

Investigations
- FBC, U&Es, blood glucose; send blood to the Meningococcal Reference Laboratory for typing
- Blood culture – Gram-negative diplococci
- CT head (rule out raised ICP)
- Lumbar puncture (NB: contraindicated in raised ICP):
  - CSF – turbid/purulent; Gram-negative diplococci; glucose < 40% of serum glucose; protein > 50 mg/dl; pressure > 25 cmH2O; raised neutrophils
  - Send CSF to the Meningococcal Reference Laboratory for typing
- Nasopharyngeal swab for meningococcal carriage
- Skin scraping or aspiration from petechial lesions

NB: Administration of benzylpenicillin **must not** be delayed in order to take blood and/or CSF

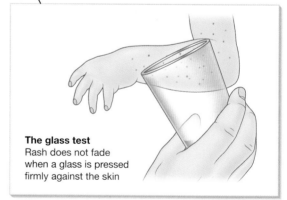

The glass test
Rash does not fade when a glass is pressed firmly against the skin

Infection Prevention and Control at a Glance, First Edition. By Debbie Weston, Alison Burgess and Sue Roberts.
© 2017 John Wiley & Sons, Ltd. Published 2017 by John Wiley & Sons, Ltd.

Invasive meningococcal disease, presenting as meningitis, septicaemia or both, has a dramatic clinical presentation and rapid disease progression. Annual rates of invasive disease in the UK are between 2 and 6 per 100 000 population, with a 10% case fatality (HPA, 2012e). Long-term complications for survivors include visual disturbances, hearing loss, limb amputation, seizures and brain damage. National guidance on the management on meningococcal disease is available from Public Health England / Department of Health ('The Green Book), and NICE at www.gov.uk/government/collections/immunisation-against-infectious-disease-the-green-book and www.nice.org.uk/guidance/cg102. **Meningococcal meningitis and septicaemia are notifiable diseases.**

The organism

Neisseria is the only pathogenic Gram-negative coccus and the bacterial cause of invasive meningococcal disease (*Neisseria meningitidis*, also known as the meningococcus) and gonorrhoea (*Neisseria gonorrhoeae*). It grows in pairs (diplococci), is bean-shaped and has concave sides facing inwards. The lipopolysaccharide (LPS) capsule is the most important virulence factor, and meningococci can be segregated into 13 different serogroups according to their capsular antigens (Ala' Aldeen, 2007); five are associated with invasive disease. The meningococcus produces lipid A (endotoxin) (see Chapter 4), and as the bacterial load in the bloodstream increases rapidly, lipid A is shed in large amounts from both living and dead bacteria. It causes the blood vessels to haemorrhage and is responsible for the petechial rash that develops, as well as septic shock (Ala' Aldeen, 2007)

Epidemiology

Meningococcal serogroups A, B and C have historically accounted for approximately 90% of cases. A and C in particular are associated with epidemics in the sub-Saharan meningitis belt (Africa), extending from Senegal to Ethiopia. Y accounts for very few cases in the UK. W-135 has caused international outbreaks, most notably among pilgrims attending the Hajj in Mecca. However, since 2009, there has been a continued increase in MenW cases in the UK due to clonal expansion of a single hypervirulent strain associated with **clonal** complex 11, which was previously associated with the large outbreak of MenC in the 1990s (PHE, 2015d). In the UK, babies and young children are vaccinated against MenC at 3 months (primary vaccine) and 12–13 months (booster). A second booster is given at the age of 13–15 and, as of 2014, to university students under the age of 25. Details of the vaccination programme, including the new MenB vaccine (developed but not at the time of writing on the immunisation schedule), are available at http://www.nhs.uk

The pathogenesis of infection
Carriage versus infection

The meningococcus is a normal inhabitant of the nasopharynx. Between 5 and 11% of adults, and up to 2% of adolescents, are estimated to have asymptomatic carriage, which is associated with the production of antibodies; systemic immunity develops within 14 days of acquisition. One per cent of the population are estimated to carry an invasive strain. Invasive disease primarily occurs in individuals who are newly 'infected' with the meningococcus or in carriers with weakened immune defences.

The incidence is highest in children under the age of 5, with peak incidence in those under the age of 1 year. Infants under 6 months of age are protected by maternal antibodies that cross the placenta during pregnancy. Infants and children lose this protection between 6 months and 2 years of age and are slow to develop their own antibodies. There is therefore a 'window period' in which they are at increased risk of infection. As the meningococcus inhabits the nasopharynx, it can be acquired through contact with oral and respiratory secretions (excluding saliva).

Meningitis

The blood–brain barrier (an intricate network of endothelial cells lining the small blood vessels of the brain) prevents the direct entry of microorganisms, because tight junctions between the endothelial cells prevent the free exchange of substances between the blood and the brain. However, if microorganisms have entered the circulation from other body sites, the central nervous system can be invaded. The meningococcus uses pili to attach to the microvilli of the non-ciliated epithelial cells on the nasopharyngeal surface. It then enters the microvilli, passing through the cell and into the submucosa. From there it is transported via the bloodstream to the ventricles of the brain where it directly infects the choroid plexus, which has an exceptionally high blood flow (Ryan and Drew, 2010c). Cerebrospinal fluid (CSF), secreted by the epithelial cells within the choroid plexus, also becomes infected and the meningococci are lysed into the subarachnoid space. Cell wall toxins induce inflammation of the meninges and stimulate cytokine release, giving rise to physiological and physical manifestations of headache, fever and raised intracranial pressure (ICP).

Meningococcal septicaemia

Meningococci entering the circulation initiate a massive inflammatory response, stimulating the release of inflammatory mediators such as tumour necrosis factor (TNF) and interleukin-1 (IL-1), along with neutrophils, monocytes and platelets, producing signs of septicaemia / septic shock (see Chapters 6, 7 and 25).

Figure 39.1 describes the clinical features of meningitis and meningococcal septicaemia and the laboratory investigations required.

Infection control management

• Intramuscular / intravenous benzylpenicillin prior to admission or on admission.
• Isolation in a single room until the patient has received 24 hours of antibiotic therapy.
• Masks are not required unless aerosol-generating procedures are undertaken (i.e. resuscitation, airway management).
• Chemoprophylaxis for healthcare contacts is not routinely required unless staff participated in an aerosol-generating procedure without wearing a mask, and should only be prescribed / taken on the advice of a consultant microbiologist / Public Health England.
• Household contacts of the patient will be identified by Public Health England, and oral chemoprophylaxis prescribed by the GP.
• Meningococci do not survive outside the nasopharynx, so cross-infection arising from the environment does not occur.

40 Norovirus

Figure 40.1 Norovirus management

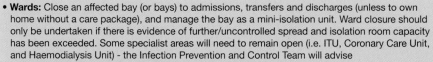

Admission avoidance
- Advice to members of the public and care home staff on the importance of remaining hydrated with oral fluids as tolerated
- Admission to hospital should only be considered if the individual is at risk of complications that cannot be addressed through simple re-hydration
- Triage patients presenting in A&E promptly and discharge with advice on remaining hydrated

Report symptomatic patients and staff
- Notify the Infection Prevention and Control Team or local Health Protection (Public Health) Team as appropriate
- Symptomatic members of staff must not work until they have been symptom free for 48 hours
- Record patient symptoms (frequency/severity/duration); fluid intake and output; 4-hourly vital signs; ensure daily medical review for hospital inpatients; seek GP review for elderly residents in care homes if there are concerns around maintaining adequate hydration
- Do not administer laxatives or anti-diarrhoeal agents (i.e. loperamide)

Management of cases with wards/care home
- **Wards:** Close an affected bay (or bays) to admissions, transfers and discharges (unless to own home without a care package), and manage the bay as a mini-isolation unit. Ward closure should only be undertaken if there is evidence of further/uncontrolled spread and isolation room capacity has been exceeded. Some specialist areas will need to remain open (i.e. ITU, Coronary Care Unit, and Haemodialysis Unit) - the Infection Prevention and Control Team will advise
- **Care homes:** Where possible, confine symptomatic residents to their own room and away from communal areas

Infection control precautions
- Hand washing with soap and water in between patient contacts (NB: must continue to use alcohol handrub at the point of care in accordance with the '5 Moments')
- Appropriate use of PPE; designated commode/other patient equipment for isolation rooms/cohort bays; display appropriate signage re. bay/ward/home closure
- Remove bowls of fruit and opened packets of food (e.g. biscuits, chocolates); cover water jugs and change water frequently
- Non-urgent investigations must be cancelled by the Medical Team/GP; urgent investigations should go ahead with appropriate liaison; only essential staff should visit the ward/home; restrict visitors
- Where possible, dedicate nursing and domestic staff to side rooms and cohort bay(s)
- Clean toilets/bathrooms at least twice daily, and 'high-touch points' more frequently using an approved hypochlorite (bleach) product, as well as steam cleaning
- Ensure that a thorough deep/terminal clean of the side rooms/bay/ward is undertaken 72 hours after the onset of the last new case, or 72 hours after the last symptomatic patient has resolved (according to local policy)

First identified in 1972 as 'small round structured viruses' (SRSVs) by electron microscopy from saved stool samples originating from an outbreak of non-bacterial gastroenteritis in the town of Norwalk, Ohio, USA, in 1968 (Dolin and Treanor, 2009; Ahmad et al, 2010c), noroviruses have emerged as a major pathogen in community and healthcare settings over the last five decades.

There were 72 993 laboratory confirmed cases of noroviruses in England and Wales during the period 2000–2012 (PHE, 2013 k), and 676 hospital outbreaks were reported in 2014 via the Public Health England Hospital Norovirus Outbreak Reporting Scheme (HNORS); 93% of these resulted in bay and ward closures. At the peak of norovirus activity in the community, 3000 patients per year are admitted to hospitals in England, accounting for 0.3% and 0.1% of emergency admissions in adults and elderly patients respectively (Houstein et al, 2009).

The virus

Norovirus belongs to the virus family *Caliciviridae*; the name is derived from the Latin word *calyx*, meaning goblet or cup, in reference to the 32 cup-shaped depressions on the surface of the capsid (Dolin and Treanor, 2009; Collier et al, 2011d).

The media often report outbreaks of norovirus infection as 'winter vomiting disease', which was first described in 1929 (Vipond et al, 1999) and so named because of its seasonal incidence and the dominant symptom of vomiting. There are now at least five different norovirus genogroups (GI–GV), which are further divided into gene clusters, with most of the strains responsible for causing outbreaks residing in genogroup GII (Dolin and Treanor, 2009), and 80% of infections associated with genotype II.4 in particular. Mutations can occur during the process of viral replication, giving rise to mutations within the viral genome, which can assist the virus to evade host immune response mechanisms (Harris et al, 2011). This leads to the emergence of new strains that may be associated with increased outbreaks, the severity of which may vary from year to year depending on which strains are in circulation and immunity within the local population (Dolin and Treanor, 2009).

Peaks in incidence have occurred globally with the emergence of new variant genotypes in 1995, 2002 and 2004 (Bull et al, 2006), and the emergence of a new strain in Australia in March 2012 – the Sydney 2012 genotype, which became the dominant strain in many countries (Eden et al, 2014).

Incubation, transmission and clinical features

Norovirus is highly contagious. The infecting dose necessary to induce symptoms is extremely small, at only 10–100 virus particles (Vipond et al, 1999). It has a short incubation period (12–48 hours) and an **attack rate** often higher than 50%, affecting both patients and staff in healthcare settings. There is no viral **prodrome** and the onset of the presenting clinical features of profuse, watery diarrhoea and / or forceful (projectile) vomiting

is abrupt. Affected individuals often report other symptoms such as nausea, headache, abdominal pain and **myalgia** once the initial symptoms have manifested themselves. It is a self-limiting infection, and most affected indivuals start to recover within 48–72 hours.

Vomiting appears to result in greater numbers of individuals becoming infected because of airborne spread, and it has been estimated that more than 30 million virus particles are released during vomiting (Patterson et al, 1997). Up to 5 billion infectious doses of norovirus may be shed by an infected person in each gram of faeces (Hall, 2012). While the virus can continue to be excreted in faeces after the symptoms have resolved, it is also thought that virus excretion can occur *before* the onset of symptoms (Goller et al, 2004), giving rise to the possibility of norovirus being transmissible prior to the onset of clinical symptoms and after resolution, potentially prolonging outbreaks.

Within the healthcare setting, outbreaks arise as a result of faecal–oral spread and person-to- person spread following the dissemination of virus particles through the air, which leads to widespread environmental contamination. Contaminated fingers can transfer norovirus onto as many as seven clean surfaces (Barker et al, 2004), and the virus can remain viable within the environment for up to 12 days (Cheesbrough et al, 1997). Food has been implicated in community outbreaks in particular, either contaminated at source (i.e. oysters harvested from water contaminated with human sewage) or by an infected food handler (HPA, 2009c).

Laboratory diagnosis

Faecal specimens should be obtained within 48 hours of the onset of symptoms and sent to the laboratory immediately for enzyme-linked immunosorbent assays to detect norovirus antigens or polymerase chain reaction (PCR) to detect norovirus nucleic acid (see Chapter 9). However, they may yield a negative result because a positive result is dependent upon the viral load and the timing of the specimen. Although a positive result is useful for epidemiological / surveillance purposes, a diagnosis of norovirus infection can be made based on the clinical features and the attack rate.

Management of outbreaks

If norovirus is 'introduced' into a closed setting, such as a hospital ward or care facility, by a patient, member of staff or a visitor, it can rapidly ignite an outbreak, leading to closure of bays or whole wards, or a care home, within 48–72 hours. The elderly are most frequently affected by norovirus infections with prolonged duration of symptoms, and may be more severely affected than younger 'healthy' individuals (Chadwick et al, 2000; Goller et al, 2004). Revised national *Guidelines for the management of norovirus outbreaks in acute and community health and social care settings* were published in 2012 (HPA/Norovirus Working Party, 2012), and the key principles of outbreak prevention / management are described in Figure 40.1.

41 Pandemic influenza

Figure 41.1 Characteristics of the past four influenza pandemics

Pandemic year of emergence and common name	Area of origin	Influenza A virus subtype (type of animal genetic introduction/recombination event)	Estimated productive number ****	Estimated case fatality	Estimated attributable excess mortality worldwide	Age groups most affected
1918 'Spanish flu'	Unclear	H1N1 *(unknown)	1.2–3.0	2–3%	20–50 million	Young adults
1957–1958 'Asian flu'	Southern China	H2N2 (avian)**	1.5	< 0.2%	1–4 million	All age groups
1968–1969 'Hong Kong flu'	Southern China	H3N2 (avian)***	1.3–1.6	< 0.2%	1–4 million	All age groups
2009–2010 'Influenza A (H1N1)2009'	North America	H1N1 (swine)	1.1–1.8	0.02%	100 000–400 000	Children and young adults

Notes:
*The 1918 H1N1 virus is believed to have been an avian-like influenza virus derived from an unknown source (Taubenberger and Morens, 2006), possibly a swine flu strain (Reid et al, 1996). It possibly occurred as a result of an adaptive mutation, but it is not known whether this occurred over a period of months or years (WHO, 2005).
** The 1957–1958 H2N2 strain obtained genes from an avian influenza virus and the strain responsible for the 1918 pandemic (WHO, 2005).
*** The 1968–1969 virus obtained genes from an avian influenza virus and the 1957–1958 virus, which was still in circulation (WHO, 2005).
****Productive number = the number of cases that one case generates on average over the course / duration of its infectious period in an uninfected population.

Source: WHO, 2013a

Figure 41.2 Pandemic influenza virus

1 Direct transmission via adaptive change during viral replication

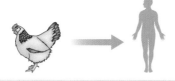

2 Genetic exchange between animal strains

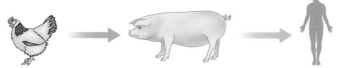

(a) Influenza A in birds can jump into another animal host (e.g. pig) and from there to humans

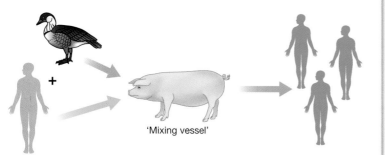

'Mixing vessel'

(b) An animal is co-infected with a human and an animal strain of influenza A. The virus recombines leading to the creation of a novel influenza virus

Figure 41.3 Avian influenza

- All birds are susceptible to avian influenza, of which there are over 100 subtypes

- Migratory birds can affect domestic flocks along flight paths

- Live bird markets in Asia have led to amplification of the virus, where the risk of exposure is significantly high during activities such as slaughter, defeathering, butchering and preparation of the carcass for cooking
- Human cases of avian influenza are linked to direct contact with infected poultry, dead or dying birds, or surfaces and objects contaminated by bird faeces

- 1 gram of faeces from a bird infected with A/H5N1 contains sufficient virus particles to kill 1 million birds (DH, 2002a)

Infection Prevention and Control at a Glance, First Edition. By Debbie Weston, Alison Burgess and Sue Roberts.
© 2017 John Wiley & Sons, Ltd. Published 2017 by John Wiley & Sons, Ltd.

Pandemics of influenza, regarded by many experts as **the most significant global public health emergency caused by a naturally occurring pathogen**, have been reported since the 16th century and are associated with high morbidity, excess mortality and social and economic disruption (WHO, 2005). The 'swine flu' pandemic of 2009–2010 was relatively mild, despite killing 457 people in the UK and an estimated 100 000–400 000 globally (WHO, 2013a). It did not fulfil its true pandemic potential (the swine flu A/H1N1/2009 'pandemic' virus is now a seasonal influenza strain) but it gave the world a scare.

The problem with pandemic influenza

The word pandemic is derived from the Greek words *pan*, meaning 'all', and *demos*, meaning 'people'. It is essentially a worldwide epidemic or outbreak of an infectious disease (not restricted to influenza) to which there is little, or no, immunity. Influenza viruses exhibit enormous pandemic potential.

• They have the ability to jump the species barrier, from an animal reservoir to a human host, and cause severe infections in humans, as evidenced by the last four pandemics (see Figure 41.1).

• Their behaviour cannot be predicted (compare the 1918 'Spanish flu' H1N1 pandemic and the A/H1N1/2009 'swine flu' pandemic as examples), and their real **pathogenic** potential can only be estimated as the **mortality rate**, severity of illness and pattern of spread can vary greatly; **until a flu virus starts circulating, its full effects will not be known.**

• Pandemics tend to occur in **waves**, with each wave affecting different age groups and different geographical areas. Mortality can increase during the second wave.

• **Global spread** is likely to occur quickly, within a matter of months, given the expansion of international air travel, so once cases have been detected in one country, pandemic influenza will have started to arrive in many more.

• **People of all ages** will be susceptible to pandemic flu, not just those in the 'at risk' groups, and although it is likely to cause the same symptoms as 'ordinary flu', these are likely to be more severe.

• **Vaccination** against seasonal influenza will offer no protection against a pandemic strain. There will be no vaccine available until the subtype of influenza virus is identified.

The role of antigenic shift

Major changes to the HA and NA surface antigens lead to the creation of a new virus. Antigenic shift (see Chapter 35) can occur as a sudden, adaptive change during replication of a normal virus, or from genetic exchange between a human and an animal strain of influenza A (see Figure 41.2). **Adaptive change** occurs when a circulating animal influenza virus undergoes a spontaneous mutation and develops the ability to cause infection in humans through animal to human contact. Strains of **avian influenza** (see Figure 41.3) have undergone adaptive antigenic shift twice in recent years. **A/H5N1** influenza first emerged in birds in China in 1996, and the first human cases were reported one year later. Since 2003, it has given rise to 694 human cases and 402 deaths in 16 countries (http://www.who.int).

A/H7N6 has been responsible for 486 cases and 185 deaths since April 2013.

Genetic exchange can occur in two ways. An animal (bird or pig) co-infected with both a human *and* an animal strain can serve as a 'mixing vessel' for the virus, allowing it to genetically 're-combine' or 're-assort' itself and create a new influenza virus capable of causing disease in humans. With A/H5N1, given that the virus can already infect humans and has been doing so for a number of years, it is not improbable that a human could become co-infected with both A/H5N1 *and* a human influenza virus and therefore act as the mixing vessel. Genes can also recombine between different strains. The **A/H1N1/2009** pandemic was caused not by the emergence of a new strain of influenza, but by a triple reassortment North American swine influenza virus, with genes derived from human, swine and avian influenza A viruses, (including the 1918 pandemic virus) that in turn had acquired genes for Eurasian strains of influenza (Collier et al, 2011c). **A/H5N8**, which caused a major outbreak of bird flu in Ireland in 1983, has since re-emerged in 2014 as a new reassortment of highly pathogenic avian influenza, with A/H5N1 as its 'parent' virus. Having been circulating in Asia since 2010, it began to cause significant concern during 2014 with outbreaks reported in October and November 2014 in Germany, Holland and the UK. No human cases of A/H5N8 have occurred to date but it has become increasingly pathogenic and is being closely monitored by the World Health Organization, Public Health England, the Centers for Disease Prevention and Control (Atlanta) and the Department of the Environment and Rural Affairs (DEFRA).

Pandemic influenza preparedness planning

Interim pandemic influenza risk management guidelines were published by WHO in 2013 in response to lessons learnt from the 2009 pandemic (WHO, 2013a), and set out the global preparedness and response arrangements (WHO, 2013b). Within the UK, a report into the UK response to the 2009 pandemic was published in 2010 (Hine, 2010) and preparedness planning is ongoing (hampered slightly by organisational changes to the NHS and the response to the Ebola crisis in West Africa in 2014–2015). The UK plans can be viewed at www.england.nhs.uk/ourwork/eprr/pi

The routine day to day running and operational issues that govern the provision of healthcare services within primary and secondary care will be required to change significantly in order to accommodate the exceptional infection control arrangements that will be in place. The severe acute respiratory syndrome (SARS) outbreak in 2003 caught everyone by surprise and gave the world a wake-up call, and there were significant lessons to be learnt regarding the implementation of, and compliance with, infection control measures (Cameron et al, 2006). The 2009 pandemic put everyone to the test, and '…the threat of another influenza pandemic is such that it remains the top risk on the UK Cabinet Office National Risk Register of Civil Emergencies (2013 edition) and continues to direct significant amounts of emergency preparedness activity on a global basis' (NHS England, 2013).

42 Salmonella

Figure 42.1 Salmonella species bacteria

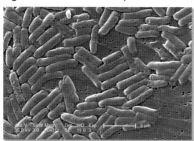

Source: U.S. Centers for Disease Control and Prevention; photo credit: Janice Haney Carr

Figure 42.2 Characteristics of Salmonella bacteria

- Family: Enterobacteriaceae
- Gram-negative rods, motile, non-sporing flagella
- Non-capsulate except for *Salmonella typhi*
- Toxin-producing
- Capable of aerobic and anaerobic respiration

Source: Mims et al, 2004

Figure 42.3 The story of Mary Mellon

- An asymptomatic carrier of typhoid
- Employed as a cook in the New York area
- 1900–1906: Infected more than 50 people (3 of whom died)
- 1906: George Soper (typhoid investigator) identified Mary as the source
- 1907–1910: Mary was quarantined
- 1910: Mary was employed as a laundress, but later returned to her preferred occupation of cook
- 1915: Mary was implicated in a second major outbreak of typhoid
- Quarantined again – this time for the remainder of her life

Source: Newsom, 2009c

Figure 42.4 A risk factor for Salmonella – red-eared slider turtles

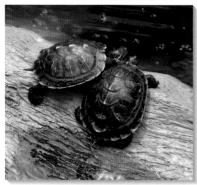

Source: U.S. Centers for Disease Control and Prevention; photo credit: Eric Grafman

Figure 42.5 Clinical features of Salmonella

- Abrupt onset
- Diarrhoea
- High fever: 38–39°C for 48 hours
- Abdominal cramps
- Nausea, vomiting rare
- Headache
- Myalgia
- Bacteraemia may occur
- Self-limiting

Source: PHE, 2014d

Figure 42.6 Infection prevention and control precautions

In the hospital

- **Isolation:** Until patient has been free of diarrhoea for a minimum of 48 hours, and preferably passed a formed stool
- **Personal protective equipment (PPE):** Gloves and aprons are required for direct contact with faeces
- **Hand hygiene:** Hand washing should be implemented (refer to Chapter 14 for more information on hand hygiene)
- **En suite toilet** preferred or designated commode
- **Decontamination of isolation room:** The room must be thoroughly cleaned daily according to local Trust Guidelines
- **Clinical waste:** Correct disposal
- **Equipment:** Designated/cleaned as per local guidelines

NB: As part of general management it is important to ensure that fluids and electrolytes are replaced in dehydrated patients.

In the community

- Surveillance of cases/management of outbreaks is undertaken by Public Health England (PHE), and followed up by an Environmental Health Officer (EHO)
- Cases will need to be excluded from school/nursery until free of symptoms for 48 hours
- Exclusion of food handlers from work is usually necessary

Infection Prevention and Control at a Glance, First Edition. By Debbie Weston, Alison Burgess and Sue Roberts.
© 2017 John Wiley & Sons, Ltd. Published 2017 by John Wiley & Sons, Ltd.

almonella (see Figure 42.1) was first discovered in 1885 by Theobald Smith, an American scientist who (as was customary at the time) named it in honour of his Bureau Director, veterinary pathologist Daniel Salmon (Niemi, 2009). There are over 2500 species of Salmonella, *Salmonella typhimurium* and *Salmonella enteritidis* being the most common (PHE, 2014d). Salmonella is the *second most common* cause of food poisoning in the UK after Campylobacter (see Chapter 28), is more common in the summer months, and accounts for approximately 80 deaths annually in the UK. Certain types of Salmonella are responsible for causing **typhoid** and **paratyphoid** (known as **enteric fever**), but these are *almost exclusively* acquired abroad through the ingestion of contaminated food and water (PHE, 2014d). Salmonella species are found in the intestinal tracts of many different animals, including birds, but fruit and vegetables can also become contaminated if in contact with livestock, manure or untreated water (PHE, 2014d). Some people are asymptomatic carriers of Salmonella and outbreaks of Salmonella food poisoning are therefore common. Salmonella is a **notifiable** disease (see Chapter 2).

Figure 42.2 describes the characteristics of Salmonella.

Historically important Salmonella outbreaks

Probably the most famous asymptomatic 'carrier' of *Salmonella typhi* was Mary Mellon, otherwise known as 'Typhoid Mary', who was an Irish immigrant working in the New York area as a cook. Mary worked for several different families and is thought to have infected *at least* 50 people, but possibly in excess of 100, several of whom died (Newsom, 2009c). In spite of being identified by investigator George Soper, and forcibly imprisoned for many years, before finally agreeing to give up cooking to work in a laundry, she later changed her name and continued working as a cook, infecting more people (Figure 42.3). A more recent but significant outbreak of *Salmonella typhimurium* occurred in 1984 at Stanley Royd psychiatric hospital in West Yorkshire. A total of 355 patients (19 of whom died) and 106 staff were affected. This led to the first ever public enquiry into the running of a hospital and resulted in the removal of crown immunity from NHS premises (Weston, 2008).

Risk factors, transmission, incubation period and clinical signs and symptoms

Those most at risk include children under the age of 5 years, the elderly and immunocompromised individuals. Infection occurs most commonly by ingestion of Salmonella via contaminated food or water. The source is usually of animal origin, such as beef, poultry, unpasteurised milk or eggs, although sometimes it is contaminated vegetables. It is also frequently caused by cross-contamination between surfaces and tools used in cooked and infected uncooked food areas, and inadequate thawing of frozen foods. Another source is contact with exotic pets. Reptiles such as turtles, lizards and snakes are particularly likely to harbour Salmonella (see Figure 42.4), which means that children are at an increased risk of infection if hand-washing is inadequate

(PHE, 2014e). Person-to-person spread by the faecal–oral route (see Chapter 14) is common, especially from food handlers not washing their hands after going to the toilet.

The incubation period is 12–72 hours, and the duration of illness is typically 4–7 days.

Figure 42.5 lists the clinical signs and symptoms of Salmonella.

Complications

The most common complications are dehydration and electrolyte imbalance. A small percentage of people will go on to develop Reiter's syndrome (joint pain, irritation of eyes, painful urination), which may last for months or years, and sometimes becomes chronic (CDC, 2009). Other complications may be the onset of irritable bowel syndrome, temporary lactose intolerance, and rarely persistent diarrhoea syndromes.

Diagnosis and treatment

Diagnosis is by polymerase chain reaction (PCR) (see Chapter 9), confirmed by stool culture.

For most people specific treatment is not required and the only advice for affected individuals is to drink more fluids for the duration of the diarrhoea. Symptoms may be particularly severe in babies less than 6 months of age who may require hospitalisation to correct dehydration / electrolyte imbalance.

Antibiotics are **not** given routinely **unless** there is evidence of invasive disease as they do not shorten the illness, may prolong carrier status, and contribute to the problem of antimicrobial resistance. However, antibiotics may be given in those at high risk of bacteraemia including infants less than 6 months and those who are immunocompromised. In addition, antibiotics are sometimes given to asymptomatic carriers if they are food handlers or work in nurseries. Antibiotics are also used to treat individuals with *Salmonella typhi* and *Salmonella paratyphi*. The use of anti-diarrhoeal medication is controversial but generally not recommended as it prolongs the transit time of the bacteria in the bowel. Vaccines are available to protect against typhoid and paratyphoid for those who plan to travel abroad.

Infection prevention and control precautions

Figure 42.6 describes the required infection control precautions for hospitalised patients. Individuals can generally return to work 48 hours after symptoms have resolved. Testing of stools is not routinely required for clearance but may be required for food handlers before they can return to work.

Prevention of Salmonella infection

The risk of acquiring Salmonella food poisoning can be reduced by adhering to the following rules: ensure that meat is well cooked, not pink in the middle, and that eggs are cooked until the yolk is set; avoid contamination of cooked and uncooked meats and kitchen utensils; wash hands before handling different food items, before eating and drinking and after going to the toilet, and after handling pets.

43 *Staphylococcus aureus* and MRSA

Figure 43.1   Panton–Valentine leukocidin (PVL) associated *Staphylococcus aureus*

Key points
- Panton–Valentine leukocidin (PVL) is a toxin that destroys white blood cells and is a virulence factor in some strains of *Staphylococcus aureus*.
- Strains of PVL-SA have emerged in the UK and worldwide, producing a new pattern of disease.
- In the UK the PVL genes are carried by < 2% of clinical isolates of *Staphylococcus aureus* (MSSA and MRSA).
- PVL has been strongly associated with virulent, transmissible strains of *Staphylococcus aureus* including community-associated (CA) MRSA.
- Strains of *S. aureus* encoding the PVL genes were first recognised in staphylococcal skin abscesses.
- In the 1950s and 1960s a phage type 80/81 strain spread widely; this PVL-MSSA strain proved to be highly successful in the UK and abroad, causing widespread illness (mostly boils and abscesses in previously healthy individuals in the community, hospitalised patients and healthcare workers).
- To date, most PVL strains in the UK have been MSSA; however, a major problem has emerged in North America with CA-MRSA, most of which produce PVL. The USA300 clone is now spreading in hospitals in the USA.

Clinical features of PVL-SA
- PVL-SA predominantly causes skin and soft tissue infection, but can also cause invasive infection.
- The most serious invasive infection is necrotising haemorrhagic pneumonia. This is associated with a high mortality and often follows a 'flu-like' illness. It may affect previously healthy young people residing in the community.

Risk factors for PVL-SA
The risk factors for PVL-SA seen in the UK correspond to those described for CA-MRSA in North America. These include compromised skin integrity, skin-to-skin contact, and sharing of contaminated items such as towels. Worldwide experience suggests that closed communities with people in close contact are higher risk settings for transmission of staphylococcal infections.
In North America the following settings have been identified as higher risk for transmission from an individual colonised or infected with CA-MRSA:
- households
- close contact sports, e.g. wrestling, American football, rugby, judo
- military training camps
- gyms
- prisons

CDC guidance refers to risk factors for PVL-related infection as '5 C's':
1 Contaminated items
2 Close contact
3 Crowding
4 Cleanliness
5 Cuts and other compromised skin integrity

Source: HPA, 2008

Table 43.1   Hospital-associated MRSA versus community-associated MRSA

	Hospital-associated MRSA	Community-associated MRSA
Typical patients	Elderly, debilitated and/or critically ill or chronically ill	Young healthy people, students, athletes, military service personnel
Infection site	Wounds/invasive devices Often causes bacteraemia	Often spontaneous skin, cellulitis, abscesses
Transmission	Within healthcare settings; little spread among household	Community-acquired; may spread in close community settings, e.g. families, sports teams, via pets
Diagnosis is typically made	In an inpatient setting	In an outpatient setting
Medical history	History of MRSA colonisation / infection, recent surgery, admission to hospital or nursing home, antibiotics, renal dialysis, permanent indwelling catheter, skin ulcers, diabetes	No significant history
Virulence factors	Community spread limited. PVL genes absent	Spreads readily in community, PVL genes present, predisposition to necrotising skin and soft tissue infection
Antibiotic susceptibility	Choice of agents – limited antibiotics	Currently more susceptible to antibiotics* * From the North American literature; many points resonate with experience thus far in the UK.

Source: HPA, 2008

Infection Prevention and Control at a Glance, First Edition. By Debbie Weston, Alison Burgess and Sue Roberts.
© 2017 John Wiley & Sons, Ltd. Published 2017 by John Wiley & Sons, Ltd.

Figure 43.2 Best practice recommendations for the prevention and management of MRSA

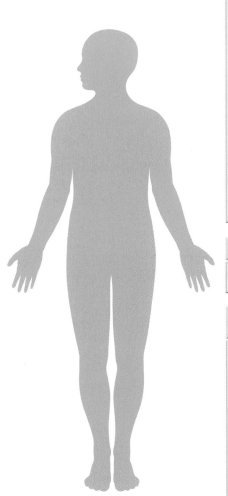

Box 1 MRSA screening

Body sites to screen:
- nose
- groin/perineum
- other sites as appropriate, e.g. wounds, indwelling device entry sites, throat, etc. The frequency of (repeat) screening should be determined locally and made explicit in local guidance. Follow-up screening should be undertaken at least 48 hours after antibiotic and antiseptic therapy have been completed (DH, 2014).

Box 2 Identification of patients known to have MRSA

The admission assessment should include the facility to check for existing MRSA colonisation/infection, ideally electronically, e.g. patient tagging

Box 3 Patient isolation

Patients should be isolated/cohorted according to local policy.

Box 4 Surgical/invasive procedures

Prior to any planned invasive procedure, efforts should be made to minimise the risk of infection through topical and systemic decolonisation and prophylactic antimicrobial therapy, as appropriate. Patients should be managed normally through theatre with standard precautions.

Box 5 Patient information

The implications of MRSA colonisation, infection and treatment should be explained to the patient at the time of diagnosis and ideally prior to being isolated. The patient's care should not be compromised as a result of having MRSA.

Box 6 Cleaning and decontamination

High standards of environmental cleaning are an important factor in reducing the environmental reservoir for MRSA and therefore its spread, including:
- high standards of cleaning in areas occupied by patients with MRSA
- enhanced cleaning following patient transfer/discharge
- high standards of patient equipment cleaning/decontamination
- disposal of contaminated waste and used linen protocols

Box 10 MRSA screening criteria for acute and elective admissions admitted to NHS hospitals in England

- All patients previously identified as colonised with or infected by MRSA
- High-risk specialties/units. High-risk specialties are defined as vascular, renal dialysis, neurosurgery, cardiothoracic surgery, haematology/oncology/bone marrow transplant, orthopaedics/trauma, and all intensive care units (adult/paediatric ICUs, neonatal intensive care units, high dependency units, coronary care units) (DH, 2014)

Box 7 Transfer and discharge of MRSA colonised or infected patients

- Transfer of patients between wards and departments should be minimised without compromising other aspects of care, including rehabilitation
- The receiving area should be notified of the patient's MRSA status in advance of the transfer to minimise contact with other patients
- Lesions should be covered with an impermeable dressing
- PPE – for patient contact, plastic aprons should be worn
- Gloves should only be worn if staff transporting the patient have skin abrasions
- The trolley or chair used to transport the patient should be cleaned after use
- Linen should be managed as infected
- Staff should decontaminate their hands following contact with the patient and trolley/wheelchair, etc.

Box 8 Ambulance transportation

- Standard precautions
- High standards of cleaning/decontamination

Box 9 MRSA decolonisation/suppression therapy

Nasal decolonisation using topical agents should be used with other forms of intervention such as skin decolonisation with 4% chlorhexidine gluconate aqueous solution.

Skin decolonisation/suppression therapy:
- Bathe daily for 5 days. Skin should be moistened first with water and the antiseptic detergent should be applied thoroughly to all areas before rinsing
- Mupirocin should not be used for prolonged periods or used repeatedly as this will promote resistance
- Hair should be washed with the antiseptic detergent – twice weekly
- After each course of treatment, clean clothing, bedding and towels should be provided
- For patients with eczema or other skin conditions attempts should be made to treat underlying skin conditions on the advice of a dermatologist

Nasal decolonisation/suppression therapy:
- Mupirocin 2% in a paraffin base to the inner surface of the nostril (anterior nares) 3 times a day for 5 days. The patient should be able to taste the mupirocin at the back of the throat after application
- Mupirocin should not be used for prolonged periods or used repeatedly as resistance may be encouraged
- Three weekly screens before staff can be considered to be clear of MRSA. Systemic antibiotics may be used to clear persistent carriage

Staphylococcus aureus

For more than a century *Staphylococcus aureus* has been recognised as a major cause of infection that commonly involves the skin. *S. aureus* is a Gram-positive coccus (see Chapter 3) first discovered in the 1880s. It is found in about a third of the population, commonly colonising human skin and mucosa, for example under the arms, groin, skin folds, hairline, perineum, umbilicus and anterior nares without any obvious signs and symptoms. *S. aureus* can cause invasive disease, particularly if there is an opportunity for the bacteria to gain entry to the body, for example through broken skin, which includes skin-penetrating medical procedures such as surgery and the use of indwelling medical devices which provide a portal of entry for the bacteria (Coia et al, 2006).

Illnesses associated with *S. aureus* range from mild to life threatening, and include superficial skin infections, wound infections, infected eczema, septic arthritis / osteomyelitis, endocarditis, food poisoning, pneumonia (see Chapter 32), bacteraemia, sepsis (see Chapter 25) and toxic shock syndrome.

An individual becomes clinically infected if the organism invades the skin or deeper tissues and multiplies, resulting in a localised or **systemic** response (RCN, 2005). Clinical infection with *S. aureus* occurs either from the patient's own resident bacteria (if he or she is an asymptomatic carrier colonised with *S. aureus*) or by cross-infection from another person, who could be an asymptomatic carrier or someone with a clinical infection.

Virulence factors

S. aureus is an important organism as it has the additional ability to produce toxins (see Chapter 4). The virulence of *S. aureus* is defined by a large repertoire of virulence factors including toxins aimed at evading elimination by the host and those with the ability to create **biofilms** (see Chapters 20 and 30). Many *S. aureus* toxins damage biological membranes leading to cell death (Otto, 2014). Panton–Valentine leukocidin (PVL) is a toxin that destroys white blood cells and is a virulence factor in some strains of *S. aureus* (see Figure 43.1).

Meticillin-resistant *Staphylococcus aureus* (MRSA)

Most strains of *S. aureus* are sensitive to the more commonly used antibiotics and can be effectively treated; these are known as meticillin-sensitive *Staphylococcus aureus* (MSSA). However, some strains are more resistant than others. Those resistant to the antibiotic meticillin are termed meticillin-resistant *Staphylococcus aureus* (MRSA). The resistance of the bacterium to first-line antibiotics, such as penicillins, makes infection with MRSA more difficult to treat, which can represent a particular risk to immunocompromised patients.

In the UK, 1–3% of the total population are colonised with MRSA. Although the majority of patients who acquire MRSA are colonised, about one third of patients (depending on the patient population) develop infection (Coia et al, 2006). Factors predisposing to superficial colonisation include procedures involving direct hands-on care, especially in surgical, renal dialysis and critical care units. Carriage may be short or long term (PHE, 2014g). Infection can develop into an MRSA bloodstream infection which is associated with 10–20% mortality. MSSA and MRSA only differ in their degree of antibiotic resistance; MRSA is not considered to be any more virulent than MSSA, as was once thought to be the case (PHE, 2014g).

MRSA and antibiotic resistance (see Chapter 11)

Staphylococcal resistance to penicillin was first described in 1961, after the widespread introduction of penicillin in the 1940s to treat infection (Jevons, 1961). Since the introduction of penicillin, the overuse and misuse of antibiotics has supported natural bacterial evolution by helping microbes become resistant to drugs developed to target infections. Resistance is due to the production by *S. aureus* of a penicillinase (beta-lactamase) enzyme. In order to combat this, new antibiotics that were not easily destroyed by this enzyme were introduced in the 1960s. Meticillin, a forerunner of flucloxacillin, a narrow-spectrum beta-lactam antibiotic of the penicillin class, was one example. Although meticillin is no longer used to treat patients, it is still used for susceptibility testing to flucloxacillin.

During the late 1970s and early 1980s, strains of *S. aureus* resistant to multiple antibiotics, including meticillin and gentamicin, were increasingly responsible for outbreaks of hospital infection worldwide and **clonal** spread (Schaefler et al, 1981; Pavillard et al, 1982). MRSA has the potential to thrive in the hospital setting due to its propensity to spread and colonise debilitated patients, the limited treatment options for the treatment of systemic MRSA infections, and because an environment exists where the extensive use of antibiotics promotes the survival of bacteria that are resistant.

In England and Wales the spread of MRSA was well controlled until the 1990s; between 1989 and 1991 only 1.6% of *S. aureus* bacteraemias were meticillin resistant (Cookson, 1999). However, meticillin resistance rates increased steadily throughout the 1990s, accompanied by significant increases in the percentages of isolates resistant to erythromycin, clindamycin, ciprofloxacin, gentamicin, trimethoprim and rifampicin (Speller et al, 1997). The prevalence of meticillin resistance among strains of *S. aureus* causing bloodstream infections (bacteraemia) in the UK between 1990 and the early 2000s increased from 2% to more than 40%, which triggered the introduction of mandatory surveillance of MRSA bacteraemia in 2001. During the 1990s, two particular strains of MRSA with enhanced **epidemic** potential (EMRSA-15 and EMRSA-16) emerged in the UK causing excess **morbidity** and **mortality**. As the unprecedented incidence of MRSA increased over recent decades, it became the subject of considerable public concern and media attention, and MRSA was labelled the first 'superbug'. As a result, the control of MRSA became a political priority.

Epidemiology of MRSA

Public Health England (PHE) has carried out mandatory enhanced surveillance of MRSA bacteraemia since October 2005, and of MSSA bacteraemia since January 2011 for NHS acute trusts; patient-level data of all MRSA and MSSA bacteraemias are reported monthly to PHE. The introduction of mandatory reporting in England of MRSA bloodstream infection in 2001 was followed in 2004 by the setting of target reductions for all NHS hospitals. The original target of a 50% reduction in MRSA bloodstream infection was largely considered to be unachievable; however, subsequently there has been a very significant decline in morbidity and mortality related to MRSA infection in England. Annual MRSA bacteraemia rates fell from 17.7 (April 2005–March 2006) to 3.2 cases per 100 000 bed days (April 2011–March 2012) (DH, 2014). Significant reductions have also been observed in surgical site infections (see Chapter 24) where MRSA was reported as the causative microorganism (from 27% in 2004–2006 to only 4% in 2011–2012).

The number of death certificates in England and Wales mentioning MRSA infection has also decreased year on year since 2006 (DH, 2014). From April 2013, all NHS organisations reporting cases of MRSA bacteraemia have been required to complete a post infection review (PIR) as part of the NHS requirement to have a zero tolerance approach to MRSA bloodstream infections. The purpose of the PIR is to identify how a case of MRSA bloodstream infection occurred and to identify actions that will prevent it reoccurring (NHS England, 2014c).

Since 1986, national polices for the control and reduction of MRSA transmission in hospitals have been developed. The first set of guidance was published by a joint working party of the British Society for Antimicrobial Chemotherapy (BSAC), and the Hospital Infection Society (HIS) (HIS/BSAC, 1986), and has since been reviewed several times (Duckworth et al, 1998; Coia et al, 2006, DH, 2014). The approach to the control of the spread of MRSA largely focuses on patient screening to provide a means of identifying both patients and staff who may be at risk of infection and / or involved in the transmission of the organism (PHE, 2014g). Other key areas of focus are the administration of decolonisation / suppression therapy and source isolation of affected patients, particularly in high-risk areas, maintaining a clean environment, and the provision of adequate staff, in particular nursing staff, to implement the measures required. MRSA surveillance and antimicrobial stewardship are also important areas of focus (see Chapter 10). Control measures have been shown to be effective, resulting in reduced mortality and healthcare costs. MRSA control measures have advantages additional to those of just controlling MRSA as they accentuate the awareness of the importance of healthcare associated infection and support the containment of other antibiotic-resistant bacteria (Rubinovitch and Pittet, 2001). As a general rule, patients should be managed according to the type of ward / department in which they are cared for, the resources available, and the level of risk that is posed to them and to others of acquiring MRSA infection (Coia et al, 2006).

Surveillance – information for action

Surveillance is the systematic collection of data and its analysis, interpretation and dissemination for action (Coia et al, 2006). Surveillance facilitates the early recognition of changes in patterns of infection, identifying the size of the problem, monitoring trends and comparing rates, evaluating the effectiveness of the intervention, identifying areas for further investigation or research, re-enforcing best practice and influencing organisational leaders. This, allied to the setting of targets and performance indicators, has been used by the government to highlight unacceptably high rates of MRSA bacteraemia and to drive NHS Trusts to take action. MRSA surveillance generally focuses on MRSA screening results highlighting healthcare acquired cases and outbreak situations.

Screening and decolonisation

MRSA control strategies are based on screening patients to identify those who are colonised or infected with MRSA to allow segregation and therefore protect against transmission. It is also necessary to protect those who are colonised who may be at risk of developing infection; this is particularly important in the acute hospital environment where invasive treatments such as the insertion of invasive devices and surgical procedures provide the opportunity for MRSA colonisation to develop into infection. MRSA decolonisation (suppression) therapy refers mainly to the use of topical agents such as nasal ointment and body wash / shampoo to eliminate or reduce nasal and skin carriage.

Decolonisation regimes are only 50–60% effective for long-term clearance but as soon as the procedure is implemented the presence and shedding of MRSA are reduced significantly and the risk of the patient infecting themselves or transmitting MRSA to another patient is much reduced (DH, 2006). The effectiveness of decolonisation is likely to be reduced in the presence of wounds, skin lesions and foreign bodies such as urinary catheters. All patients identified as MRSA positive must receive decolonisation therapy (DH, 2014).

Until April 2009, national guidance in England recommended targeted screening of patients in high-risk specialties. From April 2009 and December 2010, respectively, the Department of Health (DH) in England introduced mandatory screening of all elective and emergency admissions. This decision was based on a DH impact assessment that modelled the cost-effectiveness of different screening and decolonisation strategies in preventing MRSA bacteraemias (bloodstream infections), wound infections and deaths. The DH impact assessment committed to a review of this policy and the National One Week (NOW) study was commissioned in 2011 (Fuller et al, 2013). The most recent DH guidance is based on this study, advocating admission screening to high-risk specialties and all patients previously identified as colonised with or infected by MRSA (DH, 2014).

Staff screening

Screening of staff is not recommended routinely. However, screening of nurses, doctors, physiotherapists, other allied health professionals and non-clinical support staff is indicated if transmission on a ward / department continues despite active control measures, or if epidemiological aspects of an outbreak are unusual. Screening should include asking staff about skin lesions. If these are present, the member of staff should be referred for screening and for consideration of dermatological treatment by the Occupational Health Department. Only staff members with colonised or infected hand lesions should be off work while receiving treatment for clearance. MRSA clearance for staff generally requires three weekly negative screens following the completion of antimicrobial therapy (Coia et al, 2006).

Hand hygiene, cleaning and decontamination

Transient contamination of healthcare workers' hands is widely believed to be the predominant method by which MRSA is transmitted to patients, therefore high standards of hand hygiene should be adhered to when caring for all patients, especially those with MRSA (WHO, 2009) (see Chapter 14). Patients with MRSA will shed skin scales into the environment which will lie dormant in dust particles. The ability of MRSA to survive in dust demonstrates the need for dust minimisation and the requirement for high standards of environmental cleaning, waste disposal and linen management in clinical areas in healthcare environments that may be frequented by patients colonised with MRSA (Coia et al, 2006). In addition enhanced standards of terminal cleaning are required after patient transfer / discharge. Standard source isolation procedures should be instituted for affected patients.

Antimicrobial stewardship

The inappropriate or unnecessary use of antibiotics should be avoided to reduce the likelihood of the emergence and spread of MRSA strains with reduced susceptibility to glycopeptides, vancomycin and teicoplanin. Antimicrobial stewardship programmes have been shown to result in significant reductions in MRSA colonisation and infection rates (Frank et al, 1997; Fukatsu et al, 1997).

Treatment options

The most prevalent epidemic MRSA strains in the UK remain susceptible to several antibiotics, including glycopeptides. However, MRSA strains showing reduced susceptibility to vancomycin have been reported. Despite this situation, there are several agents that are appropriate for the treatment of MRSA infections and new agents continue to be developed and introduced (PHE, 2014g).

Figure 43.2 summarises the best practice recommendations for the prevention and management of MRSA.

44 Tuberculosis

Figure 44.1 Initial stages in the pathogenesis of TB infection

- Inhalation of TB bacilli via droplet nuclei – implant into alveoli in the middle and lower lung fields
- Attacked and engulfed by non-specific alveolar macrophages (see Chapter 6)
- Phagocytosis will destroy some TB bacilli, but others will survive and replicate within the macrophages. Most of the 'infected' macrophages will die, releasing a new generation of bacilli and cell debris – cycle of infection, bacterial replication and host cell death
- Local inflammatory lesion (Ghon focus) develops in the middle or lower lung field and develops into a granuloma, which consists of infected macrophages, lymphocytes and fibroblasts
- The granuloma walls off and isolates the site of infection
- Macrophages within the granuloma are metabolically active and consume oxygen – the centre of the granuloma becomes necrotic, creating a hostile environment
- The majority of the bacilli within the granuloma die, bacterial replication is inhibited, infection is arrested, and over time the granuloma becomes calcified
- 90–95% of initial infections do not progress to active, clinical disease, and therefore individuals may be asymptomatic and unaware that they contracted TB

Figure 44.2 Individuals at risk of developing TB

- People with HIV
- People who are immunocompromised (i.e. receiving chemotherapy or steroids)
- Drug abusers and alcoholics
- Rough sleepers/those in night shelters/bed and breakfast dwellers
- Immigrants (South-East Asia, the Middle East, South and Central America, Africa, Eastern Europe)
- Close contacts of infectious cases
- The very young and elderly

Figure 44.3 Individuals with latent TB who are at risk of developing active TB

- HIV positive
- Injecting drug users
- Have received a solid organ transplant
- Have had a jejunoileal bypass
- Have chronic renal failure or are receiving haemodialysis
- Have had a gastrectomy
- Are receiving anti-tumour necrosis factor
- Have silicosis

Source: NICE, 2011

Figure 44.4 Clinical features of TB

Non-specific (general) features
- Generally 'unwell'
- Anorexia and weight loss
- Fever and drenching night sweats
- Enlarged lymph glands

Respiratory symptoms
- A chronic cough – which may have been unresponsive to a course of antibiotics – becoming more productive
- Shortness of breath
- Chest pain
- Haemoptysis

Figure 44.6 Risk factors for the acquisition/development of developing MDR-TB

- Previous drug treatment for TB
- HIV positive
- Contact with a known case of MDR-TB
- Birth in a foreign country
- Residence in London
- Failure of clinical response to treatment
- Prolonged sputum smear (at 4 months) or culture positive (at 6 months) while on treatment

Source: NICE, 2011

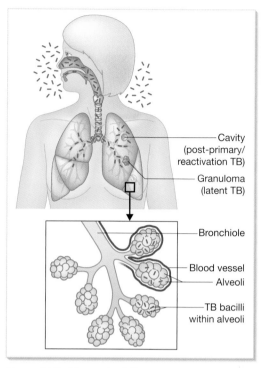

Cavity (post-primary/reactivation TB)

Granuloma (latent TB)

Bronchiole

Blood vessel

Alveoli

TB bacilli within alveoli

Figure 44.5 Diagnosing TB

Latent TB
- Mantoux test – an intradermal injection of tuberculin purified protein derivative (PPD) that results in an induration at the injection site which is 'read' 48–72 hours later (see PHE, 2013l)
- T-SPOT – a single blood test that detects the response by effector T cells to specific antigens which are not present in the BCG vaccination

Active TB
- Posterior-anterior chest x-ray – evidence of shadows, lesions, cavities and calcifications. As shadows and lesions may be indicative of other diseases such as lung cancer, more detailed images of the lung fields can be provided by chest CT/MRI scan
- Multiple sputum specimens – at least 3, including one early morning specimen. Ideally these should be obtained before TB therapy is started, or within 7 days of treatment starting
- Induction of sputum or bronchial washings and aspirate if the patient is unable to expectorate
- In order to diagnose TB at other body sites, whole body CT/MRI scans may be indicated, along with:
  - urine
  - CSF
  - pleural fluid
  - lymph node biopsy
  - tissue biopsy
  - pus
  - gastric aspirate
- A diagnosis of TB may be made post mortem from clinical specimens

Infection Prevention and Control at a Glance, First Edition. By Debbie Weston, Alison Burgess and Sue Roberts.
© 2017 John Wiley & Sons, Ltd. Published 2017 by John Wiley & Sons, Ltd.

Figure 44.7 Patient in hospital when diagnosis is made (drug-sensitive TB)

- Isolation in a single room (negative-pressure if available – see Chapter 21) until 2 full weeks of anti-TB treatment is completed or the patient is discharged (whichever is the soonest)
- Risk assessment for MDR-TB (rapid diagnostic tests for rifampicin resistance if MDR-TB is suspected)
- Local PHE Health Protection Team notified (see Chapter 2)
- Daily review by Chest Team/Respiratory (TB) Physician
- FFP3 Respirator masks are only required to be worn by staff if MDR-TB is suspected/confirmed, or if an aerosol-generating procedure (AGP) is undertaken (see Chapter 16)
- Patient to wear a surgical face mask if s/he is required to leave the room until 2 weeks of treatment has been completed

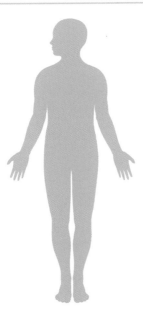

Figure 44.8 Patient in a community setting when diagnosis is made (i.e. by GP)

- Urgent referral to Chest Team/Respiratory (TB) Physician (to be seen with 2 weeks of diagnosis)
- The patient should only be admitted to hospital if their clinical condition warrants admission; otherwise s/he should remain in their place of residence. Advice on the infection control management of patients with TB in various community settings is covered in the NICE Guidance (NICE, 2011)
- Risk assessment for MDR-TB (rapid diagnostic tests for rifampicin resistance if MDR-TB is suspected)
- Anti-TB treatment to commence – consider need for directly observed therapy (DOT) if there are concerns about compliance/adherence
- Local PHE Health Protection Team notified (see Chapter 2)

Figure 44.9 Treatment (2HRZE / 4HR)

Initial 2 month phase (2HRZE) – aims to reduce the bacterial population as quickly as possible so that the patient becomes non-infectious as quickly as possible, and to prevent the emergence of drug resistance (Pratt et al, 2005)

(H) Isoniazid – the principal 'killing' drug; destroys all replicating bacilli in the pulmonary cavity; side effects include peripheral neuropathy in patients with HIV, diabetes, malnutrition, alcohol dependence and chronic renal failure

(R) Rifampicin – targets less active bacilli within macrophages and inflammatory lesions; also sterilises pulmonary cavities. Side effects include transient disturbances in renal function; affects the efficacy of the oral contraceptive pill

(Z) Pyrazinamide – assists rifampicin with targeting the less active bacilli within macrophages and inflammatory lesions. Side effects: can induce liver toxicity and may need to be discontinued; only prescribed for 2 months

(E) Ethambutol - assists the action of isoniazid. Side effects include visual disturbances (loss of acuity, colour blindness), and an eye examination must be undertaken before commencing treatment

Second (continuation) phase – 4 months treatment with (H) isoniazid and (R) rifampicin

Figure 44.10 Contact tracing (active case finding)

This is conducted according to the 'stone in the pond' principle (NICE, 2011). Closest contacts (those with the most exposure – typically household contacts) are found and assessed first, and offered screening for latent TB. If sufficient latent TB is identified in close contacts, another layer of contacts are identified and screened, and so on. In the community, this is undertaken by the local PHE Health Protection Team and the Community TB Team. **Full details in relation to active case finding in different community settings are provided in the NICE Guidance (NICE, 2011).**

In a healthcare setting, the Infection Prevention and Control Team and the Occupational Health Department will identify patient and staff contacts. Generally, this will involve identifying those individuals with 8 hours or more cumulative contact with the index case and/or who are immunocompromised. 'At risk' individuals will be contacted and offered screening for latent TB. Contacts who are identified as having been exposed to the index case but are not deemed to be at risk and who do not require screening will be written to, informed of their exposure, and advised of the clinical symptoms of TB and the action to take should they develop symptoms

Tuberculosis (TB) is the second commonest cause of death in the world after HIV / AIDS, and although the incidence is declining year on year, in 2013 it was estimated that nine million people globally developed the disease and there were 1.5 million deaths (WHO, 2015b). In the UK, 7892 cases were notified to Public Health England (PHE, 2014f), giving an incidence of 12.3 per 100<ths>000 population. TB disproportionately affects deprived communities, with 70% of all cases in the UK being isolated from 40% of the most deprived areas. Large urban cities such as London, Leicester, Birmingham, Luton, Manchester and Coventry all have three times the national average of TB cases (PHE, 2014f). Although TB can affect any body site, **respiratory TB** is the most common form of the disease, accounting for almost 60% of cases in the UK (PHE, 2013l). Respiratory TB is defined in the NICE Guidance as active TB that is affecting any of the following:

- lungs
- pleural cavity
- mediastinal lymph nodes
- larynx.

The diagnosis and management of TB is complex. National guidance on the *Clinical diagnosis and management of tuberculosis, and measures for its prevention and control* was revised by the National Institute for Health and Clinical Excellence (NICE) in 2011 and 2016. **The Guidelines cover: diagnosis; the management of respiratory and non-respiratory TB; monitoring, adherence and treatment completion; risk assessment and infection control; management of latent TB; BCG vaccination; active case finding (contact tracing); and the prevention of infection in specific settings).** The updated Guidelines can be accessed at http://www.nice.org.uk/guidance/NG33.

The organism

Mycobacteria are slender, **obligate**, aerobic Gram-positive rods (bacilli) with no capsule. They are motile, non-spore forming and divide once every 16–24 hours, forming visible colonies on solid agar 3–6 weeks (Ryan and Drew, 2010d). The bacterial cell wall consists of 60% lipids, and the Ziehl–Neelsen stain technique is used to identify the waxy bacterial cell wall. There are over 80 species of Mycobacteria. Those which are human pathogens belong to a group of organisms known as the *Mycobacterium tuberculosis* complex (MTC), consisting of *Mycobacterium tuberculosis, M. bovis, M. africanum* and *M. microti. M. tuberculosis* is the principal cause of infectious tuberculosis in humans, pulmonary disease being the most clinically significant illness.

Opportunistic Mycobacteria

Some species of Mycobacteria are environmental opportunists isolated from water, soil, dust, milk, animals and birds (i.e. *M. kansasii, M. xenopi, M. chelonae, M. scrofulaceum, M. ulcerans, M. abscessus*). Although they are of low virulence and low grade pathogenicity, they can cause a wide range of opportunistic infections in immunocompromised individuals, particularly those with HIV infection or pre-existing chronic pulmonary disease. Human-to-human transmission is very rare, and even if an environmental mycobacterum is isolated from the sputum, the normal notification and contact tracing procedures that would be initiated in the event of infection with *M. tuberculosis* do not apply.

The pathogenesis of infection
The initial infection

Figure 44.1 describes the initial stages in the pathogenesis of infection. The primary site of TB infection is usually the lung, and takes place through the inhalation of TB bacilli, which are expelled in small droplets of moisture from infected individuals through coughing, talking and sneezing. These airborne droplets contain just a few viable bacilli but, as they are released into the air, water evaporates from the surface of the droplets and they become much smaller, forming droplet nuclei with a more concentrated bacterial count. Droplet nuclei can float in room air for several hours and it has been estimated that a single droplet is sufficient to initiate pulmonary infection in a susceptible individual (Plorde, 2004).

Figure 44.2 lists general patient risk factors for developing TB.

Latent and post-primary (reactivation) TB

Latent TB occurs when the individual's immune system has successfully overcome the initial infection (Figure 44.1). It is described as 'a state of persistent immune response to stimulation by *Mycobacterium tuberculosis* antigens without evidence of clinically manifested TB' (www.who.int/tb/challenges/ltbi/en) and one third of the world's population (two billion people) is estimated to have latent TB 'infection' (NICE, 2011).

Not all of the bacilli within the alveolar macrophages within the granuloma (see Figure 44.1) are destroyed; 'persisters' can survive for months to years, and active clinical disease can subsequently develop. Of individuals with latent TB, 5–10% will go on to develop active (symptomatic) infection (**post-primary, or reactivation, TB**), with the majority of these becoming symptomatic within five years of the initial infection (www.who.int/tb/challenges/ltbi/en). There are certain individuals with latent TB who are at **particular risk** of going onto develop active TB, and these are described in Figure 44.3. The granuloma becomes more necrotic and develops into a tuberculoma that eventually erodes into the bronchi and forms cavities in the lung. The oxygen-rich environment of the lung facilitates the growth of the bacilli, which can be found in huge numbers in the cavity walls (Pratt et al, 2005). From there, the bacilli gain access to the sputum and the individual becomes symptomatic.

Extra-pulmonary TB

Although the lung is the main focus, bacilli may be transported within the macrophages through the lymphatic system to the lymph nodes draining the affected site, where they may be disseminated via blood and lymph tissue to the liver, spleen, bone, brain and kidneys, giving rise to clinical disease affecting any of these organs. This is known as extra-pulmonary, non-respiratory or 'closed' TB, and is generally not considered to be infectious, although active pulmonary disease must be excluded. TB that is widely disseminated throughout the body is known as **miliary TB.** Extra-respiratory disease and disseminated tuberculosis are more commonly seen in HIV-positive patients compared to other patient groups, and may coexist alongside other opportunistic infections.

Figure 44.4 describes the clinical features of extra-pulmonary and respiratory disease. Figure 44.5 describes the investigations required in order to diagnose latent and active TB.

Multi-drug resistant (MDR) TB

As with any antimicrobial agent, bacteria can develop resistance (see Chapter 11), and Mycobacteria are no exception. Multi-drug resistant (MDR) TB is defined by the WHO as resistance to at least rifampicin (the main 'killing', or bactericidal, drug) and isoniazid (the 'sterilising' drug). NICE (2011) defines resistance to TB drugs as 'a level of resistance to four times or greater the concentration of drug required to inhibit a fully susceptible organism'. In 2013, it was estimated that 480 000 individuals worldwide developed MDR-TB, of whom 210 000 died. MDR-TB has developed because of:

• inadequate treatment of drug-sensitive strains, i.e. inadequate dose / duration

• poor patient compliance, i.e. lack of understanding regarding the duration of treatment, self-discontinuation of treatment due to side effects or when symptoms resolve.

Although it is no more infectious than drug-sensitive TB, and the pathogenesis of infection is the same, **the implications are greater in relation to treatment and patient outcomes**. Whereas an individual with drug-sensitive respiratory TB would be considered to be non-infectious after 2 weeks of anti-TB therapy (although treatment will last a minimum of 6 months), treatment for an individual with MDR respiratory TB may take up to two years and will consist of multiple antimicrobial agents with side effects.

The complexities of treatment and the need for prolonged close monitoring of their response to treatment mean that individuals with MDR-TB require admission to hospital. They may require isolation in a negative-pressure isolation room (see Chapter 21) for **many months**. Healthcare staff must be aware of the psychological impact of such prolonged enforced isolation, and work with the Chest / Respiratory Team, the local Public Health England Health Protection Team and the Infection Prevention and Control Team to plan how any risks of exposure / cross-infection can be mitigated in order to allow, for example, supervised walks for the patient outside.

All patients with suspected or confirmed TB must have a documented **risk assessment** undertaken for the likelihood of acquiring or developing MDR-TB (see Figure 44.6).

Extensively drug resistant (XDR) TB is defined as MDR-TB plus resistance to any fluoroquinolones *and* at least one of three injectable second-line drugs – capreomycin, kanamycin and amikacin (www.who.int/tb/challendes/mdr/xdr/en).

It has been reported in 100 countries worldwide and makes up 9% of the 480 000 individuals who were diagnosed with MDR-TB in 2013 (WHO, 2015b). In underdeveloped countries, and countries where there is a high prevalence of individuals living with HIV, XDR-TB poses a significant risk, and it was identified as a **global** threat to public health in 2006.

TB and HIV

Immunocompromised individuals are at increased risk of developing TB as an **opportunistic** infection, with those who are HIV positive being 26 – 31 times more likely to develop tuberculosis in a given year than those who are HIV negative (http://www.who.int). TB and HIV have been described as 'fatally synergistic' (http://www.tballiance.org). Approximately 90% of HIV-positive individuals co-infected with TB die within months of contracting it, as the suppression of the immune system with HIV rapidly accelerates the progression of TB from latent infection to active disease. TB is harder to diagnose in someone who is HIV positive as it can present in a non-specific, or atypical way, leading to misdiagnosis and a delay in treatment with rapidly fatal consequences.

Extra-respiratory disease and disseminated tuberculosis are more commonly seen in HIV-positive patients compared to other patient groups, and may coexist alongside other opportunistic infections.

Infectivity

Individuals with active (symptomatic) respiratory TB will generally be deemed to be infectious from the point at which they develop a cough, and a diagnosis of infectious respiratory tuberculosis is made if 5000–10 000 acid-fast bacilli are detected in 1 ml of sputum (Pratt et al, 2005; Fitzgerald et al, 2009). Bacilli will continue to be observed in sputum specimens, but an individual with 'ordinary' drug-sensitive respiratory TB will not be considered to be infectious if s/he has completed 2 weeks of anti-TB therapy. When investigating a case of infectious respiratory TB in either a healthcare or a community setting and identifying close contacts for screening (**active case finding**), determining the period of infectivity is key to establishing how far back (weeks to months) contact tracing needs to go, and who needs to be traced and screened.

The management of patients with respiratory TB

Figures 44.7 and 44.8 describe the management of patients in hospital and community settings, Figure 44.9 describes the treatment regimen, and Figure 44.10 describes the principles of contact tracing (active case finding).

Prevention of TB

Details of the BCG immunisation programme, which is no longer part of the 'schools ' immunisation programme but is instead based on an assessment of individuals at risk, can be found at www.gov.uk/government/collections/immunisation-against-infectious-disease-the-green-book

New entrants to the UK are identified from Port of Arrival reports, new registrations with primary care, entry to education (including university) and links with statutory and voluntary groups working with new entrants (NICE, 2011). In prisons and remand centres, a health questionnaire is completed on entry to the prison system, and all prisoners receiving treatment for latent or active TB have their medication administered and directly observed (DOT – directly observed therapy) in order to ensure compliance. Healthcare workers receive pre-employment screening via the Occupational Health Department in accordance with the NICE (2011) Guidance.

Staff working in healthcare settings in particular should always have an 'index of suspicion' with regard to TB for any patient presenting with the symptoms described in Figure 44.4. Differential diagnoses can include asthma, chest infection and lung cancer.

45 Varicella zoster

Figure 45.1 Presentation of varicella zoster virus (chickenpox) vesicles

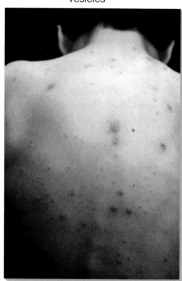

Source: U.S. Centers for Disease Control and Prevention; photo credit: CDC

Figure 45.4 Characteristics of varicella zoster virus

- Virus family: Herpesviridae
- Type: Double-stranded DNA (dsDNA)
- Enveloped virus: Yes
- Shape: Icosahedral
- Size: 180–200 nm
- Nucleocapsid: Icosahedral

Figure 45.2 Presentation of typical varicella zoster virus (chickenpox) vesicles

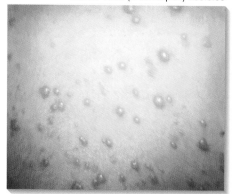

Source: U.S. Centers for Disease Control and Prevention; photo credit: Joe Miller

Figure 45.3 Presentation of shingles

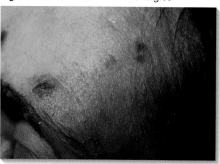

Source: U.S. Centers for Disease Control and Prevention; photo credit: CDC/Heinz F. Eichenwald, MD

Figure 45.5 Infection prevention and control precautions

In hospital

- Patients with varicella zoster infection must be nursed in isolation with **standard precautions** until lesions dry. They must not be nursed near immunocompromised individuals
- Only immune individuals may enter the room to visit or undertake care
- **Non-immune healthcare workers** with significant contact > 15 minutes must avoid contact with high-risk patients for 8–21 days after contact and may be offered the vaccine.
- Risk assessment of patients and staff exposed to case and identification of vulnerable contacts who may require varicella zoster immunoglobulin (VZIG)

In the community

- Individuals with chickenpox should be excluded from nursery, school or work until the vesicles have crusted over. For shingles, exclusion is only required if the rash is weeping and cannot be covered over
- Individuals with chickenpox or shingles must be advised to avoid contact with the following groups of people:
  - people who are immunocompromised
  - A pregnant woman
  - infants 4 weeks or less

Infection Prevention and Control at a Glance, First Edition. By Debbie Weston, Alison Burgess and Sue Roberts.
© 2017 John Wiley & Sons, Ltd. Published 2017 by John Wiley & Sons, Ltd.

Varicella zoster virus (VZV) causes a **systemic** viral infection. It was not recognised as an infectious agent until 1875 when Rudolf Steiner inoculated volunteers with vesicular fluid from an infected individual; the volunteers went on to develop the disease. In 1909 Von Bokay made the observation that chickenpox and herpes zoster were related infections, although this was not proven until the 1920s and 1930s. However, it was not until 1954 that Thomas Weller successfully isolated VZV from both varicella zoster and herpes zoster lesions. This was followed much later in 1972 by the development of a chickenpox vaccine by Japanese virologist Michiaki Takahashi, and in 2006 by the herpes zoster vaccine (CDC, 2015).

VZV causes two distinct diseases: primary disease in the form of **chickenpox** (see Figures 45.1 and 45.2), and secondary disease in the form of herpes zoster, more commonly referred to as **shingles** (Jumaan and Lavanchy, 2008) (see Figure 45.3). Man is the only reservoir. Primary infection with VZV (chickenpox) usually leads to life-long immunity which generally prevents a second attack of chickenpox (although occasionally there is a second occurrence), but the virus remains **latent** in the body and reactivation of the virus at a later stage in life results in herpes zoster (shingles) (Hawker et al, 2012). It is *not* possible to 'catch' shingles from someone with chickenpox, but individuals who have never had chickenpox (i.e. those who have no immunity to VZV) may acquire chickenpox from someone with shingles. Chickenpox is **highly contagious** with **epidemics** occurring every 1–2 years, usually in winter to early spring. Outbreaks are common in nurseries, schools and other institutional settings. In temperate climates at least 90% of the population will have had chickenpox by the age of 15 years, and 95% by young adulthood. Shingles occurs in approximately 10–20% of the population (Jumaan and Lavanchy, 2008).

Chickenpox is *not* notifiable in England or Wales. For ease of understanding in this chapter the two diseases caused by VZV will be referred to simply as 'chickenpox' and 'shingles'.

Characteristics of VZV

Figure 45.4 describes the characteristics of VZV.

Pathogenesis of infection

Chickenpox: In primary infection VZV enters the body through the respiratory tract and conjunctiva and is believed to replicate at the site of entry in the nasopharynx and in regional lymph nodes. Approximately 4–6 days after infection a primary **viraemia** occurs and the virus is disseminated to other organs, such as the liver, spleen and sensory ganglia. The virus then replicates in the viscera, and this is followed by a secondary viraemia and viral infection of the skin which causes the characteristic eruption of the vesicles (CDC, 2015). During primary infection VZV enters sensory nerve endings and establishes latent infection in sensory neurones in dorsal root ganglia.

Shingles: Secondary infection reactivation usually occurs at the sites of the original varicella lesions – most commonly the thoracic, cervical and ophthalmic dermatomes. The lesions of shingles, however, are unilateral because the reactivation is a localised event in a single dorsal root ganglion, most often involving the trunk or the fifth cranial nerve (Hawker et al, 2012). Lesions are histologically identical to those of chickenpox, but are deeper and more closely aggregated (Jumaan and Lavanchy, 2008).

Mode of transmission

Chickenpox and shingles: The most common mode of transmission of VZV is believed to be person to person from infected respiratory tract secretions, including saliva, and via respiratory contact with airborne droplets. It may also occur by direct contact or inhalation of aerosols from vesicular fluid from both chickenpox and shingles skin lesions (CDC, 2015). Approximately 96% of susceptible people exposed to VZV will develop primary chickenpox (Hawker et al, 2012). The virus in shingles lesions is transmitted in the same way but has a lower rate of transmission (Jumaan and Lavanchy, 2008).

Incubation period

Chickenpox: The incubation period is about 16 days but ranges from 7 to 24 days (Hawker et al, 2012). The period of infectivity begins 1–2 days before the rash appears and continues until all lesions are crusted over (average 5 days), although people who are immunosuppressed may be infectious for much longer (Jumaan and Lavanchy, 2008).

Shingles: This is much less infectious than chickenpox. The period of communicability is 1–2 days before the individual develops a rash until the lesions are dry.

Risk factors for VZV infection

Chickenpox: Susceptibility to chickenpox is universal among those not previously infected or vaccinated but the disease is more common in children under 10 years (PHE, 2013m). The main concern lies in the fact that certain groups of people are at a *greater risk of serious complications*, for example those who are immuno compromised, undergoing chemotherapy, have HIV, or are on high-dose corticosteroids. Those who smoke, have severe lung or cardiovascular disease, or have undergone organ transplants or splenectomy are also more vulnerable to infection (Hawker et al, 2012). Pregnant women are *not at greater risk of infection but for non-immune women there is particular risk to the foetus* in weeks 13–20 of pregnancy with **congenital varicella syndrome** seen in 1–2% of cases (Hawker et al, 2012). In addition, if a pregnant woman is infected a few days before or after delivery, the infant is exposed without the protection of maternal antibodies and can suffer serious disease.

Shingles: Individuals are more likely to develop shingles if they are immunosuppressed, had intrauterine exposure to VZV or had chickenpox under 18 months of age. Shingles occurs mainly in the elderly population and the incidence is related to increasing age (PHE, 2013m).

Clinical signs and symptoms
Chickenpox

Infection in healthy children is generally mild and self-limiting, but adults may have more severe disease with a higher incidence of complications (CDC, 2015). Signs and symptoms are as follows:

Mild prodromal illness: This may occur with fever up to 38.9 °C (102 °F) for 2–3 days, headache, nausea, anorexia, general malaise and myalgia.

Rash: Small, erythematous macules that appear on scalp, face, trunk and proximal limbs, progressing over 12–14 hours to papules, clear vesicles (which are intensely itchy) and pustules. **Vesicles** can occur on the palms and soles, and mucous membranes can also be affected with painful and shallow oral or genital ulcers. Vesicles appear in crops so stages of development of the rash may vary on different parts of the body. **Crusting** occurs within 1–4 days, and crusts fall off after 1–2 weeks.

In the immunosuppressed and those with malignancies, extensive chickenpox lesions may appear outside the main dermatome affected (Jumaan and Lavanchy, 2008).

Shingles

VZV reactivates in the affected sensory root ganglions approximately 2–4 days prior to the eruption of the erythematous vesicular rash. It takes a few days for the virus to travel down peripheral nerves and multiply in the skin. There may be paraesthesia and severe pain accompanied by fever and malaise (CDC, 2015). The rash lasts 7–10 days and heals in 2–4 weeks, but the pain, particularly in the elderly, may persist long after the initial lesions have healed (Hawker et al, 2012).

Complications

Chickenpox: The risk of complications from chickenpox varies with age. Complications are infrequent among healthy children and occur much more frequently in children older than 15 years of age and in infants younger than 1 year of age (CDC, 2015). Secondary bacterial infections of skin lesions with Staphylococcus or Streptococcus (see Chapters 43 and 36) are the most common cause of hospitalisation, including infection with invasive group A Streptococcus. Varicella pneumonia is usually viral but may be bacterial and is more common in those who smoke or have severe lung or cardiovascular disease. Immunocompromised individuals have a high risk of pneumonia, encephalitis, disseminated disease and haemorrhagic complications (CDC, 2015). Another complication is Reye's syndrome, which occurs almost exclusively in children who have taken aspirin during the acute stage of the disease.

Shingles: Complications occur in approximately 30% of shingles cases (Jumaan and Lavanchy, 2008). The most common complication is severe pain or post-herpetic neuralgia (PHN), particularly in the elderly. This may last for 30–90 days after the rash has resolved, but can persist for months or years (Jumaan and Lavanchy, 2008). VZV may also cause permanent damage such as cranial nerve palsy (and contralateral hemiplegia). Ophthalmic zoster involving the upper eyelid, forehead and scalp may lead to serious visual impairment (Jumaan and Lavanchy, 2008). Patients with shingles may also have disseminated disease with generalised skin lesions.

Method of diagnosis for VZV

Laboratory confirmation is rarely required as the clinical features for both chickenpox and shingles are *so specific* (Hawker et al, 2012). VZV is most often isolated from vesicle fluid from both chickenpox and shingles lesions. Blood for serology (VZV IgG) is also useful in terms of demonstrating immunity and determining past infection.

Treatment of VZV infection

Chickenpox: Treatment is not recommended for healthy individuals. Symptomatic relief includes paracetamol for pain or fever, soothing baths, calamine lotion on spots, and antihistamines with the aim of preventing scratching and secondary infection (NICE, 2015). Antiviral drugs are not given routinely but may be given to immunocompromised individuals or if there is a risk of complications.

Shingles: Antiviral agents are usually recommended because they help to reduce the incidence, duration and severity of the pain but they must be started within 72 hours of the rash appearing. Symptomatic treatment is as for chickenpox.

Vaccination for VZV

Chickenpox: In the UK, the chickenpox vaccine (which is a live vaccine containing a small amount of weakened VZV) is *not* part of the routine vaccination schedule. It is generally recommended for healthy susceptible contacts of immunocompromised individuals, non-immune healthcare workers and laboratory workers (PHE, 2013m).

Shingles: The shingles vaccine is similar to that for chickenpox but not identical. It confers protection for approximately 5 years. The UK varicella zoster (shingles) vaccine is currently administered routinely to those aged 70 and is also offered as part of a catch-up programme to eligible individuals until their 80th birthday (PHE, 2013m). Vaccine effectiveness declines with increasing age, especially over the age of 80 years (CDC, 2015)

Varicella zoster immunoglobulin (VZIG)

Varicella zoster immunoglobulin (VZIG) prophylaxis should be offered to all vulnerable contacts who are susceptible and have had significant exposure. This includes pregnant women, neonates and immunocompromised individuals.

Infection prevention and control precautions

The recommended infection prevention and control requirements are described in Figure 45.5.

Glossary

acidosis Increased acidity in the blood / body tissues.

adsorption (attachment) The adhesion of atoms, ions or molecules from a gas, liquid or dissolved solid to a surface. For example it may refer to the adhesion of a virus to a cell, or the adhesion of bacteria to surfaces.

antigen/antigenic A 'substance' that stimulates that the immune system into generating a response.

aqueous humor Gelatinous clear fluid that fills the space in the front of the eye between the lens and the cornea.

arthralgia Joint pain.

aseptic meningitis Inflammation of the meninges surrounding the brain that is not caused by a bacterial infection.

attack rate The proportion of individuals who become ill after exposure to infection.

autonomic dysreflexia A life-threatening medical emergency occurring in individuals with a spinal cord injury above the level of the sixth thoracic vertebrae (T6), occurring as the result of an 'irritating' stimulus below the level of the injury (e.g. constipation / faecal impaction or a full bladder / blocked urinary catheter.

bacteraemia The presence of bacteria in the blood (blood is sterile).

biofilm Biofilms are densely packed communities of microbial cells that grow on living or inert surfaces excreting a slimy, glue-like substance that enables them to anchor themselves.

blepharitis A chronic condition of the eyelids that arises when the glands around the eyelashes become blocked and infected.

chemoprophylaxis The use of drugs to prevent infection or disease.

clonal A clone is a group of identical cells that share a common ancestry, meaning that they are derived from the same cell.

colonised Adherence of microorganisms to the skin or mucosal surfaces without any obvious adverse effects on the host (individual) (no clinical signs of infection).

commensal(s) Part of the 'normal' bacterial flora; they are different species of bacteria that 'live' together and benefit from each other, and generally do not cause disease or infection in the host, although they may have disease potential in certain situations (i.e. if the host is immunocompromised).

co-morbidities Additional disorders / illness / disease, including chronic conditions.

congenital varicella syndrome Congenital abnormalities seen in babies born to mothers infected with varicella zoster virus during early pregnancy (up to 20 weeks gestation). These include encephalitis, hydrocephalus (abnormal build-up of CSF in the ventricles of the brain), visual defects, spinal cord defects, underdevelopment or incomplete development of the upper / lower extremities, growth retardation, and defects of the gastrointestinal and genitourinary tracts.

conjunctiva / conjunctival The mucous membrane covering the front of the eye and lining the eyelids.

conjunctivitis Inflammation of the conjunctiva.

cytokines Non-antibody proteins or mediators that influence other cells.

desiccation The state of extreme dryness. In the absence of water, microorganisms cannot grow or reproduce, but can remain viable for years. When water is made available to them, their resume their growth and cellular division.

disseminated intravascular coagulation (DIC) An inappropriate activation of the blood clotting cascade.

dysuria Pain or difficulty passing urine.

EDTA Ethylenediamine tetraacetic acid – used as an anticoagulant to prevent blood samples from clotting.

encephalitis / encephalopathy Inflammation, damage or malfunction of the brain.

endemic Regularly found amongst a particular group of people, or in a certain area / region.

enteric Intestinal.

epidemic Occurrence of an illness or disease within a community or population at a particular time.

epidemiology The study of the incidence, distribution / pattern and causes of infection and infectious diseases.

eukaryote Cell with a nucleus, nuclear membrane and organelles ('little organs').

extended spectrum beta-lactamases (ESBLs) Enzymes 'expressed' by Gram-negative bacteria that render bacteria multi-antibiotic resistant – to cephalosporins and penicillins predominantly, but also to other antibiotics.

furunculosis A deep infection of the hair follicle.

glomerulonephritis Damage to the tiny filters inside the kidneys (the glomeruli), often caused by the immune system attacking healthy body tissue. In severe cases, glomerulonephritis may cause visible blood in the urine, swelling of the legs (oedema) or other parts of the body.

glycocalyx A glycoprotein (protein and carbohydrate) polysaccharide (carbohydrate containing sugar molecules) covering or coat.

glycopeptide-resistant enterococci (GRE) Enterococci are commensals of the bowels in humans and animals; GRE are enterococci that have acquired resistance to glycopeptide antibiotics (vancomycin).

Guillain–Barré syndrome An autoimmune condition in which the immune system 'attacks' the peripheral nervous system, leading to extreme muscle weakness and paralysis. The exact cause is unknown but it is often preceded by an acute bacterial or viral infection.

haematuria Blood in the urine.

helminth A parasitic worm.

hyperkeratotic / hyperkeratosis Thickening of the outermost layer of the epidermis (stratum corneum).

hypoxia Deprivation of an adequate supply of oxygen.

incidence The occurrence, rate or frequency of an illness or disease.

incubation period The period (time) between exposure to an infection / disease and displaying symptoms.

index case The first identified case / person in a population of individuals with the same infection / disease.

inocula A substance used for inoculation (a virus, toxin or immune serum).

invasiveness Ability to enter the body and spread in the tissues.

keratitis Inflammation of the cornea of the eye.

Lancefield antigens Antigenic characteristics of streptococci are based on the C-carbohydrate in the bacterial cell walland named after Rebecca Lancefield, an American microbiologist.

latent Dormant or hidden; present, but not visible; capable of developing or emerging.

lyse / lysis Disintegration of a cell caused by cell wall or membrane rupture.

maculopapular rash A rash characterized by a flat, red area on the skin that is covered with small confluent bumps. It may only appear red in lighter-skinned people. The term 'maculopapular' is a compound: macules are small, flat, discoloured spots on the surface of the skin; papules are small, raised bumps.

morbidity The state of being diseased or unhealthy.

mortality / mortality rate Death / the number of deaths in a particular population due to a particular cause or over a specific period of time.

myalgia Pain in a muscle / group of muscles.

myocarditis Inflammation of the myocardium, the middle and thickest layer of the heart wall.

nephritis Inflammation of the kidneys.

neutropenia / neutropenic Increased susceptibility owing to abnormally low levels of neutrophils (white blood cells) in the bloodstream.

nucleocapsid The nucleic acid and its surrounding protein coat or capsid; the basic unit of a virion structure (Prescott et al, 2005c).

obligate Able to exist only in a certain environment; for example, obligate aerobe, or obligate anaerobe.

opportunistic Infections that arise as a result of the host's weakened immunity / altered body defences, that would otherwise not normally occur.

papilloedema Swelling of the disc of the optic nerve (where the nerve meets the eye) caused by raised intracranial pressure.

pathogen / pathogenic The ability to cause disease.

pericarditis Inflammation of the pericardium, the membrane (sac) that encloses the heart and the roots of the great blood vessels.

petechiae Red or purple spots under the skin caused by broken blood capillaries.

photophobia Extreme sensitivity to light, causing pain.

positive / negative sense In virology the genome of an RNA virus can be said to be either positive sense 'plus strand', or negative sense 'minus strand'. Whether a virus is positive or negative sense can be used as a basis for classifying viruses.

prions Proteinaceous infectious particles (PrP); the causative agents of the transmissible spongiform encephalopathies, causing scrapie in sheep and goats, BSE in cattle, and CJD in humans. They are thought to be naturally occurring proteins derived from normal body proteins which undergo a rare spontaneous process, affecting normal protein synthesis in the individual and creating microscopic vacuoles (holes) in the grey matter of the brain. They do not induce an immune response and have no detectable nucleic acid.

prodrome / prodromal illness Early symptoms of illness / infection; often non-specific.

prokaryote A cell that does not contain a nucleus or organelles ('little organs').

protozoa / protozoal Single-celled microscopic animals with no cell wall.

pruritic Itchy, giving the urge to scratch.

purulent Containing, discharging or causing the production of pus.

resident bacteria: Bacteria that 'live' or reside in / on certain parts of the body.

self / non-self antigens Markers on cell walls and tissues that identify whether or not the cell belongs to the host or whether it is 'foreign' (i.e. has originated from elsewhere).

seroconversion The development of specific antibodies in response to a specific agent (infection).

skin squames Flakes of dead skin tissue.

spasticity Muscle overactivity arising as a consequence of brain or spinal cord injury, which can result in contracture of muscles.

subacute sclerosing panencephalitis A rare and chronic form of progressive brain inflammation caused by a persistent infection.

synergistic Working together.

systemic System wide; affecting the whole body.

thrombocytopenia A deficiency in the platelets in the blood that causes bleeding into the tissues, bruising and slow clotting after injury.

transverse myelitis Acute inflammation of a segment of the spinal cord.

ubiquitous Found everywhere.

vector A living organism, usually an animal or an arthropod (insect or tick) that transfers an infectious microbe from one host to another.

vesicles Small blisters.

viraemia The presence of a virus in the blood.

virion A complete virus particle that represents the extracellular phase of the virus life cycle; at the simplest, it consists of a protein capsid surrounding a single nucleic acid molecule (Prescott et al, 2005c).

virulent / virulence Extremely infectious or malignant; a measure of an organism's ability to cause severe disease / infection.

References

Abad C., Fearday A., Safdar N. (2010). Adverse effects of isolation in hospitalised patients: a systematic review. *Journal of Hospital Infection* 76 (2): 97–102.

Adair C.G., Gorman S.P., Feron B.M. et al (1999). Implications of endotracheal biofilm for ventilator-associated pneumonia. *Intensive Care Medicine* 25: 1072–1076.

Ahmad N., Ray C.G., Drew W.L. (2010a). Retroviruses: Human T-Lymphotropic Virus, Human Immunodeficiency Virus, and Acquired Immune Deficiency Syndrome. In: Ryan K., Ray C.G. (Eds) *Sherris Medical Microbiology*. Fifth Edition. McGraw Hill, London: pp. 305–326.

Ahmad N., Ray C.G., Drew W.L. (2010b). Influenza, Parainfluenza, Respiratory Syncytial Virus, Adenovirus, and Other Respiratory Viruses. In: Ryan K.J., Ray C.G. (Eds) *Sherris Medical Microbiology*. Fifth Edition. McGraw Hill, London: pp. 167–188.

Ahmad N., Ray C.G., Drew W.L. (2010c). Viruses of Diarrhoea. In: Ryan K.J., Ray C.G. (Eds) *Sherris Medical Microbiology*. Fifth Edition. McGraw Hill, London: pp. 271–278.

Ala'Aldeen D.A.A. (2007). Neisseria and Moraxella. In: Greenwood D., Slack R., Peutherer J., Barer M. (Eds) *Medical Microbiology. A Guide to Microbial Infections: Pathogenesis, Immunity, Laboratory Diagnosis and Control*. Seventeenth Edition. Churchill Livingstone, London: pp. 251–259.

American Thoracic Society and the Infectious Diseases Society of America (2004). Guidelines for the management of adults with hospital-acquired, ventilator-associated and healthcare-associated pneumonia. *American Journal of Respiratory and Critical Care Med* 171: 388–416.

Barer M. (2007). Bacterial growth, physiology and death. In: Greenwood D., Slack R., Peutherer J., Barer M. (Eds) *A Guide to Microbial Infections, Pathogenesis, Immunity, Laboratory Diagnosis and Control*. Seventeenth Edition. Churchill Livingstone, London: pp. 38–51.

Barker J., Vipond I.B., Bloomfield S.F. (2004). Effects of cleaning and disinfection in reducing the spread of norovirus contamination via environmental surfaces. *Journal of Hospital Infection* 58 (1): 42–49.

Barrett R. (2010). Behind barriers: patients' perceptions of source isolation for methicillin-resistant 'Staphylococcus aureus' (MRSA). *Australian Journal of Advanced Nursing* 28 (2): 53–59.

Betsy T.D.C., Keogh R.N. (2012a). Prokaryote Cells and Eukaryotic Cells. In: *Microbiology De-Mystified. Hard Stuff Made Easy*. McGraw-Hill, London: pp. 65–88.

Betsy T.D.C., Keogh R.N. (2012b). Viruses, Viroids and Prions. In: *Microbiology De-Mystified. Hard Stuff Made Easy*. McGraw-Hill, London: pp. 193–206.

Bonten M.J., Hayden M.K., Nathan C., et al. (1996). Epidemiology of colonisation of patients and environment with vancomycin-resistant Enterococci. *Lancet* 348: 1615–1619.

Boyce J.M., Potter-Bynoe G., Opal S.M., Dziobek L. Medeiros A.A. (1990). A common-source outbreak of Staphylococcus epidermidis infections among patients undergoing cardiac surgery. *Journal of Infectious Diseases* 161 (3): 493–499.

Bray M., Chertow D.S. (2015). Epidemiology and pathogenesis of Ebola virus disease. Available at: http://www.uptodate.com/contents/epidemiology-and-pathogenesis-of-ebola-virus-disease

Briggs M., Wilson S., Fuller A. (1996). The principles of aseptic technique in wound care. *Professional Nurse* 11 (12): 805–810.

British HIV Association (2012). *BHIVA Guidelines for the Treatment of HIV-1 Infected Adults with Antiretroviral Therapy 2012*. British HIV Association, London.

Buggy D. (2000). Can anaesthetic management influence surgical wound healing? *Lancet* 356 (9227): 355–357.

Bull R.A., Tu E.T., McIver C.J., Rawlinson W.D., White P.A. (2006). Emergence of a new norovirus genotype II.4 variant associated with global outbreaks of gastroenteritis. *Journal Clinical Microbiology* 44 (2): 327–333.

Burgess C.M., Wolverson A.S., Dale M.T. (2005). Cervical epidural abscess: a rare complication of intravenous cannulation. *Anaesthesia* 60 (6): 605–608.

Burton G.W., Duben-Engelkirk P.G. (2004). Pathogenesis of Infectious Disease. In: *Microbiology for the Health Sciences*. Lippincott, Williams and Wilkins, Philadelphia: pp. 360–379.

Cameron P.A., Schull M., Cooke M. (2006). The impending influenza pandemic: lessons from SARS for hospital practice. *Medical Journal of Australia* 185 (4): 188–189.

Carling P.C., Parry M.F., Von Beheren S.M. (2008). Identifying opportunities to enhance environmental cleaning in 23 acute care hospitals. *Infection Control and Hospital Epidemiology* 29: 1–7.

Centers for Disease Control and Prevention (2002). Guideline for Hand Hygiene in Health-Care Settings. Recommendations of the Healthcare Infection Control Practices advisory committee and the HICPAC/SHEA/APIC/IDSA Hand Hygiene Force. *Morbidity and Mortality Weekly Report* 51 RR-16:1-48. Available at: http://www.cdc.gov/mmwr/PDF/rr/rr5116.pdf

Centers for Disease Control and Prevention (2012). *Principles of Epidemiology in Public Health Practice, third edition. An Introduction to Applied Epidemiology and Biostatics*. Office of Workforce and Career Development, Atlanta, GA. Available at: http://www.cdc.gov/ophss/csels/dsepd/SS1978/SS1978.pdf

Centers for Disease Control and Prevention (2009). Salmonellosis. Available at: http://www.cdc.gov/nczved/divisions/dfbmd/diseases/salmonellosis/#prevent

Centers for Disease Prevention and Control (2015). *Epidemiology and Prevention of Vaccine-Preventable Diseases.* Thirteenth Edition Public Health Foundation, Washington D.C.

Chadwick P.R., Beards G., Brown D. et al (2000). Report of the Public Health Laboratory Service Viral Gastro Enteritis Working Group: Management of hospital outbreaks of gastro-enteritis due to small round structured viruses. *Journal of Hospital Infection* 45 (1): 1–10.

Cheesbrough J.S., Barkess-Jones L., Brown D.W. (1997). Possible prolonged environmental survival of small round structured viruses. *Journal of Hospital Infection* 35 (4): 325–326.

Coia J.E., Duckworth G.J., Edwards D.I., Farrington M., Fry C., Humphreys H., Mallaghan C., Tucker D.R.; Joint Working Party of the British Society of Antimicrobial Chemotherapy; Hospital Infection Society; Infection Control Nurses Association (2006). Guidelines for the control and prevention of meticillin-resistant Staphylococcus aureus (MRSA) in healthcare facilities. *Journal of Hospital Infection* 64 (1): 97–98.

Coia J.E., Ritchie L., Adisesh A. et al, The Healthcare Infection Society Working Group on Respiratory and Facial Protection (2013). Guidance on the use of respiratory and facial protection equipment. *Journal of Hospital Infection* 85: 170–182.

College of Emergency Medicine and the UK Sepsis Trust (2014). *Sepsis: A Toolkit for Emergency Departments.* Available at: http://sepsistrust.org/wp-content/uploads/2015/08/1409306451EMToolkit2104FINAL.compressed.pdf

Collier L., Kellam P., Oxford J. (2011a). Retroviruses and HIV. In: *Human Virology.* Fourth Edition. Oxford University Press, Oxford: pp. 223–236.

Collier L., Kellam P., Oxford J (2011b). The blood-borne hepatitis C virus. In: *Human Virology.* Fourth Edition. Oxford University Press, Oxford: pp. 201–217.

Collier L., Kellam P., Oxford J. (2011c). Orthomyxoviruses and influenza. In: *Human Virology.* Fourth Edition. Oxford University Press, Oxford: pp. 101–109.

Collier L., Kellam P., Oxford J. (2011d). Gastroenteritis viruses. In: *Human Virology.* Fourth Edition. Oxford University Press, Oxford: pp. 110–120.

Cook D.J., Walter S.D., Cook R.J. et al (1998). Incidence of and risk factors for ventilator-associated pneumonia in critically ill patients. *Annals of Internal Medicine* 129 (6): 433–440.

Cookson B.D. (1999). Nosocomial antimicrobial resistance surveillance. *Journal of Hospital Infection* 43; Supplement S97–103.

Coppage C.M. (1961). *Hand Washing in Patient Care* [Motion picture]. US Public Health Service, Washington, DC.

Craven D.E., Chroneou A. (2009). Nosocomial Pneumonia. In: Mandell G.L., Bennett J.E., Dolin R (Eds) *Mandell, Douglas and Bennett's Principles and Practice of Infectious Diseases.* Seventh Edition. Churchill Livingstone, London. Available at: http://expertconsult.com

Cunningham J.B., Kernohan W.G., Sowney, R. (2005) Bed occupancy and turnover interval as determinant factors in MRSA infections in acute settings in Northern Ireland. *Journal of Hospital Infection* 61 (3): 189–193.

Dancer S.J. (2010). Control of transmission of infection in hospitals requires more than clean hands. *Infection Control Hospital Epidemiology* 31 (9): 958–960.

Daniels R., Nutbeam T., McNamara G., Galvin C. (2011). The sepsis six and the severe sepsis resuscitation bundle: a prospective observational cohort study. Emergency Medicine Journal 28 (6): 507–512.

Darouiche R.O., Wall M.J. Jr., Itani K.M. et al (2010). Chlorhexidine-alcohol versus povidone-iodine for surgical-site antisepsis. *New England Journal of Medicine* 362 (1): 18–26.

Deen G.F., Knust B., Broutet N. et al (2015). Ebola RNA persistence in semen of Ebola virus disease survivors – Preliminary Report. *New England Journal of Medicine.* Available at: www.nekm.org/doi/full/10.1056/NEJMoa1511410

Department of Health (2002). *Getting Ahead of the Curve. A Strategy for Combating Infectious Diseases (Including Other Aspects of Health Protection). A report by the Chief Medical Officer.* DH, London.

Department of Health (2004) *Towards Cleaner Hospitals and Lower Rates of Infection: A Summary of Action.* DH, London.

Department of Health (2006). *Screening for Meticillin-resistant Staphylococcus aureus (MRSA) colonisation: A strategy for NHS trusts: a summary of best practice.* DH, London. Available at: http://webarchive.nationalarchives.gov.uk/20130107105354/

Department of Health (2007a). *Hospital organisation, specialty mix and MRSA.* DH, London

Department of Health (2007b). *Taking Blood Cultures: A Summary of Best Practice.* DH, London.

Department of Health (2007c). *High Impact Intervention No.5. Care Bundle for Ventilated Patients.* DH, London.

Department of Health (2010). High-Impact Intervention – care bundle to reduce the risk from Clostridium difficile in: *Saving Lives: reducing infection, delivering clean safe care.* DH, London

Department of Health (2011a). *Annual Report of the Chief Medical Officer 2011. Volume 2. Infections and the rise of antimicrobial resistance.* DH, London.

Department of Health (2011b). *High impact Intervention care bundle peripheral intravenous cannula.* DH, London

Department of Health (2011c). *High Impact Intervention care bundle to prevent surgical site infection.* DH, London

Department of Health (2013a). *Decontamination Health Care Technical Memorandum 01-5. Decontamination on primary care dental practices.* DH, London.

Department of Health (2013b). *Department of Health Choice Framework for local Policy and Procedures 01-01-Management and decontamination of surgical instruments (medical devices) used in acute care.* DH, London.

Department of Health (2013c). *Department of Health Choice Framework for local Policy and Procedures 01-06 – Decontamination of flexible endoscopes.* DH, London

Department of Health (2014). *Implementation of modified admission MRSA screening guidance for NHS.* Department of Health expert advisory committee on Antimicrobial Resistance and Healthcare Associated Infection (ARHAI). DH, London.

Department of Health (2015). *The Health and Social Care Act 2008. Code of Practice on the prevention and control of infections and related guidance.* DH, London.

Department of Health Advisory Committee on Antimicrobial Resistance and Healthcare Associated Infection / Health Protection Agency (2010). *Advice on Carbapenemase Producers: Recognition, infection control and treatment.* HPA, London.

Department of Health Advisory Committee on Antimicrobial Resistance and Healthcare Associated Infections (ARHAI) (2011). *Antimicrobial Stewardship. Start Smart-Then Focus. Guidance for antimicrobial stewardship in hospitals (England)*. DH, London.

Department of Health Advisory Committee on Dangerous Pathogens / Health and Safety Executive (2015). *Management of Hazard Group 4 viral haemorrhagic fevers and similar human infectious diseases of high consequence*. ACDP, London.

Department of Health and Health Protection Agency (2008). *Clostridium difficile Infection: How to deal with the problem*. DH/HPA, London.

Department of Health and Health Protection Agency (2013). *Prevention and control of infection in care homes – an information resource*. DH, London.

Department of Health / Department of the Environment, Food and Rural Affairs (2013). *UK Five Year Antimicrobial Resistance Strategy 2013 to 2018*. DH, London.

Department of Health/Public Health Laboratory service Joint Working Group (1994). *Clostridium difficile Infection Prevention and Management*. Department of Health / Public Health Laboratory Service. London 362 (1): 18–26.

Department of Health/UK Health Departments (1998). *Guidance for Clinical Health Care Workers: Protection against infection with blood-borne viruses*. DH, London.

Dolin R., Treanor J.J. (2009). Noroviruses and Other Caliciviruses. In: Mandell G.L., Bennett J.E., Dolin R (Eds) *Mandell, Douglas, and Bennett's Principles and Practice of Infectious Diseases*. Seventh Edition. Churchill Livingstone, London. Available at: http://expertconsult.com

Donowitz G.R. (2009). Acute Pneumonia. In: Mandell G.L., Bennett J.E., Dolin R.D (Eds) *Mandell, Douglas, and Bennett's Principles and Practice of Infectious Diseases*. Seventh Edition. Churchill Livingstone, London. Available at: http://expertconsult.com

Duckworth G., Cookson B., Humphreys H., Heathcock R. (1998). Revised methicillin-resistant Staphylococcus aureus infection control guidelines for hospitals. Report of a Working Party of the British Society for Antimicrobial Chemotherapy, the Hospital Infection Society and the Infection Control Nurses Association. *Journal of Hospital Infection* 39: 253–290.

Dunn L. (2005). Pneumonia: classification, diagnosis and nursing management. *Nursing Standard* 19 (42): 50–54.

Eberhard M., Ndowa F., Watson J. (2008). Scabies. In: Heyman D.I. (Ed) *Control of Communicable Diseases Manual*. Nineteenth Edition. American Public Health Association, Baltimore.

Eden J.E., Hewitt J., Lim K.L. et al (2014). The emergence and evolution of the novel epidemic norovirus GII.4 variant Sydney 2012. *Virology* 450–451: 106–113.

Engelkirk P.G., Duben-Engelkirk J.D. (2011). Containing microbial growth in vivo using antimicrobial agents. In: *Burtons' Microbiology for the Health Sciences*. Ninth Edition. Lippincott, Williams and Wilkins, Baltimore: pp. 140–157.

Esposito S., Purrello S.M., Bonnet E. et al (2013). Central venous catheter-related biofilm infections: An up-to-date focus on meticillin-resistant Staphylococcus aureus. *Journal of Global Antimicrobial Resistance* 1 (2): 71–78.

European Centre for Disease Prevention and Control (2014*). ECDC Rapid Risk Assessment. Circulation of drifted influenza A (H3N2) viruses in the EU/EAA*. 22nd December 2014.

Fitzgerald D., Sterling T.R., Haas D.W. (2009). Mycobacterium tuberculosis. In: Mandell G.L., Bennett J.E., Dolin R.D (Eds) *Mandell, Douglas, and Bennett's Principles and Practice of Infectious Diseases*. Seventh Edition. Churchill Livingstone, London. Available at: http://expertconsult.com

Foca M., Jacob K., Whittier S., Della L. P., Factor S., Rubenstein D., Saiman L. (2000). Endemic Pseudomonas aeruginosa infection in a neonatal intensive care unit. *New England Journal of Medicine* 343 (10): 695–700.

Food Standards Agency (2014) Campylobacter. Available at: https://www.food.gov.uk/science/microbiology/ campylobacterevidenceprogramme

Frank M.O., Batteiger B.E., Sorensen S.J., et al. (1997). Decrease in expenditures and selected nosocomial infections following implementation of an antimicrobial-prescribing improvement program. *Clinical Performance and Quality Health Care* 5: 180–188.

Fukatsu K., Saito H., Matsuda T., Ikeda S., Furukawa S., Muto T. (1997). Influences of type and duration of antimicrobial prophylaxis on an outbreak of methicillin-resistant Staphylococcus aureus and on the incidence of wound infection. *Archives of Surgery* 132: 1320–1325.

Fuller C., Robotham J., Savage J. et al (2013). *The National One Week Prevalence Audit of Universal Meticillin-Resistant Staphylococcus aureus (MRSA) Admission Screening 2012*. Available at: www.ucl.ac.uk/medicine/documents/doh-now-report-2013

Gallant P, Schultz A.A. (2006). Evaluation of a visual infusion phlebitis scale for determining appropriate discontinuation of peripheral intravenous catheters. *Journal of Infusion Nursing* 29 (6): 338–345.

Garbino J., Bernard J-E., Uckay I., Fonseca S.M., Sax H. (2004). Impact of positive legionella urinary antigen test on patient management and improvement of antibiotic use. *Journal of Clinical Pathology* 57 (12): 1302–1305.

Garner J.S., Favero M.S. (1986). Guideline for Handwashing and Hospital Environmental Control. *Infection Control* 7 (4): 231–243.

Gilmour D. (1999). Redefining aseptic technique. *Journal of Community Nursing* 13 (7): 22–26.

Girou E., Legrand P., Soing-Altrach S. et al (2006). Association between hand hygiene compliance and methicillin resistant Staphylococcus aureus prevalence in a French rehabilitation hospital. *Infection Control and Hospital Epidemiology* 27 (10): 1128–1130.

Gladwell M. (2000). *How Little Things Can Make a Big Difference*. Little, Brown & Co, Boston.

Gladwin M., Trattler B. (2006a). Bacterial Taxonomy. In: *Clinical Microbiology Made Ridiculously Simple*. Third Edition. Medmaster Inc, Miami: pp. 1–7.

Gladwin M., Trattler B. (2006b). Cell Structures, Virulence Factors and Toxins. In: *Clinical Microbiology Made Ridiculously Simple*. Third Edition. Medmaster Inc, Miami: pp. 8–15.

Gladwin M., Trattler B. (2006c). Virus Replication and Taxonomy. In: *Clinical Microbiology Made Ridiculously Simple*. Third Edition. Medmaster Inc, Miami: pp. 161–170.

Gladwin M., Trattler B. (2006d). Haemophilus, Bordetella and Legionella. In: *Clinical Microbiology Made Ridiculously Simple*. Third Edition. Medmaster Inc, Miami: pp. 68–72.

Golden S.H., Peart-Vigilance C., Kao W.H., Brancati F.L. (1999). Perioperative glycaemic control and the risk of infection complications in a cohort of adults with diabetes. *Diabetes Care* 22: 1408–1414.

Goller J.L., Dimitriadis A., Tan A., Kelly H., Marshall J.A. (2004). Long-term features of norovirus gastroenteritis in the elderly. *Journal of Hospital Infection* 58 (4): 286–291.

Gordon F.M., Schultz M.E., Huber R.A., Gill J.A. (2005). Reduction in nosocomial transmission of drug-resistant bacteria after introduction of an alcohol-based hand rub. *Infection Control and Hospital Epidemiology* 26 (7): 650–653.

Graham C (2010). Investigation of Urine Samples. In: Ford M. (Ed.) *Medical Microbiology*. Oxford University Press, Oxford: 117–141.

Griffiths P., Renz A., Rafferty A.M. (2008). *The Impact of Organisation and Management Factors on Infection Control in Hospitals: A Scoping Review.* Royal College of Nursing / Kings College London.

Hall A.J. (2012). Norovirus: The Perfect Human Pathogen? *Journal of Infectious Diseases.* Available at: http://www .oxfordjournals.or/our_journals/jid/preditorial.pdf (accessed 10th June 2012).

Harris J.P., Allen D.J., Ituriza-Gomara M. (2011). Norovirus: changing epidemiology, changing virology. The challenges for infection control. *Journal of Infection Prevention*12 (3): 102–106.

Hart C.A. (2007). Arenaviruses and filoviruses. In: Greenwood D., Slack R., Peutherer J., Barer M.R. (Eds) *Medical Microbiology. A Guide to Microbial Infections: Pathogenesis, Immunity, Laboratory Diagnosis and Control.* Seventeenth Edition. Churchill Livingstone, London: pp. 536–544.

Hasham S., Matteucci P., Stanley P., Hart N. (2005). Necrotising fasciitis. *British Medical Journal* 330: 830–833.

Hawker J., Begg N., Blair I., Reintjes R., Weinberg J., Ekdahl K. (2012). *Communicable Disease Control and Health Protection Handbook.* Third Edition). Wiley-Blackwell, Oxford.

Health and Safety Executive (2000). *Legionnaires' disease. The control of legionella bacteria in water systems: Approved Code of Practice and guidance.* Available at: http://www.hse.gov.uk/ pubns/books/l8.htm

Health and Safety Executive (2006) identifying and evaluating the social and psychological impact of workplace accidents and ill health incidents on employees. Sudbury: HSE Books. Research Report 464. Available at: http;//www.hse.gov.uk/ research/rrdf/rr464.pdf

Health and Safety Executive (2013). *Information Sheet 7 – Health and Safety (Sharps Instruments in Healthcare) Regulations 2013.* Available at: http://www.hse.gov.uk/ pubns/hsis7.pdf

Health and Safety Executive (2015). *Methods of decontamination.* Available at: http://www.hse.gov.uk/biosafety/blood-borne- viruses/methods-of-decontamination.htm

Health Protection Agency (2008) *Guidance on the diagnosis and management of PVL-associated staphylococcus aureus infections (PVL-SA) in England. Report prepared by the PVL sub-group of the steering group on Healthcare Associated Infection.* HPA, London.

Health Protection Agency (2009a). *Review of the major outbreak of E.coli O157 in Surrey, 2009. Report of the Independent Investigation Committee, June 2010.* HPA, London.

Health Protection Agency (2009b). *Clostridium difficile Fact Sheet.* Available at: https://www.gov.uk/government/uploads/ system/uploads/attachment_data/file/339322/Clostridium_ difficile_fact_sheet.pdf

Health Protection Agency (2009c). *Foodborne illness at the Fat Duck restaurant. Report of an investigation of a foodborne outbreak of norovirus among diners at The Fat Duck restaurant, Bray, Berkshire, in January and February 2009.* HPA, London.

Health Protection Agency (2012a). *English National Point Prevalence Survey on Healthcare Associated Infections and Antimicrobial Use, 2011.* HPA, London.

Health Protection Agency (2012b). *Eye of needle: United Kingdom surveillance of significant occupational exposures to bloodborne viruses in health care workers.* HPA, London.

Health Protection Agency (2012d). *Public Health Management of Pertussis – HPA Guidelines for the Public health Management of Pertussis Incidents in Healthcare Settings.* HPA, London.

Health Protection Agency (2012e). *Guidance for public health management of meningococcal disease in the UK.* Health Protection Agency Meningococcal and Haemophilus Forum. HPA, London.

Health Protection Agency and the Department of Health (2011). *Prevention of infection and communicable disease control in prisons and places of detention. A manual for healthcare workers and other staff.* HPA/DH, London.

Health Protection Agency / Norovirus Working Party (2012). *Guidelines for the management of norovirus outbreaks in acute and community health and social care settings.* HPA, London.

Heymann D.L (2015). *Control of Communicable Diseases Manual. An Official Report of the American Public Health Association.* Twentieth Edition. APHA, Washington, DC.

Hine D. (2010). *The 2009 Influenza Pandemic. An Independent Review of the UK Response to the 2009 Influenza Pandemic.* DH, London.

Hirsch T., Spielmann M., Zuhail B. (2008). Enhanced susceptibility to infections in a diabetic wound model. Available at: http://www.biomedcentral.com/1471-2482/8/5

Hodges K., Gill R. (2010). Infectious diarrhoea: cellular and molecular mechanisms. *Gut microbes* 1 (1): 4–21.

Hood J., Edwards G.F.S. (2007). Legionella. In: Greenwood D., Slack R., Peutherer J., Barer M. (Eds) *Medical Microbiology. A Guide to Microbial Infections: Pathogenesis, Immunity, Laboratory Diagnosis and Control.* Seventeenth Edition. Churchill Livingstone, London: pp. 332–335.

Hooton M. (2010). Nosocomial Urinary Tract Infections. In: Mandell G.L., Bennett J.E., Dolin R.D. (Eds) Mandell's Principles and Practices of Infectious Diseases. Sixth Edition. Churchill Livingstone, Elsevier. Expert Consult online: http://expertconsult.com

Hospital Infection Society / British Society for Antimicrobial Chemotherapy (1986). Report of a combined Working Party of the Hospital Infection Society and British Society for Antimicrobial Chemotherapy. Guidelines for the control of meticillin-resistant Staphylococcus aureus. *Journal of Hospital Infection* 7: 193–201.

Houstein T., Harris J.P., Pebody R., Lopman B.A. (2009). Hospital admissions due to norovirus in adults and elderly patients. *Clinical Infectious Diseases* 49 (12): 1890–1892.

Hoy R.F. (2012). Respiratory problems: occupational and environmental exposure. *Australian Family Physician* 41 (11): 856–860.

Infusion Nurses Society (2006). *Infusion Nursing Standards of Practice.* J.P. Lippincott, Hagerstown, MD.

Jackson A. (1998). Infection Control – a battle in vein: infusion phlebitis. *Nursing Times* 94 (4): 68–71.

Jacobsen S.M., Stickler D.J., Mobley H.L.T., Shirtliff M.E. (2008). Complicated catheter-associated urinary tract infections due to Escherichia coli and Proteus mirabilis. *Clinical Microbiology Reviews* 21 (1): 26–59.

Jevons P.C. (1961). Resistant Staphylococci. *British Medical Journal* 1: 124.

Johnson A.P., Pearson A., Duckworth G. (2005). Surveillance and epidemiology of MRSA bacteraemia in the UK. *Journal of Antimicrobial Chemotherapy* 56: 455–462.

Judson S., Prescott J., Munster V. (2015). Understanding Ebola virus transmission. *Viruses* 7 (2): 511–521.

Jumaan A., Lavanchy D. (2008). Chickenpox / Herpes Zoster. In: Heymann D.L. (Ed) *Control of Communicable Diseases Manual*. Nineteenth Edition. American Public Health Association, Baltimore: pp. 540–543.

Kampf G., Ostermeyer C., Heeg P. (2005). Surgical hand disinfection with a propanol-based hand rub: equivalence of shorter application times. *Journal of Hospital Infection* 59: 304–310. Available at: http://www.ncbi.nlm.nih.gov/pubmed/15749318

Kieninger A.N., Lipsett P.A. (2009). Pneumonia: pathophysiology, diagnosis and treatment. *Surgical Clinics of North America* 89 (2): 439–461.

Leggett H.C., Cornwallis C.K., West S.A. (2012). Mechanisms of pathogenesis, infectious dose and virulence in human parasites. *PLoS Pathogens* 8 (2). Available at: e1002512. doi:10.1371/journal.ppat.1002512

Lewis S.J., Heaton K.W. (1997). Stool form scale as useful guide to intestinal transit time. *Scandinavian Journal of Gastroenterology* 32 (9): 920–924.

Lim W.S., Baudonin S.V., George R.C. et al (2009). Guidelines for the management of community-acquired pneumonia in adults: update 2009. *Thorax* 64, Suppl III: iii1–iii55.

Loudon I. (2013). Ignaz Phillip Semmelweis' studies of death in childbirth. JLL Bulletin: Commentaries on the history of treatment evaluation. Available at: http://www.jameslindlibrary.org/articles/ignaz-phillip-semmelweis-studies-of-death-in-childbirth/

Loveday H.P., Wilson J.A., Pratt R.J. et al (2014). National Evidence-Based Guidelines for Preventing Healthcare-Associated Infections in NHS Hospitals in England. *Journal of Hospital Infection* 86S1: S1–S70.

Macklin D. (2003). Phlebitis, a painful complication of peripheral IV catheterization that may be prevented. *American Journal of Nursing* 103 (20): 55–60.

Maki D.G. (1976). Lister revisited: surgical antisepsis and asepsis. *New England Journal of Medicine* 249: 1286–1287.

Mandell L.A., Wunderink R.G., Anzueto A. et al (2007). *Infectious Diseases Society of America / American Thoracic Society Consensus Guidelines on the Management of Community Acquired Pneumonia in Adults*. Available at: https://www.thoracic.org/statements/resources/mtpi/idsaats-cap.pdf

Mangram A.J., Horan T.C., Pearson M.L., Silver L.C., Jarvis W.R. (1999). Guideline for the prevention of surgical site infection. *Infection Control and Hospital Epidemiology* 20 (4): 247–278.

Marchetti M.G., Kampf G., Finzi G., Salvatorelli G. (2003). Evaluation of the bactericidal effect of five products for surgical hand disinfection according to prEN 12054 and prEN 12791. *Journal of Hospital Infection* 54 (1): 63–67.

Marples R.R., Towers A.G. (1979) A laboratory model for the investigation of contact transfer of micro-organisms. *Journal*

of Hygiene (London) 82: 237–248. Available at: http://www.ncbi.nlm.nih.gov/pubmed/429788

Masterton R.G., Galloway A., French G. et al (2008). Guidelines for the management of hospital-acquired pneumonia in the UK: Report of the Working Party of Hospital-Acquired Pneumonia of the British Society for Antimicrobial Chemotherapy. *Journal of Antimicrobial Chemotherapy* 62: 5–34.

Medicines and Healthcare Products Regulatory Agency (MHRA) Microbiology Advisory Committee to Department of Health (2010).Sterilization, disinfection and cleaning of medical equipment. *The MAC Manual Part I*. Medicines and Healthcare Products Regulatory Agency (MHRA) Microbiology Advisory Committee to Department of Health. London. Available at: http://naep.org.uk/members/documents/MHRAMACPart1.pdf

Medicines and Healthcare Products Regulatory Agency (2004). *Reusable Nebulisers*. MDA/2004/020. MHRA, London.

Mims C., Dockrell H.M., Goering R.V., Roitt I., Wakelin D., Zuckerman M. (2004a). Microbes and Parasites. In: *Medical Microbiology*. Updated Third Edition. Elsevier Mosby, St Louis: pp. 7–10.

Mims C., Dockrell H.M., Goering R.V., Roitt I., Wakelin D., Zuckerman M. (2004b). The bacteria. In: *Medical Microbiology*. Updated Third Edition. Elsevier Mosby, St Louis: pp. 11–28.

Mims C., Dockrell H.M., Goering R.V., Roitt I., Wakelin D., Zuckerman M. (2004c). The Pathological Consequences of Infection. In: *Medical Microbiology*. Updated Third Edition. Elsevier Mosby, St Louis: pp. 183–197.

Mims C., Dockrell H.M., Goering R.V., Roitt I., Wakelin D., Zuckerman M. (2004d). The Viruses. In: *Medical Microbiology*. Updated Third Edition. Elsevier Mosby, St Louis: pp. 29–36.

Mims C., Dockrell H.M., Goering R.V., Roitt I., Wakelin D., Zuckerman M. (2004e). The Cellular Basis of Adaptive Immune Responses. In: *Medical Microbiology*. Updated Third Edition. Elsevier Mosby, St Louis: pp. 99–110.

Mims C., Dockrell H.M., Goering R.V., Roitt I., Wakelin D., Zuckerman M. (2004f). Vaccination. In: *Medical Microbiology*. Updated Third Edition. Elsevier Mosby, St Louis: pp. 513–538.

Mims C., Dockrell H.M., Goering R.V., Roitt I., Wakelin D., Zuckerman M. (2004g). Pathogen Parade. In: *Medical Microbiology*. Updated Third Edition. Elsevier Mosby, St Louis: pp. 567–629.

Mims C., Dockrell H.M., Goering R.V., Roitt I., Wakelin D., Zuckerman M. (2004h). Infections of the Skin, Soft Tissue, Muscle and Associated Systems. In: *Medical Microbiology*. Updated Third Edition. Elsevier Mosby, St Louis: pp. 567–629.

Mims C., Dockrell H.M., Goering R.V., Roitt I., Wakelin D., Zuckerman M. (2004i). Upper Respiratory Infections. In: *Medical Microbiology*. Updated Third Edition. Elsevier Mosby, St Louis: pp. 201–216.

Mosby (2013). *Mosby's Dictionary of Medicine, Nursing and Health Professions*. Ninth Edition. Mosby, St Louis.

Nairns R., Helbert M. (2005a). Basic Concepts and Components of the Immune System. In: *Immunology for Medical Students*. Mosby, London: pp. 3–19.

Nairns R., Helbert M. (2005b). Antigen and Antibody Structure. In: *Immunology for Medical Students*. Mosby, London: pp. 23–30.

Nairns R., Helbert M. (2005c). Antigen Processing and Presentation. In: *Immunology for Medical Students* Mosby, London: pp. 71–78.

Nairns R., Helbert M. (2005d). Constitutive Defences Including Complement. In: *Immunology for Medical Students*. Mosby, London: pp. 157–166.

Nairns R., Helbert M. (2005e). Infections and Vaccines. In: *Immunology for Medical Students*. Mosby, London: pp. 207–213.

Nash A.A., Dalziel R.G., Fitzgerald J.R. (2015). Microbial Strategies in Relation to Immune Response. In: *Mims' Pathogenesis of Infectious Diseases*. Elsevier, London (Kindle version).

National Institute for Health and Care Excellence (2012). *Infection: Prevention and control of healthcare-associated infections in primary and community care*. National Clinical Guideline Centre, London.

National Institute for Health and Care Excellence (2014a). *Clinical Knowledge Summaries. Diarrhoea Antibiotic Associated*. National Institute for Health and Care Excellence, London. Available at: http://cks.nice.org.uk/diarrhoea-antibiotic-associated

National Institute for Health and Care Excellence (2014b). *Pneumonia in adults: diagnosis and management*. National Clinical Guideline Centre, London.

National Institute for Health and Care Excellence (2015). *Clinical Knowledge Summaries. Chickenpox*. National Institute for Health and Care Excellence, London. Available at: http://cks.nice.org.uk/chickenpox

National Institute for Health and Care Excellence (2016). *Sepsis: recognition, diagnosis and early management*. NICE guideline. Available at: http://Nice.org.uk/guidance/ng51

National Institute for Health and Clinical Excellence (2008) *Surgical site infection: prevention and treatment. NICE clinical guidelines 74*. NICE, London. Available at: https://www.nice.org.uk/guidance/cg74

National Institute for Health and Clinical Excellence (2011). *Tuberculosis. Clinical diagnosis and management of tuberculosis, and measures for its prevention and control. NICE Clinical Guideline 117*. NICE / National Collaborating Centre for Chronic Conditions and Centre for Clinical Practice at NICE, London.

NHS England (2013). *Pandemic Influenza. NHS Guidance on the current and future preparedness in support of an outbreak*. NHS England, London.

NHS England (2014a). *Factsheet: Implementation of the 'Sepsis Six' care bundle*. Available at: https://www.england.nhs.uk/wp-content/uploads/2014/02/rm-fs-10-1.pdf

NHS England (2014b). *Patient Safety Alert. Resources to support the prompt recognition of sepsis and the rapid initiation of treatment*. Alert reference number: NHS/PSA/R/2014/015.

NHS England (2014c). *Guidance on the reporting and monitoring arrangements and post infection review process for MRSA bloodstream infections*. Version 2. NHS England, London. Available at: http://www.england.nhs.uk/wp-content/uploads/2014/04/mrsa-pir-guid-april14.pdf

Neidhardt F.G. (2004). Bacterial Genetics. In: Sherris J.C., Ryan K.J., Ray G.C. (Eds) *Medical Microbiology: An Introduction to Infectious Diseases*. Fourth Edition. McGraw-Hill, London: pp. 53–75.

Newsom S. (2009a). The Life of Edward Jenner. In: *Infections and Their Control. A Historical Perspective*. Sage Publications, London: pp. 71–80.

Newsom S. (2009b). Semmelweis and Handwashing. In: *Infections and their Control, a Historical Perspective*. Sage Publications, London: pp. 7–12.

Newsom S. (2009c). Typhoid fever: another continuing problem. In: *Infections and their Control, a Historical Perspective*. Sage Publications, London: pp. 125–134.

Niemi S.M. (2009). Theobald Smith – Brief life of a pioneering comparative pathologist: 1859–1934. *Harvard Magazine*, July–August 2009. Available at: http://harvardmagazine.com

Nursing and Midwifery Council (2015). *The Code. Professional Standards of Behaviour and Practice for Nurses and Midwives*. NMC, London.

Otter J.A., Yezli S., French G.L. (2011). The role played by contaminated surfaces in the transmission of nosocomial pathogens. *Infection Control and Hospital Epidemiology* 32 (7): 687–699.

Otter J.A., Yezli S., Salkeld J.A. G., French G.L. (2013). Evidence that contaminated surfaces contribute to the transmission of hospital pathogens and an overview of strategies to address contaminated surfaces in hospital settings. *American Journal of Infection Control* 41 (5 suppl): S6–S11.

Otto M. (2014). Host–microbe interactions in bacteria Staphylococcus aureus toxins. *Current Opinion in Microbiology* 17: 32–37.

Parliamentary and Health Service Ombudsman (2013). *Time to Act. Severe sepsis: rapid diagnosis and treatment saves lives*. Available at: www.ombudsman.org.uk/time-to-act

Passaretti C.L., Otter J.A., Reich N.G. et al (2013). An evaluation of environmental decontamination with hydrogen peroxide vapour for reducing the risk of patient acquisition of multidrug-resistant organisms. *Clinical Infectious Disease* 56(1): 27–35.

Patel K.S., Patel A.K., Chaudhary H.H., Aal L.B., Parmar J.N., Patel V.R., Sen D.J. (2014). Pathogenesis of Ebola virus: A deadly viron hosted by bats. *World Journal of Pharmaceutical Sciences*. Available at: http://www.wjpsonline.org

Patrick D.R., Findon G., Miller T.E. (1997). Residual moisture determines the level of touch-contact associated bacteria transferred following handwashing. *Epidemiology and Infection* 119: 319–325.

Patterson W., Haswell P., Fryers P.T., Green J. (1997). Outbreak of small round structured virus gastroenteritis arose after kitchen assistant vomited. *Communicable Disease Report* 7; Review 7: R101–R103.

Pavillard R., Harvey K., Douglas D. et al (1982). Epidemic of hospital-acquired infection due to methicillin-resistant Staphylococcus aureus in major Victorian hospitals. *Medical Journal of Australia* 1: 451–454.

Pelag A.Y., Hooper D.C. (2010). Hospital-acquired infections due to gram-negative bacteria. *New England Journal of Medicine* 362 (19): 1804–1813.

Pittet D., Hugonnet S., Harbarth S., Mourouga P., Sauvan V., Touveneau S., Perneger T.V. (2000). Effectiveness of a hospital wide programme to improve compliance with hand hygiene. *Lancet* 356: 1307–1312.

Plorde J.J. (2004). Mycobacterium. In: Sherris J.C., Ryan K.J., Ray G.C. (Eds) *Medical Microbiology: An Introduction to Infectious Diseases*. Fourth Edition. McGraw-Hill, London: pp. 439–456.

Plowman R., Graves N., Griffin M. et al (2000). *The Socio-economic Burden of Hospital Acquired Infection*. Public Health Laboratory Service, London.

Pratt R.J., Pellowe C.M., Loveday H.B., Robinson M., Smith G.W and the Epic Guidelines Development Team (2001). The epic Project: Developing National Evidence-Based Guidelines for Preventing Healthcare Associated Infections. *Journal of Hospital Infection* 47 (suppl): S1–S82.

Pratt R.J., Grange J.M., Williams V.G. (2005). The treatment of tuberculosis and other mycobacterial diseases. In: *Tuberculosis: A Foundation for Nursing and Healthcare Practice*. Hodder Arnold, London: pp. 149–167.

Prescott L.M., Harley J., Klein D.A. (2005a). Prokaryotic Cell Structure and Function. In: *Microbiology*. Sixth Edition. McGraw-Hill, New York: pp. 39–72.

Prescott L.M., Harley J.P., Klein D.A. (2005b). Human Diseases caused by Bacteria. In: *Microbiology*. Sixth Edition. McGraw-Hill, New York: pp. 873-875.

Prescott L.M., Harley J.P., Klein D.A. (2005c). Human Diseases caused by Viruses. In: *Microbiology*. Sixth Edition. McGraw-Hill, New York: pp. 845-873.

Price P.B. (1939). Ethyl alcohol as a germicide. *Archives of Surgery* 38: 528-542.

Public Health England (2013a). *Inoculation of Culture Media for Bacteriology. UK standards for microbiology investigation*. Q5. Issue 1.3. PHE, London.

Public Health England (2013b). *Guidance – List of Zoonotic Diseases* PHE, London. Available at: http://www.gov.uk/government/publications/list-of-zoonotic-diseases/list-of-zoonotic-diseases

Public Health England (2013c). Immunity and How Vaccines Work. *The Green Book. Immunisation against Infectious Disease*. PHE, London. Available at: http://www.gov.uk/government/collections/immunisation-against-infectious-disease-the-green-book

Public Health England (2013d). *Protocol for the surveillance of surgical site infection. Surgical site infection surveillance service*. Version 6. PHE, London. Available at: ttps://www.gov.uk/government/uploads/system/uploads/attachment_data/file/364412/Protocol_for_surveillance_of_surgical_site_infection_June_2013.pdf

Public Health England (2013e). *Acute trust toolkit for the early detection, management and control of carbapenemase-producing Enterobacteriaceae*. PHE, London.

Public Health England (2013f). *Updated guidance on the management and treatment of Clostridium difficile infection*. PHE, London. Available at: https://www.gov.uk/government/uploads/system/uploads/attachment_data/file/321891/Clostridium_difficile_management_and_treatment.pdf

Public Health England (2013g). Chapter 25: Pneumococcal. In: *Immunisation against Infectious Diseases (The Green Book)*. PHE/DH, London. Available at: http://www.gov.uk/government/collections/immunisation-against-infectious-disease-the-green-book

Public Health England (2013h). Chapter 19. Influenza. In: *Immunisation against Infectious Diseases (The Green Book)*. PHE/DH, London. Available at: http://www.gov.uk/government/collections/immunisation-against-infectious-disease-the-green-book

Public Health England (2013i). Legionnaires' disease in England and Wales. PHE/DH, London.

Public Health England (2013j). German measles. In: *Immunisation against Infectious Diseases (The Green Book)*. PHE/DH, London. Available at: http://www.gov.uk/government/collections/immunisation-against-infectious-disease-the-green-book

Public Health England (2013k). Norovirus: annual figures 2000–2012. Available at: www.gov.uk/government/statistics/norovirus-annual-figures-2000-to-2012

Public Health England (2013l). Tuberculosis. In: *Immunisation against Infectious Diseases (The Green Book)*. PHE/DH, London. Available at: http://www.gov.uk/government/collections/immunisation-against-infectious-disease-the-green-book

Public Health England (2013m). Varicella. In: *Immunisation against Infectious Diseases (The Green Book)*. PHE/DH, London. Available at:http://www.gov.uk/government/collections/immunisation-against-infectious-disease-the-green-book

Public Health England (2014a). *Communicable Disease Outbreak Management. Operational Guidance*. PHE, London.

Public Health England (2014b). *HIV in the United Kingdom: 2014* Report. PHE, London

Public Health England (2014c) *Annual Epidemiological Commentary: Mandatory MRSA, MSSA and E. coli bacteraemia and C. difficile infection data, 2013/14*. PHE, London

Public Health England (2014d). *Salmonella: guidance, data and analysis* http://www.gov.uk/government/collections/Salmonella-guidance-data-and analysis

Public Health England (2014e). *Reducing the risks of Salmonella infection from reptiles* http://www.gov.uk/government/publications/Salmonella-reducing-infection-from-reptiles

Public Health England (2014f). *Tuberculosis in the UK Report*. PHE, London

Public Health England (2014g). *UK Standards for Microbiology Investigations Investigation of specimens for screening for MRSA*. London. UK.

Public Health England (2015a). *Staining Procedures. UK Standards for Microbiology Investigations*. TP39. Issue 2.1. PHE, London.

Public Health England (2015b). *Toolkit for managing carbapenemase-producing Enterobacteriaceae in non-acute and community settings*. PHE, London.

Public Health England (2015c). *PHE Guidance on use of antiviral agents for the treatment and prophylaxis of influenza (2014-15)*. PHE, London.

Public Health England (2015d). Continued increase in meningococcal group W (MenW) disease in England. *Health Protection Report*. 9 (7). 27 February.

Public Health England (2016). Guidelines for the Public Health management of Pertussis in England (produced by the Pertussis Guidelines Group). PHE, London.

Public Health England / Department of Health Expert Advisory Committee on Antimicrobial Resistance and Healthcare Associated Infection (2013). *Antimicrobial prescribing and stewardship competencies*. PHE, London.

Public Health England / NHS England (2014). *Patient Safety Alert. Stage 3: Directive. Legionella and heated birthing pools filled in advance of labour in home settings*. NHS/PSA/D/2014/011.

Ray C.G., Ryan K.J., Drew W.L (2010a). Urinary Tract Infections. In: Ryan K.J., Drew W.L (Eds). *Sherris Medical Microbiology*. Fifth Edition. McGraw Hill, London: pp. 939–944.

Reid A.H., Fanning T.G., Hultin J.V., Taubenberger J.K. (1999). Origin and evolution of the 1918 "Spanish" influenza virus hemaglutlin gene. *Procdings of the National Academy of Sciences of the United States of America (PNAS)* 96 (4): 1651–1656.

Riggs M.M., Sethi A.K., Zabarsky T.F. et al (2007). Asymptomatic carriers are a potential source for transmission of epidemic and non-epidemic clostridium difficile strains among long-term care facilities residents. *Clinical Infectious Diseases* 45: 992–998.

Robinson J. (2001). Urethral catheter selection. *Nursing Standard* 7 (15): 39–42.

Rothberg M.B., Haessler S.D., Brown R.D. (2008). Complications of viral influenza. *American Journal of Medicine* 121: 258–264.

Rotter M. (1999). Hand Washing and Hand Disinfection. Chapter 87. In: Mayhall C.G. (Ed) *Hospital Epidemiology and Infection Control*. Second Edition. Lippincott Williams & Wilkins, Philadelphia.

Rowley S. (2000). Aseptic Non-Touch Technique. In: Hubbard S., Trigg E. (Eds) *Practices in Children's Nursing*. Churchill Livingstone, Edinburgh. Rowley S., Clare S., Macqueen S., Molyneux R. (2010). ANTTv2: An updated Practice Framework for Aseptic Technique. *British Journal of Nursing*, Intravenous Supplement, 19 (5).

Rowley S., Clare S., Macqueen S., Molyneux R. (2010) ANTT v2: An updated practice framework for aseptic technique. Available at: https://www.ucc.ie/en/media/academic/epidemiologyandpublichealth/pdfdocs/ANTT2010article.pdf

Royal College of Nursing (2005) *Methicillin-resistant Staphylococcus aureus (MRSA) Guidance for nursing staff*. RCN, London. Available at: http://www.nhs.uk/conditions/mrsa/documents/rcn%20mrsa%20guidelines.pdf

Royal College of Nursing (2010). *Standards for Infusion Therapy*. Third edition. RCN, London. Available at: http://www.bbraun.it/documents/RCN-Guidlines-for-IV-therapy.pdf

Royal College of Nursing (2012a). *Essential Practice for Infection Prevention and Control. Guidance for Nursing staff*. RCN, London.

Royal College of Nursing (2012b). *Tools of the trade. RCN guidance on glove use and the prevention of contact dermatitis*. RCN, London.

Royal College of Nursing (2012c). *Catheter care. RCN guidance for Nurses*. RCN, London.

Royal College of Nursing (2013a). *Guidance to support the implementation of The Health and Safety (Sharp Instruments in Healthcare Regulations) 2013*. RCN, London. Available at: https://www.rcn.org.uk/__data/assets/pdf_file/0008/418490/004135.pdf

Royal College of Nursing (2013b). *The management of diarrhoea in adults. RCN guidance for staff*. RCN, London.

Rubinovitch B., Pittet D. (2001). Screening for methicillin-resistant *Staphylococcus aureus* in the endemic hospital: what have we learned? *Journal of Hospital Infection* 47: 9–18.

Ryan K.J., Drew W.L. (2010a). Antimicrobial Agents and Resistance. In: Ryan K.J., Ray C.G (Eds). *Sherris Medical Microbiology*. Fifth Edition. McGraw Hill, London: pp. 403–428.

Ryan K.J., Drew W.L. (2010b). Streptococci and Enterococci. In: Ryan K.J., Ray C.G. (Eds) *Sherris Medical Microbiology*. Fifth Edition. McGraw Hill, London: pp. 443–470.

Ryan K.J., Drew W.L. (2010c). Neisseria. In: Ryan K.J., Ray C.G. (Eds) *Sherris Medical Microbiology*. Fifth Edition. McGraw Hill, London: pp. 535–550.

Ryan K.J., Drew W.L. (2010d). Mycobacteria. In: Ryan K.L., Drew W.L. (Eds) *Sherris Medical Microbiology*. Fifth Edition. McGraw Hill, London: pp. 489–506.

Sartor C., Jacomo V., Duvivier C., Tissot-Dupont H., Sambuc R., Drancourt M. (2000). Nosocomial *Serratia marcescens* infections associated with extrinsic contamination of a liquid non-medicated soap. *Infection Control and Hospital Epidemiology* 21 (3): 196–199.

Schaefler S., Jones D., Perry W. et al (1981). Emergence of gentamicin- and methicillin-resistant Staphylococcus aureus strains in New York City hospitals. *Journal of Clinical Microbiology* 13: 754–759.

Scottish Intercollegiate Guidelines Network (2002). *SIGN 59: Community Management of Lower Respiratory Tract Infections*. SIGN, Edinburgh.

Scottish Intercollegiate Guidelines Network (2012). *Management of Suspected Bacterial Urinary Tract Infections in Adults. A National Clinical Guideline*. SIGN Publication 88. SIGN, Edinburgh.

Siegel J.D., Rhinehart E., Jackson M., Chiarello L. and the Healthcare Infection Control Practices Advisory Committee (2007*). Guidelines for Isolation Precautions: Preventing Transmission of Infectious Agents in Healthcare Settings*. Available at: http://www.cdc.gov/ncidod/dhqp/pdf/isolation2007.pdf

Simmons B.P. (1981). Guideline for Hospital Environmental Control. Section 1. Antiseptics, Handwashing, and Handwashing Facilities. In: Centers for Disease Control and Prevention (CDC; Ed.) *CDC Hospital infections program (HIP) guidelines for Prevention and Control of Nosocomial Infections*. CDC, Atlanta, GA: pp. 6–10.

Singh Y.D. (2012). Pathophysiology of community-acquired pneumonia. *Journal of the Association of Physicians of India* 60 (Suppl): 7–10.

Skyman E., Sjostrom H.T. (2009). Patients' experiences of being infected with MRSA at a hospital and subsequently source isolated. *Scandinavian Journal of Caring Sciences* 24 (1): 101–107.

Speller D.C., Johnson A.P., James D., Marples R.R., Charlett A., George R.C. (1997). Resistance to methicillin and other antibiotics in isolates of Staphylococcus aureus from blood and cerebrospinal fluid, England and Wales, 1989-95. *Lancet*. 350: 323–325.

Steer J.A., Lamagni T., Healy B. et al (2012). Guidelines for prevention and control of group A streptococcal infection in acute healthcare and community settings. *Journal of Hospital Infection* 64: 1–8.

Surviving Sepsis Campaign (2012*). International Guidelines for Management of Severe Sepsis and Sepsis*. Available at: www.survivingsepsis.org/guidelines

Sutherland S. (2007). Orthomyxoviruses: Influenza. In: Greenwood D., Slack R., Peutherer J., Barer M. (Eds) *Medical Microbiology. A Guide to Microbial Infections: Pathogenesis, Immunity, Laboratory Diagnosis and Control*. Seventeenth Edition. Churchill Livingstone, London: pp. 489–496.

Taubenberger J., Morens D.M. (2006). 1918 Influenza: The Mother of All Pandemics. *Emergency Infectious Diseases* 12(1): 15–22.

Thibault R., Graf S., Clerc A., Delieuvin N., Hiedegger C.P., Pichard C. (2013). Diarrhoea in the ICU. *Critical Care* 17 (4): R153.

Thielman N.M., Wilson K.H. (2009). Clostridium difficile associated disease. In: Mandell G.L., Bennett J.E., Dolin R. (Eds) *Mandell, Douglas and Bennett's Principles and Practice of Infectious Diseases.* Seventh Edition. Churchill Livingstone. Expert Consult online: http://expertconsult.com

Trautner B.W., Darouiche R.O. (2004). Catheter-associated infections: pathogenesis affects prevention. *Archives of Internal Medicine* 164: 842–850.

Trick W.E., Vernon M.O., Welbel S.F., Demarais P., Hayden M.K., Weinstein R.A. (2007). Multi-center intervention program to increase adherence to hand hygiene recommendations and glove use and to reduce the incidence of antimicrobial resistance. *Infection Control and Hospital Epidemiology* 28 (1): 42–49.

Trovillion E.W., Skyles J.M., Hopkins-Broyles D., Recktenwald A., Faulkner K. et al (2011). Development of a nurse-driven protocol to remove urinary catheters. Abstract 592. SHEA 2011 Annual Scientific Meeting, April 1–4, Dallas, TX.

Turnidge J., Christiansen K. (2005). Antibiotic use and resistance – proving the obvious. *Lancet* 365 (9459): 548–549.

Van Duin D., Kaye K.S., Neuner E.A., Bonomo R.A. (2013). Carbapenem-resistant Enterobacteriaceae: a review of treatment and outcomes. *Diagnostic Microbiology and Infectious Disease* 75 (2): 115–120.

Vipond I.B., Caul E.O., Lambden P.R., Clarke I.N. (1999). "Hyperemesis hiemis": new light on an old symptom. *Microbiology Today* 26: 110–111.

Webber M.A., Piddock L.J.V. (2003). The impact of efflux pumps in bacterial antibiotic resistance. *Journal of Antimicrobial Chemotherapy* 51 (1): 9–11.

Weber D.J., Rutala W.A., Miller M.B., Huslage K., Sickbert-Bennett E. (2010). Role of hospital surfaces in the transmission of emerging healthcare-associated pathogens: Norovirus, Clostridium difficile, and Acinetobacter species. *American Journal of Infection Control* 38 (5 Suppl 1): S25–S33.

Weber D.J., Anderson D., Rutala W.A., (2013). The role of surface environment in healthcare-associated infections. *Current Opinion in Infectious Diseases* 26 (4): 338–344.

Weinstein R.A. (1991). Epidemiology and control of nosocomial infections in adult intensive care units. *American Journal of Medicine* 91 (3): S179–S184.

Weston D. (2008). Campylobacter and Salmonella. In: *Infection Prevention and Control: Theory and Practice for Healthcare Professionals.* John Wiley and Sons, Hoboken, NJ: pp. 201–214.

Weston D. (2013) Microbial Classification and Structure. In: *Infection Prevention and Control: Theory and Practice.* Second Edition. Wiley Blackwell, New York: pp. 60–79.

Whelan K., Schneider S. (2011). Mechanisms, prevention and management of diarrhoea in enteral nutrition. *Current Opinion in Gastroenterology* 27: 152–159.

Widmer A.F., Rotter M., Voss A., Nthumba P., Allegranzi B., Boyce J., Pittet D. (2010). Surgical Hand Preparation: State of the Art. *Journal of Hospital Infection* 74 (2): 112–122.

Wigglesworth N., Wilcox M.H. (2006). Prospective evaluation of hospital isolation room capacity. *Journal of Hospital Infection* 63 (2): 156–161.

Willey J.M., Sherwood L.M., Woolverton C.J. (2011). Antimicrobial Chemotherapy. In: *Prescott's Medical Microbiology.* Eighth Edition. McGraw-Hill, London: pp. 826–849.

Wilson A.P.R., Livermore D.M., Otter J.A. et al (2015). Prevention and control of multi-drug resistant Gram-negative bacteria: recommendations from a Joint Working Party. *Journal of Hospital Infection.* Available at: http://dx.doi.org/10.1016/j.jhin.2015.08.007

Wilson J. (2006). Introduction to Microbiology. In: *Infection Control in Clinical Practice.* Third Edition. Bailliere Tindall, London: pp. 3–18.

Wilson J. (2008a). A Guide to Viruses. In: *Clinical Microbiology. An Introduction for Healthcare Professionals.* Bailliere Tindall, London: pp. 185–218.

Wilson J. (2008b). The Immune Response. In: *Clinical Microbiology. An Introduction for Healthcare Professionals.* Bailliere Tindall, London: pp. 51–72.

World Health Organization (2003).Chapter 5. SARS. Lessons from a new disease. In: *The World Health Report 2003 – Shaping the Future.* WHO, Geneva.

World Health Organization (2005). *Assessing the pandemic threat.* WHO, Geneva.

World Health Organization (2008). *Managing puerperal sepsis. Education material for teachers of midwifery.* Second Edition. WHO, Geneva.

World Health Organization (2009). *WHO Guidelines on Hand Hygiene in Health care: a summary.* WHO, Geneva.

World Health Organization (2011). *Report on the Burden of Healthcare-Associated Infection Worldwide: Clean Care is Safer Care.* WHO, Geneva.

World Health Organization (2013a). *Evolution of a Pandemic. A (H1N1)2009.* April 2009–August 2010. WHO, Geneva.

World Health Organization (2013b). *Pandemic Influenza Risk Management. WHO Interim Guidance.* WHO, Geneva.

World Health Organization (2014). *Ground zero in Guinea: the outbreak smoulders – undetected – for more than 3 months. A retrospective on the first cases of the outbreak.* World Health Organisation Global Alert and Response, Geneva.

World Health Organization (2015a). *Health worker Ebola infections in Guinea, Liberia and Sierra Leone.* WHO, Geneva.

World Health Organization (2015b). *Global Tuberculosis Report 2015.* WHO, Geneva.

World Health Organization (2015c). Water-related diseases. WHO, Geneva. Available at: www.who.int/water_sanitation_health/diseases/scabies/en

Wright S.G. (1989) *Changing Nursing Practice.* Edward Arnold, London.

Yong D., Toleman M.A., Giske G.G., Cho H.S., Lee K., Walsh T.R. (2009). Characterisation of a new metallo-beta-lactamase-gene, blaNDM-1, and a novel erythromycin esterase gene carried on a unique genetic structure in Klebsiella pneumoniae Sequence Type 14 from India. *Antimicrobial Agents Chemotherapy* 53 (12): 504–505.

Zawacki A., O'Rourke E., Potter-Bynoe G., Macone A., Harbarth S., Goldmann D. (2004). An outbreak of Pseudomonas aeruginosa pneumonia and bloodstream infection associated with intermittent otitis externa in a healthcare worker. *Infection Control and Hospital Epidemiology* 25 (12): 1083–1089.

Zhijun S., Borgwardt L., Borgwardt A. (2013). Prosthesis infections after orthopaedic joint replacement: The possible role of bacterial biofilms. *Orthopaedic Reviews* 5 (2): e14.

Index

Page numbers in *italics* refer to figures, those in **bold** refer to tables.

Infection Prevention and Control at a Glance, First Edition. By Debbie Weston, Alison Burgess and Sue Roberts.
© 2017 John Wiley & Sons, Ltd. Published 2017 by John Wiley & Sons, Ltd.